Management of Early Stage Breast Cancer

Beena Kunheri · D. K. Vijaykumar
Editors

Management of Early Stage Breast Cancer

Basics and Controversies

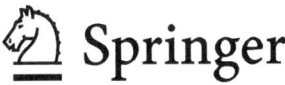 Springer

Editors
Beena Kunheri
Department of Radiation Oncology
Amrita Institute of Medical Sciences
and Research Centre
Amrita Vishwa Vidyapeetham University
Kochi
Kerala
India

D. K. Vijaykumar
Department of Breast and Gynecological
Oncology
Amrita Institute of Medical Sciences
Amrita Vishwa Vidyapeetham University
Kochi
Kerala
India

ISBN 978-981-15-6170-2   ISBN 978-981-15-6171-9   (eBook)
https://doi.org/10.1007/978-981-15-6171-9

This Springer imprint is published by the registered company Springer Nature Singapore Pte Ltd.
The registered company address is: 152 Beach Road, #21-01/04 Gateway East, Singapore 189721, Singapore

We would like to dedicate this book to

All the amazing women we have met and those we have not who battle with the dark days.

Our teachers who inspire and teach us to remain humble in our pursuit of knowledge.

Our families and special friends for the continued love and support they have selflessly given.

Foreword

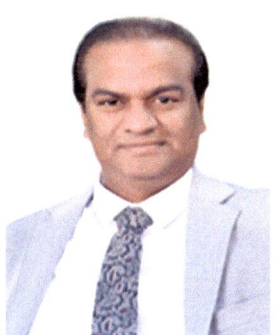

It gives me immense pleasure to write a foreword for an excellent educative exercise done by Dr. Beena and Dr. Vijaykumar.

The management of early breast cancer has always been an area of keen interest for practicing oncologists. The management schema of early breast cancer has dynamically evolved over decades. There has been a paradigm shift in the management algorithm of early breast cancer, and interestingly there are still several controversies in its management.

The book compiled, written, and authored by Dr. Beena and Dr. Vijaykumar covers every area from epidemiology, screening, various treatment modalities to rehabilitation.

Dr. Beena Kunheri has a special interest in breast cancer, and I am glad she has taken up this task and I am sure it would greatly guide practicing oncologists. Dr. Beena is a leading clinician and academic with several original publications to her credit.

Dr. D.K. Vijaykumar is an eminent oncosurgeon and has a special interest in breast cancer surgery. He is one of the pioneers in sentinel node surgery for breast cancer in India.

Although we have access to the internet, social media, smart phones, and tablet computers, I still feel that concise information on a dedicated and important topic like early breast cancer, written by experts in that field, would be quite useful and handy for an immediate reference.

I found it quite comprehensive, covering all aspects of early breast cancer. It provides valuable information and covers all the necessary components of early breast cancer management.

I congratulate Dr. Beena and Dr. Vijaykumar on this wonderfully done exercise, and I wish them good luck for their future endeavors too.

P. Vijay Anand Reddy, MBBS, MD
Director, Apollo Cancer Institute
Hyderabad, TS, India

Past President, Association of Radiation Oncologists of India
Hyderabad, TS, India

Preface

It is indeed a great pleasure to publish the first edition of this book on Early Breast Cancer. Breast cancer is the most common cancer in women in developed and developing countries like India. In India it accounts for the major proportion of oncologists' work. The incidence of breast cancer has steadily increased since the 1970s across the globe. However due to the effective implementation of screening programs, early detection, and effective treatment, breast cancer mortality has decreased in developed countries. In developing countries, early detection and improvement in overall survival are yet to be achieved.

With the rapidly advancing trends in the treatment and care of women with breast cancer, it has become increasingly difficult for busy clinicians to keep up to date with the latest guidelines and newer approaches to treatment. We have carefully chosen experts from specific fields to author each chapter so that this serves as a comprehensive textbook.

The textbook covers a broad range of topics including:

- Epidemiology
- Prevention
- Early detection and diagnosis
- Prognostic and predictive markers
- Molecular biology
- Newer pathological and molecular subtypes
- Receptor mechanism
- Genetics
- Developments in imaging modalities
- Surgical treatments
- Radiation treatments
- Drug therapies
- Advances in management including precision and personalized treatment

The closing chapter highlights the importance of psychological well-being in cancer treatment. It is included to make physicians aware of the psychosocial issues associated with breast cancer diagnosis and how best to provide psychological support for better outcomes.

We believe our book should find a place in all oncology departments as a comprehensive resource for students and oncologists helping them in their clinical decision making. We also hope our book will be a helpful specialist reference for other disciplines including pathology, radiology, pharmacology, molecular biology, genetics, surgery, and various other specialties.

It has been a wonderful opportunity to edit this book. An endeavor like this takes the help of a multitude of individuals without whom this book would not have been possible.

We are greatly appreciative of the work of all the authors for the wonderful review and their expertise.

In conclusion we want to acknowledge the thousands of women with breast cancer who have participated in the studies that have provided the information that has helped to advance the field by leaps and bounds in recent years.

Kochi, Kerala, India   Beena Kunheri
Kochi, Kerala, India   D. K. Vijaykumar

Acknowledgments

Pranams to Almighty for making this happen. We are indebted to our teachers, and this work is only a reflection of the inspiration from our teachers who offered us the grounding and foundations. Our pranams to our teachers.

Bringing out a book is harder than we thought and more rewarding than we could have ever imagined.

I along with Dr. Vijaykumar would like to thank each and every one who has helped and supported us in the planning, preparation, and completion of this textbook.

At the very outset, we express our gratitude to *Dr. Prem Nair*, Medical Director, and *Dr. (Col) Vishal Marwaha*, Principal.

We acknowledge with gratitude and affection our former Additional Medical Superintendent *Dr. Koravangattu Valsraj* (Consultant Psychiatrist, NHS, London, UK) for his guidance, invaluable suggestions, unwavering support, and encouragement throughout the preparation of this book.

It was his suggestion to add a chapter on the psychological impact of breast cancer diagnosis and treatment, making this book a truly comprehensive one.

We are thankful and indebted to *Dr. Pavithran*, Head of Dept. Medical Oncology for the invaluable suggestions and support.

We are most grateful to all the chapter contributors/authors for agreeing to be part of this project and spending their time in the midst of their busy clinical schedules.

Our special thanks to Miss. Bibin Rose Mohan (Physician Assistant) and Mrs. Sathikumari (Secretary), Department of Radiation Oncology, for their assistance and support.

We thank the publisher Springer Nature and Ms. Saanthi Shankhararaman for coordinating the project.

We wholeheartedly acknowledge both our families for their unconditional love, support, and inspiration.

Contents

Editors

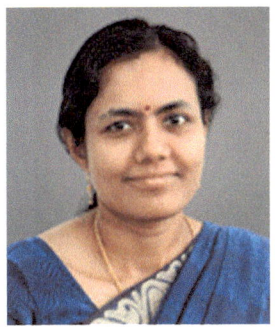

Beena Kunheri, MBBS, DMRT, DNB is currently Professor in the Department of Radiation Oncology at Amrita Institute of Medical Sciences, India. She completed her undergraduate medical training at Calicut Medical College, and her postgraduate training in Radiation Oncology at the prestigious Regional Cancer Centre, Trivandrum, under the aegis of Trivandrum Medical College.

Her areas of special interest include gynecological oncology, breast oncology, and uro-oncology, and she has authored several peer-reviewed, national and international publications and has been an invited speaker at various scientific meetings. She is also a reviewer for a number of journals. She has spent time at international oncology centers like the Royal Marsden Hospital, London; Hamad Medical Corporation, Qatar; and Heidelberg University, Germany. She is regarded as an expert and specialist in women's oncology.

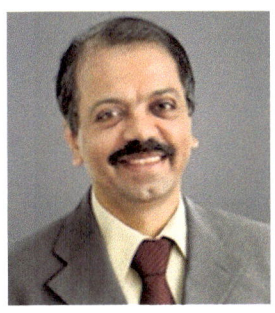

D. K. Vijaykumar, MS, MCh (Surgical Oncology) completed his MBBS and MS at BJ Medical College Pune, and his surgical oncology specialization at the Cancer Institute (WIA) Adyar, Chennai. He is currently Professor and Head of the Department of Breast and Gynecologic Oncology at Amrita Institute of Medical Sciences, India. He has worked at various major cancer centers in India, including the Regional Cancer Center, Trivandrum; Kidwai Institute, Bangalore; and Kasturba Medical College,

Manipal. His areas of interest include breast oncology and gynecologic oncology, and he has authored several peer-reviewed publications and is a reviewer for a number of oncology journals. He is also an examiner for various surgical oncology superspeciality exams.

Contributors

Sheikh Zahoor Ahmad, MBBS, MS Department of Surgical Oncology, Sher-i-Kashmir Institute of Medical Sciences, Srinagar, Jammu and Kashmir, India

Prasanth Ariyannur, MBBS, MD Molecular Oncology Laboratory, Department of Biochemistry, Amrita Institute of Medical Sciences, Amrita Vishwa Vidyapeetham, Kochi, Kerala, India

Misha J. C. Babu, MBBS, MS Department of General Surgery and Breast Clinic, Amrita Institute of Medical Sciences, Kochi, Kerala, India

Janaki P. Dharmarajan, MBBS, DMRD, DNB Department of Radiology, Amrita Institute of Medical Sciences, Kochi, Kerala, India

P. Gangadharan Department of Radiation Oncology, Amrita Institute of Medical Sciences and Research Centre, Amrita Vishwa Vidyapeetham University, Kochi, Kerala, India

Vineeta Goel, MBBS, DMRT, DNB Radiation Oncology, Max Institute of Oncology, Delhi, India

Gilsa K. Gopinadhan, MPhil (Clinical Psychology) Psycho-Oncology Division, Department of Clinical Psychology, Amrita Institute of Medical Sciences, Kochi, Kerala, India

Sanjay Hunugundmath, MBBS, DNB Deptartment of Radiation Oncology, Sahyadri Super Specialty Hospital, Pune, Maharashtra, India

Wesley M. Jose, MD, DNB (Medical Oncology) Department of Medical Oncology, Amrita Institute of Medical Sciences, Kochi, Kerala, India

Kurian Joseph, MBBS, FFRRCSI, FRCPC Cross Cancer Institute, University of Alberta, Edmonton, AB, Canada

Sruthi Kalavagunta, MBBS, MD Department of Radiation Oncology, Amrita Institute of Medical Sciences, Kochi, Kerala, India

Ashok S. Komaranchath, MD, MRCP(UK), DM, FRCP(Glas.) Aster Medcity, Kochi, Kerala, India

Shiva Kumar Siripuram, MBBS, MD JIPMER, Pondicherry, PY, India

Beena Kunheri, MBBS, DMRT, DNB Department of Radiation Oncology, Amrita Institute of Medical Sciences and Research Centre, Amrita Vishwa Vidyapeetham University, Kochi, Kerala, India

Ram Madhavan, MBBS, MD Department of Radiation Oncology, Amrita Institute of Medical Sciences, Kochi, Kerala, India

Dinesh Makuny, MBBS, DNB, MD Department of Radiation Oncology, MVR Cancer Center, Kozhikode, Kerala, India

Arun Peter Mathew, MS, MCh Division of Surgical Oncology, Department of Surgical Services, Regional Cancer Centre, Thiruvananthapuram, Kerala, India

Anjali Menon, MD Department of Radiation Oncology, Amrita Institute of Medical Sciences and Research Centre, Amrita Vishwa Vidyapeetham University, Kochi, Kerala, India

Koravangattu Valsraj, MBBS, FRCPsych, PGDAP, FHEA South London and Maudsley NHS Foundation Trust, London, UK

Amrita Institute of Medical Sciences, Kochi, Kerala, India

Haridas M, MBBS, MD Department of Radiation Oncology, Amrita Institute of Medical Sciences, Kochi, Kerala, India

Ajith Nambiar, MBBS, MD, DNB, FRCPath Department of Pathology, Amrita Institute of Medical Sciences, Kochi, Kerala, India

Vishnu R. Nambiar, MBBS, MD Department of Radiation Oncology, Baby Memorial Hospital, Calicut, Kerala, India

K. Pavithran, MD, DM, FRCP Department of Medical Oncology, Amrita Institute of Medical Sciences and Research Centre, Kochi, Kerala, India

Arun Philip, MD, DM Department of Medical Oncology, Amrita Institute of Medical Sciences, Kochi, Kerala, India

Regional Cancer Center, Thiruvananthapuram, Kerala, India

Shyama Sudha Prem, MBBS, MD JIPMER, Pondicherry, PY, India

Anand Radhakrishnan, MBBS, MD Department of Radiation Oncology, Medical College, Thiruvananthapuram, Kerala, India

Pragna Sagar Rapole, MBBS, MD JIPMER, Pondicherry, PY, India

Ajil Shaji Department of Radiation Oncology, Amrita Institute of Medical Sciences and Research Centre, Amrita Vishwa Vidyapeetham University, Kochi, Kerala, India

Deepti Sharma, MBBS, MD Max Institute of Oncology, Delhi, India

Radiation Oncology, Institute of Liver and Biliary Sciences, New Delhi, India

Sanjiv Sharma, MBBS, DNB, MD Department of Radiation Oncology, Manipal Hospital, Bangalore, India

Vijay Kumar Srinivasalu, MBBS, MD, DM Department of Medical Oncology, Amrita Institute of Medical Sciences, Amrita Vishwa Vidyapeetham, Kochi, Kerala, India

D. K. Vijaykumar, MS, MCh (Surgical Oncology) Department of Breast and Gynecological Oncology, Amrita Institute of Medical Sciences, Amrita Vishwa Vidyapeetham University, Kochi, Kerala, India

Department of Radiation Oncology, Amrita Institute of Medical Sciences and Research Centre, Amrita Vishwa Vidyapeetham University, Kochi, Kerala, India

Abbreviations

3DCRT	Three dimensional conformal radiation therapy
ABS	Association of Breast Surgery
ACR	American College of Radiology
ACT	Acceptance and Commitment Therapy
AJCC	American Joint Committee on Cancer
ALND	Axillary lymph node dissection
ALTTO Trial	Adjuvant lapatinib and or trastuzumab treatment optimisation trial
APBI	Accelerated partial breast irradiation
ASBS	American Society of Breast Surgeons
ASCO	American Society of Clinical Oncology
ASTRO	American Society for Radiation Oncology
AUS	Axillary ultrasound
BCN	Breast cancer nomogram
BCS	Breast conservation surgery
BI-RADS	Breast imaging reporting and data system
CEUS	Contrast-enhanced ultrasound
CI	Confidence interval
DBT	Digital breast tomosynthesis
DCIS	Ductal carcinoma in situ
DFS	Disease-free survival
DIBH	Deep inspiration breath hold
DSB and HR	Double strand break and homologous recombination
EBC	Early breast cancer
EBCTCG	Early Breast Cancer Trialists' Collaborative Group
EBRT	External beam radiotherapy
EGFR	Epidermal growth factor receptor
ER/PR	Estrogen/progesterone receptor
ERE	Estrogen response elements
ESTRO	European Society for Therapeutic Radiology and Oncology
FFPE	Formalin fixed paraffin embedded
FISH	Fluorescence in situ hybridization
FNAC	Fine needle aspiration cytology
HDI	Human Development Index

HER2	Human epidermal growth factor receptor 2
IARC	International Agency for Research and Cancer
ICG	Indocyanine Green
ICMR	Indian Council for Medical Research
IHC	Immunohistochemistry
ITC	Isolated tumour cells
LCIS	Lobular carcinoma in situ
LVI	Lympho vascular invasion
MAPK	Mitogen activated protein kinase
MDACC	MD Anderson Cancer Centre
MRI	Magnetic resonance imaging
MSKCC	Memorial Sloan-Kettering Cancer Center
NAC	Nipple-areolar complex
NACT	Neoadjuvant chemotherapy
NCCN	National Comprehensive Cancer Network
NICE	National Institute of Clinical Excellence
NMSC	Normal mammary stem cells
NPI	Nottingham Prognostic Index
NSABP	National Surgical Adjuvant Breast and Bowel Project
NST	No special type (Invasive carcinoma of No Special Type)
OCP	Oral contraceptive pill
OS	Overall survival
OSNA	One-step nucleic acid amplification
PARP inhibitors	Poly-ADP ribose polymerase inhibitors
PCR	Polymerase chain reaction
PET	Positron emission tomography
PFS	Progression free survival
PMRT	Post mastectomy radiation therapy
QoL	Quality of life
RCT	Randomised controlled trial
RFS	Relapse free survival
RING domain	Really interesting new gene domain
RTK	Receptor tyrosine kinase
SEER	Surveillance, epidemiology and end results
SERD	Selective estrogen receptor degrader
SERM	Selective estrogen receptor modulator
SLNB	Sentinel lymph node biopsy
SLND	Sentinel lymph node dissection
SPIO	Superparamagnetic iron oxide
TCGA	The cancer genome atlas
TNBC	Triple negative breast cancer
TNM staging	Tumour, node, metastsis
VAB	Vacuum assisted biopsy
VEGF	Vascular endothelial growth factor
VNPI	Van Nuys Prognostic Index
WHO	World Health Organisation

Breast Cancer Trends: Global and Indian Scenario

P. Gangadharan, Ajil Shaji, D. K. Vijaykumar, and Beena Kunheri

1.1   Introduction

Globally, the most common cancer in women is breast cancer. International and national variations in breast cancer incidence and its increases are amply recorded in successive volumes of the IARC publication (WHO) *Cancer Incidence in Five Continents* (CIN V). The increase of breast cancer incidence has been reported from all over the world, but in some highly industrialised countries, it has peaked and declined over the past decade [1]. Along with this, a variation of incidence rates in subsets within and between populations has been reported regularly in Globocan, in CIN volumes and in several studies [2–4]. Furthermore, populations and their progenies migrating from a low incidence country to a higher incidence country have shown an increase in incidence rates [4–8]. Studies report that breast cancer incidence is related to the Human Development Index [9–12]. There are specified modifiable and non-modifiable lifestyle factors, which influence breast cancer occurrence. The identified high-risk factors include early age at menarche, late age at menopause, small number of children, late age at first childbirth, nulliparity, nil or very little breastfeeding, post-menopausal weight gain, hormone replacement therapy, benign breast disease, etc. [13, 14]. It is important to study such observations to provide important leads for the assessment of risk factors that are essential for organising control programmes.

P. Gangadharan (✉) · A. Shaji · D. K. Vijaykumar · B. Kunheri
Department of Radiation Oncology, Amrita Institute of Medical Sciences and Research
Centre, Amrita Vishwa Vidyapeetham University, Kochi, Kerala, India
e-mail: gangadharanp@aims.amrita.edu

© Springer Nature Singapore Pte Ltd. 2021
B. Kunheri, D. K. Vijaykumar (eds.), *Management of Early Stage Breast Cancer*,
https://doi.org/10.1007/978-981-15-6171-9_1

1.2   Global Estimates and Pattern

It was estimated that in 1975 there were 5,41,200 breast cancer cases in the world [15]. Subsequent Globocan reports indicated an increase in breast cancer globally, and Globocan 2018 estimated that in 2018 a total of 2.1 million new breast cancer cases and 6,26,679 deaths due to breast cancer took place globally [16]. These were 11.6% of all cancers combined and 6.5% of all deaths. The Globocan 2018 report is from the analysis of information received from 185 countries [2].

A study of the burden of cancers and their variation across the states of India— Global Burden of Disease study 1990–2016—estimated that in India in 2016 there were 1,18,000 breast cancer cases; 98.1% of these were in females and the prevalent number of cases was 526,000 [17].

The global reports indicate that along with an increase in breast cancer incidence, a decrease in mortality has been reported in some areas over the years.

1.3   Breast Cancer Incidence: Global Variation

Cancer Incidence in Five Continents Vol. XI (IARC) reported the highest incidence of breast cancer (AAR—age-adjusted incidence rate) as 117.9/100,000 recorded among the Maori population in New Zealand, and the next lower was 116.8/100,000 among Hawaiians in Hawaii. The lowest rate of breast cancer was in Tripura, India—6.9/100,000, and the second-lowest rate was also in India in Sikkim—9.9/100,000. These were obtained by analysing the registry data (age standardised) from 343 population cancer registries from 65 countries, including a few population registry data from India.

The highest age-adjusted incidence rate of breast cancer reported globally was 17 times the lowest rate.

The 10 leading places with the highest breast cancer incidence rates and the 10 places with the lowest incidence rates are shown in Tables 1.1 and 1.2, respectively [3].

Table 1.1 The leading 10 populations with age-adjusted rates (AAR) of breast cancer greater than 100/100,000 (CIN V XI) [4]

Country	Place/population	AAR
New Zealand	Maori	117.9
USA, Hawai	Hawaiian	116.8
France, Lille	Metropole	115.4
Belgium	Belgium	109.2
Germany	Schleswig-Holstein	105.9
USA, Hawai	Japanese	105.0
Germany	Hamburg	103.8
France	Loire-Atlantique	101.8
Denmark	Denmark	101.3
Italy	Ferrara	101.3

Table 1.2 The 10 populations with the lowest AAR of breast cancer incidence (CIN V XI)

Country	Place	AAR
India	Cachar	13.9
India	Dindigul—Ambilikkai	13.0
China	Yanting County	12.7
China	Xian Ju	12.7
South Africa	Easter Cape	12.7
India	Ahmedabad	11.6
China	Jianhu County	11.6
India	Barshi—Peranda, Bhum	11.4
India	Sikkim	09.9
India	Tripura	06.9

Source: Tables 1 and 2—cancer incidence in five continents Vol. XI—IARC

An increasing incidence rate and a decreasing mortality rate observed for breast cancer by many studies in the west [16] suggest (1) a real increase in incident cases, (2) increase in detection of early staged disease and (3) optimal treatments based on biological understanding of disease manifestation and its progress. Several innovative procedures such as digital mammography, sentinel node biopsy, breast conservative surgery, advancements in medical oncology, hormonal studies, medications and their application have contributed to more effective treatment opportunities leading to increased survival rates.

Breast cancer incidence has been studied in relation to the Human Development Index (HDI) [9]. The hereditary component is less than 10% in breast cancer. The Human Development Index (HDI) is a composite measure combining indicators representing three dimensions—longevity (life expectancy at birth), knowledge (adult literacy rate and mean years of schooling) and income (World Bank). There have been four levels of HDI studied: very high HDI, high HDI, medium HDI and low HDI. Consistently, breast cancer incidence is the leading cancer in women in all of the above four groups. In cancer incidence studies, transitions to higher levels of human development cause the underlying populations to increasingly adopt behavioural and lifestyle practices that have become conventional in the prosperous and industrialised countries. An in-depth analysis is essential to identify specific lifestyle factors contributing to the association with breast cancer within HDI. In the high HDI regions apart from cancers of the female breast, lung, colorectal and prostate account for maximum cancer burden (global transition according to HDI 2008–2030) [12].

1.4 Populations Within a Nation

The great diversity of breast cancer incidence within every nation provides significant opportunities to study the epidemiology of the disease. In India, the national population census is related to geographically demarcated and administratively unified areas. Great variations in lifestyle practices exist within the country. The educational level, the life expectancy, food habits, social and religious practices, geography and the occupational involvement differ between geographical areas and population subgroups in a state and are reflected in health disparities and sickness patterns.

In India, information on the magnitude and pattern of cancer were initially reported from the hospital-based statistics [18]. These presented only frequencies relative to all cancer types seen in a hospital and did not represent the total population experience. However, the observations from the hospital data lead to more critical studies, and the population-based cancer data provided a reliable comparable picture between population groups.

In 1964, studies of cancer and its distribution in Indian hospitals reported that breast cancer among the Parsi community of Greater Bombay was more than that seen in other communities [19]. Parsees are the followers of Zoroaster who lived in Iran in the seventh century. They migrated to India after a religious conflict and landed on the west coast of India. They strictly followed the Zoroastrian religious discipline and lifestyles. They worship fire and are non-smokers.

Later on, with the availability of the population-based cancer incidence data, a high incidence of breast cancer among Parsees was confirmed. In this regard, the social factors highlighted were the following: (a) unmarried women among Parsees were more than in other communities, (b) average age at marriage among Parsees was higher than in other communities, (c) the late age of marriage caused late age at first delivery, (d) birth rate is lowered and (e) conversion of non-Parsee to Parsee faith is not permitted [20, 21].

1.5   Breast Cancer Incidence: Indian Registries

In India, the first population cancer registry (PBCR) was started by the Indian Cancer Society (ICS) in 1964 and covered only the Greater Bombay population. Later PBCRs were started in Pune, Nagpur and Aurangabad, all in the State of Maharashtra by the ICS. The National Cancer Registry Programme (NCRP) was started by the Indian Council of Medical Research (ICMR) in 1982. Three population registries (PBCR)—Mumbai, Chennai and Bangalore—and three hospital cancer registries (HBCR)—Regional Cancer Centre, Thiruvananthapuram (RCC), Post Graduate Institute Chandigarh (PGI) and Medical College Dibrugarh (MC)—were started. Several regional area populations are now covered by the population cancer registration. These are functioning apart from several hospital-based cancer registries, also organised and maintained by the National Centre for Disease Informatics and Research—NCDIR (ICMR). There are now 29 population cancer registries in India, and more are being organised. The ICMR registry system was initiated in 1982 and maintains standardised procedures for data collection and reporting according to the International Cancer Registry Standards of information collection and reporting.

In Table 1.3, crude incidence rate (CR), age-adjusted incidence rate (AAR) per 100,000 population and rank of breast cancer among all cancer in females in

Table 1.3 Crude incidence rate (CR), age-adjusted incidence rate (AAR) per 100,000 population and rank of breast cancer among all cancer in females in different PBCRs in India

PBCR (*Year*)	Breast cancer		
	CR	AAR	Rank
Bangalore *(2012)*	29.3	34.4	1
Barshi Rural *(2012–2014)*	13.2	12.4	2
Barshi Expanded *(2012)*	11.9	11.7	2
Bhopal *(2012–2013)*	28.2	33.1	1
Chennai *(2012–2013)*	40.6	37.9	1
Delhi *(2012)*	34.8	41.0	1
Mumbai *(2012)*	33.6	33.6	1
Cachar District *(2012–2014)*	11.3	12.8	1
Dibrugarh District *(2012–2014)*	12.7	13.9	1
Kamrup Urban District *(2012–2014)*	21.5	27.1	1
Sikkim State *(2012–2014)*	9.7	11.1	1
Ahmedabad Urban *(2012–2013)*	23.0	23.8	1
Aurangabad *(2012–2014)*	18.5	22.6	1
Kolkata *(2012)*	30.7	25.5	1
Kollam District *(2012–2014)*	36.3	27.7	1
Nagpur *(2012–2013)*	30.4	29.3	1
Pune *(2012–2013)*	23.4	26.4	1
Thi'puram District *(2012–2014)*	43.9	33.7	1
Tripura State *(2012–2014)*	6.6	6.9	2
Nagaland *(2012–2014)*	6.8	9.1	2
Wardha District *(2012–2014)*	20.9	18.8	1
Pasighat *(2012–2014)*	13.8	17.4	2
Patiala District *(2012–2014)*	34.2	33.1	1
Manipur (MR) State *(2012–2014)*	8.6	9.7	1
Imphal West District (2012–2014)	*16.6*	*16.2*	1
MR—Excl Imphal West (2012–2014)	*6.8*	*8.0*	1
Mizoram State (MZ) *(2012–2014)*	15.8	19.9	3
Aizwal District (2012–2014)	*24.3*	*28.0*	3
MZ Excl Aizwal (2012–2014)	*10.7*	*14.2*	4
Meghalaya *(2012–2014)*	4.3	6.7	3
East Khasi Hills District (2012–2014)	*6.3*	*8.9*	3
Naharlagun (NH) *(2012–2014)*	6.3	9.4	3
Papumpare District (2012–2014)	*17.3*	*29.2*	1
NH-Excl Papumpare District (2012–2014)	*2.8*	*4.4*	6

Source: NCRP 3 year report of PBCRs 2012–2014 [23]

different PBCRs in India are shown. The data presented are for 34 population groups, which include 7 population subgroups of the state or district (given in italics).

The crude incidence rate (CR) provides the magnitude of the problem in the population studied, and all efforts should focus on reducing this rate. The pattern of AAR enables us to study and compare the magnitude of the problem and help us to study and identify the factors associated with the risk of developing the disease as well as the outcome evaluation.

As can be seen in Table 1.3, among Indian registries, the CR is maximum in Thiruvanathapuram females, Kerala (43.9 /100.000), followed by Chennai, Tamil Nadu (40.6/100.000), Kollam, Kerala (36.3/100.000), Delhi (34.8/100.000), Patiala, Punjab (34.2/100,000) and Mumbai, Maharashtra (33.6/100,000) (source: NCRP Reports of PBCRs 2012–2014).

It may be noted that among the 27 major registration areas 19 registries have breast cancer as the leading cancer in women. These rates are observed in the population without any adjustment for age differences between the world population and local population, thus representing the load of cancer in the respective populations.

It is mentioned that the expectation of life in Kerala is more than 75 years, and the United Nations report (United Nations Population Fund UNFPA) indicate that among Indian states the percentage of persons above the age 60 years is maximum in Kerala (Caring for our elders—Early response, India Ageing Report 2017 UNFPA New Delhi) [22]. Kerala would be above the National Average of HDI as the literacy rate; expectation of life at birth and income levels are probably higher. It has been reported that Kerala has the highest HDI in India. The high crude incidence rate is a result of its association with HDI.

The age-adjusted rate is obtained by applying the age-specific rates to the age specified distribution of the world standard population. The highest reported age-adjusted incidence rate (AAR) of breast cancer was seen in Delhi followed by Chennai, Bangalore and Thiruvananthapuram district. While Delhi, Chennai and Bangalore are entirely urbanised areas, the Thiruvananthapuram district registry consists of a significant rural proportion as well (Fig. 1.1).

1.6   Observations Reported from Non-ICMR Registries in India

Apart from the cancer registries of the National Cancer Registry Programme (NCRP-ICMR), 13 population cancer registries organised by Tata Memorial Centre are functioning. Of these, four registries are in the State of Punjab. They are in Chandigarh (UT) and in the three districts—Mansa, Sangrur and SAS Nagar of Punjab State. The breast cancer incidence rates of Punjab population groups are shown in Table 1.4.

Of the third set of nine PBCRs also organised by the Tata Memorial Centre (TMC), six are in the vicinity of atomic power generating stations. The registry

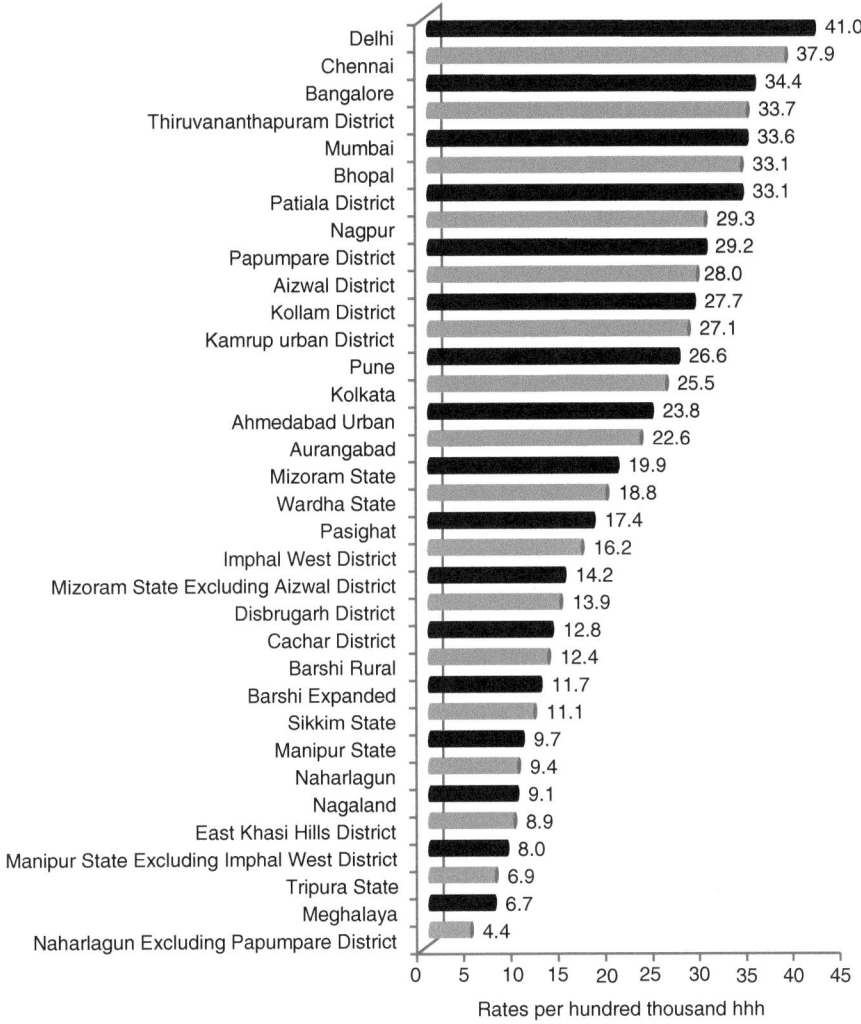

Fig. 1.1 Age adjusted incidence rates (AAR) of female breast cancer–All PBCRs in India. Source: NCRP 3 year report of PBCRs 2012–2014 [23]

Table 1.4 Breast cancer incidence rates in the districts of Punjab State and Chandigarh (UT)

SI no	Place	Year	CR	ASR	Rank[a]
1	Mansa District	2013–2014	12.3	11.5	2
2	Sangrur District	2014	13.7	13.6	1
3	SAS Nagar	2014	24.8	29.5	1
4	Chandigarh District (UT)	2014	26.7	32.7	1

[a]Rank is identified as the rank among all cancer cases in females seen in the registry area; *UT* union territory [24]

Table 1.5 Breast cancer incidence rate in cancer registries in nine centres: TMC

SI no	Place—*State*	Year	CR	ASR	Rank[a]
5	Rawatbhata—*Rajasthan*	2011–2013	6.7	7.0	2
6	Palghar—*Maharashtra*	2013–2014	9.0	9.9	1
7	Karwar—*Karnataka*	2010–2013	21.5	19.6	1
8	Kakrapara—*Gujarat*	2011–2013	8.2	8.0	2
9	Kalpakam—*Tamil Nadu*	2014–2015	30.5	29.9	1
10	Kundamkulam—*Tamil Nadu*	2014–2015	22.4	19.7	1
11	Ratnagiri—*Maharashtra*	2011–2014	13.8	11.3	1
12	SindhuDurg—*Maharashtra*	2012–2014	14.7	11.4	1
13	Visakhapatnam—*Andhra Pradesh*	2014	18.2	17.3	1

[a]Rank is identified as the rank among all cancer cases in females seen in the registry area [25]

covering Visakhapatnam Urban Area is in Andhra Pradesh. Registries in Sindhu Durgh and Ratnagiri area, which are in Maharashtra, are also organised by Tata Memorial Centre [25]. The crude and age-standardised incidence rates along with the rank of breast cancer among all cancers are shown in Table 1.5.

The registries 11, 12 and 13 are not near nuclear power generating stations.

Visakhapatnam is a busy industrial area. The ASRs are similar to those seen in the NCRP—PBCRs. It is to be noted that there will be urban–rural differences in the total incidence and age-specific breast cancer incidence curves as well.

1.7   Age Incidnce Rate Changes

1.7.1   Incidence Rate of Breast Cancer Varies over the Ages

In Fig. 1.2, the age-specific incidence of breast cancer in six centres drawn on the arithmetic grid is shown.

In the high incidence areas viz. Mumbai, Bangalore, Delhi and Chennai, the major increase of incidence in old age is after the age 40, as shown in Fig. 1.2. This is noted as the increase of incidence rates during post menopausal years, which are not seen in very low incidence areas like Barshi, Dibrugarh and Cachar, which are more rural than Chennai, Delhi, Mumbai etc. The Urban Rural lifestyle patterns are an important factor for such observed differences [26].

In Fig. 1.3, the incidence curves of breast cancer in two PBCRs of Kerala:-Thiruvananthapuram district and Kollam district are shown. These are neighbouring districts. There was a similarity in the pattern seen in both the places upto the menopausal years. The rates after age 40 are slightly higher in Thiruvananthapuram district compared to that seen in Kollam district. Kollam district has a higher percentage of rural population and cancer detection facilities in Thiruvananthapuram are much more than that seen in Kollam. The incidence rates in most rural areas differ from urban rates around 45 years age. Such urban rural age specific differences between the areas may not only relate to diagnostic opportunities but also as a resultant of lifestyle factors. Here the lifestyle impact may be the associated factor along with the diagnostic opportunities.

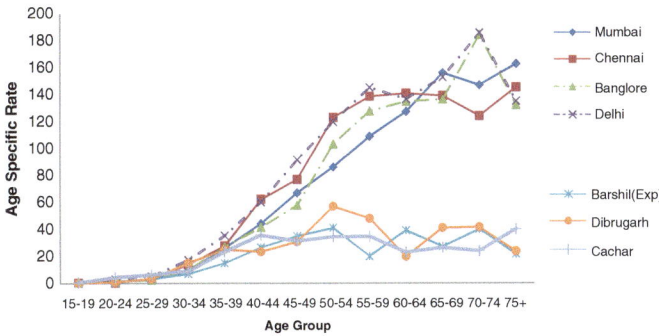

Fig. 1.2 Highest Four and lowest three PBCRs age-specific rates (per 100,000) of female breast cancer. Source: PBCR reports National Cancer Registry programme

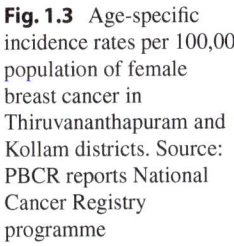

Fig. 1.3 Age-specific incidence rates per 100,000 population of female breast cancer in Thiruvananthapuram and Kollam districts. Source: PBCR reports National Cancer Registry programme

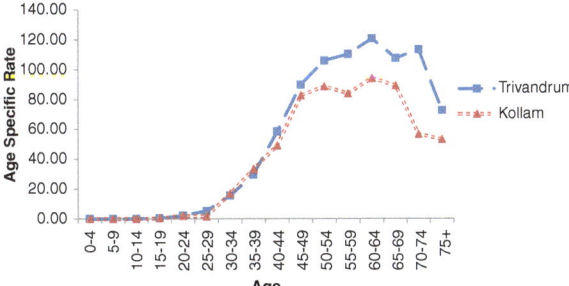

In Kollam district, there is an area—Karunagappally taluk—with high natural background radiation emitted by the monazite sand [27]. The AAR in Karunagappally taluk was 16.6 per 100,000, as reported in CIN Vol. X. In CIN Vol. XI, the Kollam district population incidence was 27.7; Karunagappally taluk is a small limited area taluk in Kollam District. In Fig. 1.3, age-specific incidence rates per 100,000 population are shown.

As noted earlier, in the urban areas, there is an increase even after the age of 45 years.

1.7.2   Breast Cancer Incidence Variation: National Estimates

An increase in breast cancer incidence was initially recorded by the Bombay Cancer Registry. Three consecutive studies recorded the increase of breast cancer incidence since the 1980s.

The National Cancer Registry programme has analysed the time trends under the NCRP registries for the period 2012–2014 and has recorded a steady increase in incidence, as shown in Fig. 1.4 [23].

It may be noted that breast cancer incidence rate has been increasing in all Indian registry areas. The NCDIR (ICMR) has estimated that in 2020 there

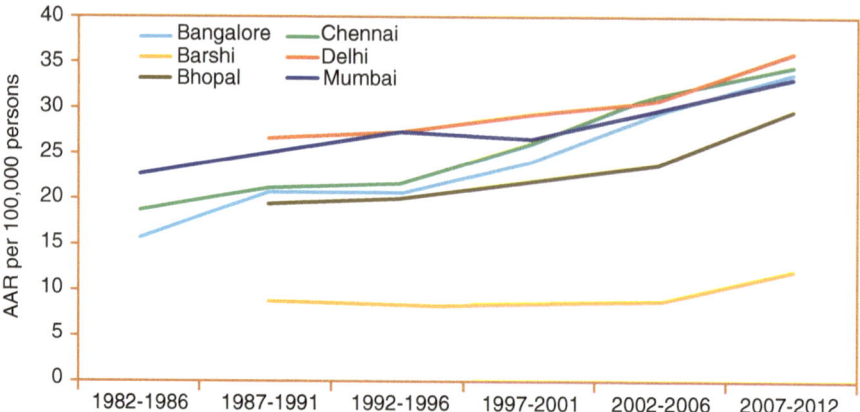

Fig. 1.4 Female breast cancer—5-year trend (trends over time in AARs). Source: Page: 109 3 year report of population based cancer registries 2012–2014, Indian Council of Medical Research

would be 1,79,790 new breast cancer in India based on the current trend in breast cancer incidence.

1.8   Migrant Study Observations

Life practices influence breast cancer incidence. Identification of the associative, causative and high-risk factors could help the control of the disease by continued studies of habits and curtailment of high-risk lifestyle practices. Comparisons with the incidence, pattern and trends of breast cancer in a native population over time and with that seen among migrants from one population to another are essential to study the sources of the differences seen in incidence and pattern. Cancer pattern changes observed after migration are mainly caused by lifestyle changes, and studies of such differences observed help us to control the disease occurrence [28].

An increase in breast cancer incidence in migrants has been reported by several studies [6–8]. Mostly, such migrations have been from low incidence countries, and the lifestyle changes tend to increase the incidence of breast cancer among migrants. A lowering of breast cancer incidence rates has not been reported among any migrant groups. However, such observation between groups may differ due to (a) differences in methodology adopted for the study, (b) lack of uniformity of opportunity of case identification, (c) changes in lifestyle among migrants after migration, (d) life expectancy of the host population, (e) susceptibility of the population for the particular cancer and (f) differences in religious and social practices followed and adhered to in the host country.

More often, people migrate from a country when they are looking for their life betterment. This higher society group migrating will be more than the lower social segment of the population. Breast cancer incidence is higher in the higher social group even before migration.

Migrants often follow the traditional practices observed in the migrated place. However, in the case of Parsees, the religious practices followed were retained even after their migration to India. Hence, the traditional practices were the contributory factor for the high incidence.

Several Indians have migrated to Singapore and Malaysia and the respective breast cancer incidence among migrated Indians are as follows.

1. Malaysian Indians (breast cancer—AAR—50.0 (CIN Vol. XI).
2. Singapore Indians (breast cancer—AAR—65.3 (Singapore Cancer Registry 2015).

In most migrant studies, such an increase in cancer incidence is noted among all migrating populations [3, 29].

The CIN volumes of IARC have several such population groups living in geographical areas with varying incidence rates. Also, in the Indian registry reports, the incidence of breast cancer varied almost tenfold between administrative states. Furthermore, there are differences between rural and urban rates. Such variations take place due to differences in cultural lifestyle practices.

A population study of migrants seen in four South Asian regions, India, Singapore and Indians in UK and USA, concluded that the incidence increase of breast cancer among migrants was due to adopting western lifestyle, especially semi-western diet, childbearing practices as in high socio-economic urban subgroups and physical activity levels [30].

As mentioned earlier, the differences observed between the disease rates could also relate to diagnostic opportunities and quality of medical certificates, including the death reporting system.

In India, variations in the occurrence of breast cancer and life habits have been observed within and between population groups. Such differences are more depending on lifestyle practices and diagnostic opportunities. In an analysis of Bombay cancer incidence data of two decades, from 1964 to 1983, a higher age-adjusted incidence (AAR) rate was observed for breast cancer in Parsees, the next lower was seen among Christians and Muslims, and the lowest rate was seen in Hindus (Kasturi Jayant, Cancers of Cervix Uteri and Breast: changes in incidence rates in Mumbai over the last two decades. Bulletin of WHO 1964) [31].

In breast cancer epidemiology, pre- and post-menopausal periods have contrasting risk levels for breast cancer occurrence. The differences in risk level observed among an urban life may be related to body size and other anthropometric measurements. Pre-menopausal and post-menopausal studies have shown that pre-menopausal weight gain is safer than post-menopausal weight increase [32].

A breast cancer incidence study from Karunagappilly, rural Kerala, observed by a nested case–control study that consumers of certain vegetables, especially tapioca consumers, experience a lowered risk [33].

1.9   Conclusion

Breast cancer incidence has an increasing trend in developed and developing nations. The urban cancer registries in India report that breast cancer is the most common cancer among females. An encouraging observation from western studies is that, even though the incidence of breast cancer is increasing, the mortality associated with the disease is decreasing. Early detection coupled with implementation of optimal treatment methods has resulted in the decrease in mortality. Public health action for prevention and early detection of breast cancer needs high emphasis like for many other cancers.

Acknowledgments   We are grateful to Ms. Thanuja Gopakumar, Ms. Suma M.S., Ms. Mini A.P. and Ms. Vipina K.P. for their assistance in preparing this manuscript.

References

1. Ravdin PM, Cronin KA, Howlader N, et al. The decrease in breast-cancer incidence in 2003 in the United States. N Engl J Med. 2007;356:1670–4. https://doi.org/10.1056/NEJMsr070105.
2. The Global Cancer Observatory. Globocan. IARC. 2018. https://gco.iarc.fr/today/home. Accessed 15 Dec 2018.
3. Cancer incidence in five continents, (CIN) Vol. I–XI. International Agency for Research on Cancer web site. http://ci5.iarc.fr/CI5I-XI.
4. Jemal A, Ward E, Thun MJ. Recent trends in breast cancer incidence rates by age and tumor characteristics among U.S. women. Breast Cancer Res. 2007;9:R28. https://doi.org/10.1186/bcr1672.
5. Ziegler RG, Hoover RN, Pike MC, et al. Migration patterns and breast cancer risk in Asian-American women. J Natl Cancer Inst. 1993;85:1819–27. https://doi.org/10.1093/jnci/85.22.1819.
6. Winter H, Cheng K, Cummins C, Maric R, Silcocks P, Varghese C. Cancer incidence in the south Asian population of England (1990–92). Br J Cancer. 1999;79(3–4):645–54. https://doi.org/10.1038/sj.bjc.6690102.
7. Grulich A, McCredie M, Coates M. Cancer incidence in Asian migrants to New South Wales, Australia. Br J Cancer. 1995;71(2):400–8. https://doi.org/10.1038/bjc.1995.82.
8. Ghumare SS, Cunningham JE. Breast cancer trends in Indian residents and emigrants portend an emerging epidemic for India. Asian Pac J Cancer Prev. 2007;8:507–12.
9. Hu K, Lou L, Tian W, Pan T, Ye J, Zhang S. The outcome of breast cancer is associated with National Human Development Index and Health System attainment. PLoS One. 2016;11:e158951. https://doi.org/10.1371/journal.pone.0158951.
10. Fidler MM, Soerjomataram I, Bray F. A global view on cancer incidence and national levels of the Human Development Index. Int J Cancer. 2016;139:2436–46. https://doi.org/10.1002/ijc.30382.
11. Khazaei S, Rezaeian S, Khazaei Z, Molaeipoor L, Nematollahi S, Lak P, et al. National Breast cancer mortality and incidence rates according to the Human Development Index: an ecological study. Adv Breast Cancer Res. 2016;5:30–6. https://doi.org/10.4236/abcr.2016.51003.
12. Bray F, Jemal A, Grey N, et al. Global cancer transitions according to the Human Development Index (2008-2030): a population-based study. Lancet Oncol. 2012;13:790–801. https://doi.org/10.1016/S1470-2045(12)70211-5.
13. Stewart BW, Wild CP, editors. World cancer report 2014. Lyon: International Agency for Research on Cancer; 2014. p. 115–23. Section 2.5, Reproductive and hormonal risk factors.

14. Veronesi U, Boyle P, et al. Breast cancer. Lancet. 2005;365:1727–39. https://doi.org/10.1016/S0140-6736(05)66546-4.
15. Parkin DM, Stjernsward J, Muir CS. Estimates of the worldwide frequency of twelve major cancers. Bull WHO. 1984;62:163–82.
16. Bray F, Ferlay J, Soerjomataram J, Siegel RL, Torre LA, Jemal A. Global Cancer Statistics 2018: GLOBOCAN estimates of incidence and mortality worldwide for 36 cancers in 185 countries. CA Cancer J Clin. 2018;68:394–424. https://doi.org/10.3322/caac.21492.
17. India State-Level Disease Burden Initiative Cancer Collaborators. The burden of cancers and their variations across the states of India: the global burden of disease study 1990-2016. Lancet Oncol. 2018;19:1289–306. https://doi.org/10.4103/jehp.jehp_156_19.
18. Khanolkar VR. Cancer in India. Acta Unio Int Contra Cancrum. 1950;V1(5):882–90.
19. Paymaster JC. Cancer and its distribution in India. Cancer. 1964;17:1026–34.
20. Paymaster JC, Gangadharan P. Cancer in the Parsi community of Bombay. Int J Cancer. 1970;5:426–31.
21. Paymaster JC, Gangadharan P. Epidemiology of breast cancer in India. J Natl Cancer Inst. 1972;48:1021–4.
22. United Nations Population Fund. 'Caring for our elders—early response'—India ageing report 2017 UNFPA. New Delhi: United Nations Population Fund; 2017.
23. Three year report of population based cancer registries. 2012–2014. www.ncdirindia.org.
24. Atul B, Thakur JS, Rajesh D, Badwe RA. Summary report of population based cancer registries Chandigarh, SAS Nagar, Sangrur and Mansa districts, Punjab State, India for the year 2013–2014: Tata Memorial Centre, Mumbai. Chandigarh: PGI; 2017.
25. Badwe RA, Ganesh B. Consolidated report: Tata Memorial Centre-Dept. of Atomic Energy Network of Cancer Registries, Tata Memorial Centre Publication, Tata Memorial Centre, Mumbai. 2019.
26. Nagrani RT, Budukh A, Koyande S, Panse NS, Mhatre SS, Badwe R. A comparative study of breast cancer incidence of urban and rural areas comprising 26 population groups concluded that living in rural areas decreases the risk of breast cancer (Rural Urban differences in breast cancer in India). Ind J Cancer. 2014;3:277–81.
27. Sebastine P, Padmavathy J, Harikrishnan K, Raghuram KN. Cancer incidence in Karunagappilly Kerala, India. X IARC:28.
28. Parkin DM, Khlat M. Studies of cancer in migrants: rationale and methodology. Eur J Cancer. 1996;32A(5):761–71.
29. Singapore Cancer Registry. Annual report 2015. National Registry of Diseases Office (NRDO).
30. Rastogi T, Devesa S, Mangtani P, et al. Cancer incidence rates among South Asians in four geographic regions: India, Singapore, UK and US. Int J Epidemiol. 2008;37(1):147–60. https://doi.org/10.1093/ije/dym219.
31. Yeole BB, Jayant K, Jussawalla K. Trends in breast cancer incidence in greater Bombay: an epidemiological assessment. Bull World Health Organ. 1990;66(2):245–9.
32. Mathew A, Gajalakshmi V, Rajan B, et al. Physical activity levels among urban and rural women in South India and the risk of breast cancer—a case control study. Eur J Cancer Prev. 2009;18(5):368–76.
33. Jayalekshmi P, Varughese SC, Kalavathi, Krishnan Nair M, Jayaprakash V, Gangadharan P, Raghu Ram KN, Suminori A. A nested case control study of female breast cancer in Karunagappally cohort in Kerala India. Asian Pac J Cancer Prev. 2009;10(2):239–44.

Role of Screening: Guidelines and Recommendations

Sanjay Hunugundmath, Anjali Menon, and Beena Kunheri

2.1 Introduction

The goal of screening is to detect breast cancer in healthy female population without any symptoms of the disease with the use of the ideal tests and imaging methods. The population needs to be stratified according to the level of risk they carry to develop breast cancer in their lifetime. This would help us determine the females who would need to be screened in order to detect cancer at early stages, who would need to undergo prophylactic treatment and chemoprevention and who would need genetic testing. Population-based screening studies with mammograms have shown that older women >40 years showed a 40% reduction in breast cancer mortality [1, 2].

This chapter will address the *risk stratification, screening tools, screening recommendations for breast cancer* and *risks and benefits of screening*.

2.2 Stratification of Breast Cancer Risk

The population is divided into mainly three groups, which would be those women with a high lifetime risk for developing breast cancer, those at moderate lifetime risk at developing breast cancer and those at average lifetime risk at developing breast cancer. There is no consensus or standardisation about the lifetime risk, and most of them are cateogarised based on history and available models.

S. Hunugundmath (✉)
Deptartment of Radiation Oncology, Sahyadri Super Specialty Hospital, Pune, Maharashtra, India

A. Menon · B. Kunheri
Department of Radiation Oncology, Amrita Institute of Medical Sciences and Research Centre, Amrita Vishwa Vidyapeetham University, Kochi, Kerala, India

© Springer Nature Singapore Pte Ltd. 2021
B. Kunheri, D. K. Vijaykumar (eds.), *Management of Early Stage Breast Cancer*, https://doi.org/10.1007/978-981-15-6171-9_2

High risk: More than 20% lifetime risk of developing breast cancer.

Moderate risk: 15–20% lifetime risk of developing breast cancer.

Average risk: Less than 15% lifetime risk of developing breast cancer. Most of the female population falls into this risk category.

Major factors that help in identifying the risk category are as follows:

1. Personal history of ovarian, peritoneal (including tubal) or breast cancer.
2. Family history of breast, ovarian or peritoneal cancer.
3. Genetic predisposition.
4. Radiotherapy to the chest between age 10 and 30 years.

An individual who has no such risk factors falls into the average-risk group. Women with a family history of breast cancer but no genetic predisposing syndromes fall into the moderate-risk group.

Following are the factors predisposing for high risk and eligible for screening as high-risk individuals [3–7]:

- Women who have a personal history of breast cancer.
- Confirmed or suspected genetic mutation known to increase the risk of breast cancer (e.g. BRCA1 or BRCA2, PTEN, TP53).
- First-degree relative of a mutation carrier (e.g. BRCA1, BRCA1), who has had genetic counselling and has declined genetic testing.
- History of previous radiotherapy to the chest between ages 10 and 30.
- Calculated lifetime risk of >20% for developing breast cancer (calculated by models such as BRCAPRO, IBIS and BOADICEA tools).
- History of previous breast biopsies for benign breast lesions, dense breasts on a mammogram (1.5- to 2-fold increased risk).
- Estrogen exposure: nulliparity, > 30 years of first childbirth, use of OCPs, earlier menarche, late menopause (1- to 1.5-fold increased risk).

2.3   Risk Prediction Models/Tools

Gail model [8, 9]: Based on an individual's risk factors of age, history of first degree relatives with breast cancer, previous benign breast diseases, late menarche and late parity, the Gail model can calculate the risk of developing breast cancer in five years and in an individual's lifetime. The Gail model is not very useful for calculating risk in individuals with a history of in situ lesions (DCIS, LCIS), invasive breast carcinomas, known genetic syndromes (BRCA1 and 2), strong family history and elderly age group.

The following online risk prediction tools have been developed for geneticists: BRCAPRO, IBIS and BOADICEA tools.

2.4   Screening Tools

1. Mammogram: film, digital, computer-aided detection and digital breast tomosynthesis.
2. Breast ultrasound (alone or in combination with a mammogram).
3. MRI breast.
4. Clinical examination and patient breast self-examination.

2.4.1   Age Categorisation for Screening

- Age 39 years and under.
- Age 40–49 years.
- Age 50–74 years.
- Age 75 years and older.

2.4.2   Screening for High-Risk Breast Cancer

Various international collaborative groups have presented guidelines [10–17] for screening women at high risk for breast cancer, often based on experts' opinions. The radiological screening tests recommended for women with a high risk of developing breast cancer include the following:

- Annual screening mammogram and annual supplemental screening breast MRI [18–22] should be scheduled 6 months apart so that the woman effectively has one screening test 6 months apart. Women who cannot undergo an MRI for any medical or other reasons should have a screening ultrasound at the same schedule as the screening MRI.
- For women with a family history of breast cancers and who are at high risk of developing breast cancers, annual mammography should start 5–10 years younger than the youngest case in the family, but no earlier than age 25 and no later than age 40. Annual clinical breast examination should start at the age of 25 years.
- Women who have had chest wall radiation below the age of 30 years should have annual mammography and screening breast MRI starting 5–10 years after radiation given, but no earlier than age 25 and no later than age 40. These women should also undergo annual clinical breast examination starting at the age of 25 years.

2.4.3   Screening of Moderate-Risk Breast Cancer

The screening of these women would be essentially similar to screening population with average risk. There are no randomised control trials focusing on this population.

Additional or supplemental imaging with either an ultrasound correlation or an MRI breast might be useful in this population if a mammogram alone is not confirmatory.

2.5   Screening for Average-Risk Breast Cancer

• Screening is not recommended below 39 years of age in view of very low positive predictive value [27].
• In the age group of 40–49 years, the physician after addressing the patient's concerns helps them decide the need for screening by counselling about the risk and benefits involved (shared decision making). The high rates of false positives, overdiagnosis, low sensitivity and specificity of breast cancer risk stratification tools and risk of radiation associated with screening are the important factors that aid decision making in patients [30]. Nelson et al., in their meta-analysis, even though statistically not significant, showed that advanced cancer is reduced with screening women aged 39–49 years [28]. Another study by Moss et al. also showed similar outcomes [29]. Based on these modest data, most of the expert groups recommend individualising the need for initiation of screening in the age group of 40–49 years after shared decision making [23–26].
• In the age group of 50–74 years, most of the breast expert groups from USA, UK, Canada and Australia recommend mammographic screening every two years (biennial) or every 3 years [23–26]. Nelson et al.'s meta-analysis [28] and other systematic reviews of RCTs [2, 29–36] over 50 years showed that there was a reduction in breast cancer mortality with screening in this age group with approximately 20% relative risk reduction. A Swedish study by Nyström et al. of four RCTs showed that the all-cause mortality was reduced with screening in this population and age-adjusted relative risk for total mortality was 0.98 [31].
• In the elderly population (above 74 years), screening is recommended once in 2 years in healthy women (only if there is life expectancy for more than 10 years) [40–42]. Various governmental study groups and task forces advise discontinuation of screening by 74 or 75 years of age [23–26]. Most of the observational data showed higher early detection rates but no change in mortality with screening [37–39].

2.6   Conclusion: Benefits and Risks of Screening

The primary benefit is reduction in mortality. The meta-analyses and systemic reviews have shown to reduce the odds of dying from breast cancer almost by 20% [43, 44]. The absolute benefit of screening is proportional to age, lower in younger women because they have a lower baseline risk of cancer. A 2016 systematic review analysed risk reduction by age: with at least 11 years of follow-up, the pooled relative risk for breast cancer mortality was 0.92 (95% CI 0.75–1.02) for women 39–49 years of age, 0.86 (0.68–0.97) for women 50–59 years of age and 0.67 (0.54–0.83) for women 60–69 years of age [28]. At this point of time, it is difficult to comment on the exact reduction in mortality, which we have seen over time is due to improved techniques of screening or improved effectiveness of therapy.

Risks associated with breast cancer screening most commonly include overdiagnosis and unnecessary investigations, which lead to patients' anxiety. Overdiagnosis ranges from 10 to 50% of all women diagnosed with breast cancer. Many studies have reported that DCIS is biologically insignificant and would never become clinically evident in the patient's lifetime. It is not possible to distinguish biologically insignificant cancers from those that will proceed to grow, metastasize and lead to the patient's death at this time. As a result, they receive some sort of local therapy, which may be unnecessary [45].

The future will depend upon the development of even more sensitive and specific screening tools, thereby reducing false positives and false negatives.

References

1. Armstrong K, Moye E, Williams S, et al. Screening mammography in women 40 to 49 years of age: a systematic review for the American College of Physicians. Ann Intern Med. 2007;146:516.
2. Nelson HD, Tyne K, Naik A, et al. Screening for breast cancer: an update for the U.S. Preventive Services Task Force. Ann Intern Med. 2009;151:727.
3. Collaborative Group on Hormonal Factors in Breast Cancer. Familial breast cancer: collaborative reanalysis of individual data from 52 epidemiological studies including 58,209 women with breast cancer and 101,986 women without the disease. Lancet. 2001;358:1389–99.
4. Pharoah PD, Day NE, Duffy S, et al. Family history and the risk of breast cancer: A systematic review and meta-analysis. Int J Cancer. 1997;71:800–9.
5. Bevier M, Sundquist K, Hemminki K. Risk of breast cancer in families of multiple affected women and men. Breast Cancer Res Treat. 2012;132:723–8.
6. Claus EB, Schildkraut JM, Thompson WD, et al. The genetic attributable risk of breast and ovarian cancer. Cancer. 1996;77:2318–24.
7. Whittemore AS, Gong G, Itnyre J. Prevalence and contribution of BRCA1 mutations in breast cancer and ovarian cancer: Results from three U.S. population-based case-control studies of ovarian cancer. Am J Hum Genet. 1997;60:496–504.
8. Gail MH, Brinton LA, Byar DP, et al. Projecting individualized probabilities of developing breast cancer for white females who are being examined annually. J Natl Cancer Inst. 1989;81:1879.
9. Gail MH, Costantino JP, Pee D, et al. Projecting individualized absolute invasive breast cancer risk in African American women. J Natl Cancer Inst. 2007;99:1782.
10. Ashton-Prolla P, Giacomazzi J, Schmidt AV, et al. Development and validation of a simple questionnaire for the identification of hereditary breast cancer in primary care. BMC Cancer. 2009;9:283.
11. Eccles DM, Evans DG, Mackay J. Guidelines for a genetic risk based approach to advising women with a family history of breast cancer: UK Cancer Family Study Group (UKCFSG). J Med Genet. 2000;37:203–9.
12. Vasen HF, Haites NE, Evans DG, et al. Current policies for surveillance and management in women at risk of breast and ovarian cancer: A survey among 16 European family cancer clinics—European Familial Breast Cancer Collaborative Group. Eur J Cancer. 1998;34:1922–6.
13. Evans DG, Lalloo F. Risk assessment and management of high risk familial breast cancer. J Med Genet. 2002;39:865–71.

14. Eisinger F, Alby N, Bremond A, et al. Recommendations for medical management of hereditary breast and ovarian cancer: The French National Ad Hoc Committee. Ann Oncol. 1998;9:939–50.
15. Møller P, Evans G, Haites N, et al. Guidelines for follow-up of women at high risk for inherited breast cancer: consensus statement from the Biomed 2 Demonstration Programme on Inherited Breast Cancer. Dis Markers. 1999;15:207–11.
16. Warner E, Heisey RE, Goel V, et al. Hereditary breast cancer. Risk assessment of patients with a family history of breast cancer. Can Fam Physician. 1999;45:104–12.
17. Metcalfe KA, Birenbaum-Carmeli D, Lubinski J, et al. International variation in rates of uptake of preventive options in BRCA1 and BRCA2 mutation carriers. Int J Cancer. 2008;122:2017–22.
18. Warner E, Plewes DB, Hill KA, et al. Surveillance of BRCA1 and BRCA2 mutation carriers with magnetic resonance imaging, ultrasound, mammography, and clinical breast examination. JAMA. 2004;292:1317–25.
19. Kriege M, Brekelmans CT, Boetes C, et al. Differences between first and subsequent rounds of the MRISC breast cancer screening program for women with a familial or genetic predisposition. Cancer. 2006;106:2318–26.
20. Leach MO, Boggis CR, Dixon AK, et al. Screening with magnetic resonance imaging and mammography of a UK population at high familial risk of breast cancer: a prospective multi-centre cohort study (MARIBS). Lancet. 2005;365:1769–78.
21. Kuhl CK, Schrading S, Leutner CC, et al. Mammography, breast ultrasound, and magnetic resonance imaging for surveillance of women at high familial risk for breast cancer. J Clin Oncol. 2005;23:8469–76.
22. Lehman CD, Blume JD, Weatherall P, et al. Screening women at high risk for breast cancer with mammography and magnetic resonance imaging. Cancer. 2005;103:1898–905.
23. US Preventive Services Task Force. Screening for breast cancer: US Preventive Services Task Force recommendation statement. Ann Intern Med. 2016;164:279.
24. Canadian Task Force on Preventive Health Care, Tonelli M, Connor Gorber S, et al. Recommendations on screening for breast cancer in average-risk women aged 40-74 years. CMAJ. 2011;183:1991.
25. NHS England Department of Health. Public health functions to be exercised by NHS England. Public Health Policy and Strategy Unit, Department of Health. 2013. www.gov.uk/government/uploads/system/uploads/attachment_data/file/192971/S7A_VARIATION_2013-14_FINAL_130417.pdf. Accessed 17 Aug 2015.
26. RACGP. Guidelines for preventive activities in general practice, breast cancer. www.racgp.org.au/your-practice/guidelines/redbook/9-early-detection-of-cancers/93-breast-cancer/.
27. Yankaskas BC, Haneuse S, Kapp JM, et al. Performance of first mammography examination in women younger than 40 years. J Natl Cancer Inst. 2010;102:692.
28. Nelson HD, Fu R, Cantor A, et al. Effectiveness of breast cancer screening: systematic review and meta-analysis to update the 2009 U.S. Preventive Services Task Force Recommendation. Ann Intern Med. 2016;164:244.
29. Moss SM, Cuckle H, Evans A, et al. Effect of mammographic screening from age 40 years on breast cancer mortality at 10 years' follow-up: a randomised controlled trial. Lancet. 2006;368:2053.
30. Independent UK Panel on Breast Cancer Screening. The benefits and harms of breast cancer screening: an independent review. Lancet. 2012;380:1778.
31. Nyström L, Andersson I, Bjurstam N, et al. Long-term effects of mammography screening: updated overview of the Swedish randomised trials. Lancet. 2002;359:909.
32. Freedman DA, Petitti DB, Robins JM. On the efficacy of screening for breast cancer. Int J Epidemiol. 2004;33:43.
33. Vainio H, Bianchini F. IARC Handbook of cancer prevention, vol 7. Breast cancer screening. Lyon: Lyon IARC Press; 2002.
34. National Cancer Institute. Breast Cancer (PDQ®): Screening. http://cancer.gov/cancertopics/pdq/screening/breast/healthprofessional. Accessed 15 Nov 2006.

35. Schopper D, de Wolf C. How effective are breast cancer screening programmes by mammography? Review of the current evidence. Eur J Cancer. 2009;45:1916.
36. Mayor S. Mammography screening reduces breast cancer deaths in Ireland, study finds. BMJ. 2017;359:j5932.
37. van Dijck JA, Holland R, Verbeek AL, et al. Efficacy of mammographic screening of the elderly: a case-referent study in the Nijmegen program in The Netherlands. J Natl Cancer Inst. 1994;86:934.
38. Van Dijck JA, Verbeek AL, Beex LV, et al. Mammographic screening after the age of 65 years: evidence for a reduction in breast cancer mortality. Int J Cancer. 1996;66:727.
39. Schonberg MA, Silliman RA, Marcantonio ER. Weighing the benefits and burdens of mammography screening among women age 80 years or older. J Clin Oncol. 2009;27:1774.
40. Oeffinger KC, Fontham ETH, Etzioni R, et al. Breast cancer screening for women at average risk: 2015 guideline update from the American Cancer Society. JAMA. 2015;314:1599.
41. Mainiero MB, Lourenco A, Mahoney MC, et al. ACR appropriateness criteria breast cancer screening. J Am Coll Radiol. 2013;10:11.
42. NCCN. NCCN clinical practice guidelines in oncology: breast cancer screening and diagnosis. Fort Washington, PA: NCCN; 2014.
43. Miller AB, Wall C, Baines CJ, et al. Twenty five year follow-up for breast cancer incidence and mortality of the Canadian National Breast Screening Study: randomised screening trial. BMJ. 2014;348:g366.
44. Yen AM, Duffy SW, Chen TH, et al. Long-term incidence of breast cancer by trial arm in one county of the Swedish two-county trial of mammogram screening. Cancer. 2012;118:5728.
45. Hayse B, Hooley RJ, Killelea BK, et al. Breast cancer biology varies by method of detection and may contribute to overdiagnosis. Surgery. 2016;160:454.

Imaging: Controversies and Interventions in Early Breast Cancer

Janaki P. Dharmarajan

3.1 Breast Imaging Evolution

The approach to breast cancer has evolved drastically over the millennia. Hippocrates of Cos (460–377 B.C.) was the first to recognise benign from malignant breast masses. Celsus (25 B.C.–50 A.D.) reported about enlarged axillary lymph nodes accompanying breast cancer cases. LeDran observed the tumour prognosis to be worse with axillary lymph node involvement and proposed tumour excision along with axillary lymph nodes. With the advent of anaesthetic techniques, asepsis and histopathological examination in eighteenth century, it was possible to know what kind of tumour we were dealing with. Though Roentgen discovered X-rays in 1895, it was only in the 1930s that radiographs were used to detect breast cancers. With the introduction of screen film techniques, better images that delineated details could be obtained. With a compression paddle, the breast could be uniformly compressed, and this reduced effective radiation dose and gave better images [1, 2]. The lesions seen on mammography could be characterised by ultrasound. With the advent of breast MRI, the exact tissue characteristics could be seen in multiple planes, thereby helping in localising the disease accurately. Tomosynthesis is a modification of mammography giving 1-mm thin reconstructed images that help delineate the margins of the mass. Along with the imaging modalities, constant progress was also made in guided interventions so as to approach the non-palpable masses.

India with a population of 1.3 billion has approximately 54% of the females in the age group of 25 years and above (2018 estimates). There is a significant increase in age-standardised incidence rate of breast cancer by 40.7% (95% UI 7.0–85.6) from 1990 to 2016. In India, patients with cancer generally have a poorer prognosis due to relatively low cancer awareness, late diagnosis and the

---

J. P. Dharmarajan (✉)
Department of Radiology, Amrita Institute of Medical Sciences, Kochi, Kerala, India
e-mail: janaki19727@aims.amrita.edu

© Springer Nature Singapore Pte Ltd. 2021
B. Kunheri, D. K. Vijaykumar (eds.), *Management of Early Stage Breast Cancer*,
https://doi.org/10.1007/978-981-15-6171-9_3

lack of or inequitable access to affordable curative services. The estimated number of incident breast cancer cases in India in 2016 was 118,000 (95% UI 107,000–130,000), 98.1% of which were in females, and the prevalent cases were 526,000 [3].

As less than 5% of the population present with early breast cancer at diagnosis, with a young female population, there is a high latent disease burden. Early detection and subsequent management hold the key towards increasing survival. With the existing resources, it is not possible to implement government-sponsored mass screening. This chapter provides information about early cancer diagnostic modalities available, what a proper breast imaging workup entails and subsequent importance of radiology staging in multidisciplinary tumour boards. In short, an algorithm will be presented regarding the approach to early breast cancers leading from diagnosis, guided interventions and subsequent management.

In early breast cancer, the disease is limited to the breast with or without spread to regional axillary lymph nodes and without distant metastases. These include potentially operable conditions with more than 80% of patients having long-term survival with a combination of surgery, chemotherapy, endocrine therapy and local radiation.

3.2 Breast Cancer Signs and Symptoms

There are no signs and symptoms in early breast cancer, and they are typically detected during screening. Clinically concerning symptoms and signs that need immediate diagnostic evaluation include the following:

- Painless lump
- Skin thickening and redness
- Nipple retraction, bleeding or ulceration
- Lump in armpit
- Persistent pain or heaviness

3.2.1 Diagnosis of Breast Cancer

- During screening before a lump has formed
- After any of the above symptoms occur

However, most of the masses detected on screening mammography and the palpable masses (almost 80%) turn out to be benign. The suspicious ones need further histopathologic analysis for diagnosis, staging and determining the extent of disease. This can be obtained either by excision/incision biopsy or by image-guided needle biopsy.

3.2.2 Staging Summary

- Stage 0 in TNM corresponds to the in situ stage that indicates the presence of abnormal cells that have not invaded nearby tissues.
- Stage I and some stage II cancers are local stage cancers that are confined only to the breast.
- Stage II or III cancers in the regional stage refer to tumour spread to surrounding tissue and nearby lymph nodes.
- Some stage IIIc and all stage IV cancers are the distant stage that refers to cancers that have metastasized to distant organs or lymph nodes above the clavicle.

3.2.2.1 Ductal Carcinoma In Situ (DCIS)
The normal epithelial cells that line the ducts are replaced by abnormal cells that expand the ducts and lobules. However, the basement membrane is intact. DCIS grows very slowly that without treatment it may not affect the women's health. However, there is no data to suggest which among the DCIS will progress to invasive cancer. It is seen that 20–53% of the untreated DCIS do progress to invasive cancer in 10 years.

3.2.2.2 Invasive Breast Cancer (BC)
Almost 80% of breast cancers extend beyond the basement membrane and are known as invasive or infiltrating cancers. They are now shown to extend into the surrounding breast parenchyma.

Screening shows an apparent increase in the detection of in situ and invasive cancers as they are discovered almost 3 years before they become manifest.

The stage at diagnosis influences BC survival, and the overall 5-year relative survival rate is as follows:

- Localised disease: 99%
- Regional disease: 85%
- Distant-stage disease: 27%

Tumour size within each stage also directly influences survival. The 5-year relative survival in women with regional disease is as below:

- 95% for tumors size of equal to or less than 2.0 cm
- 85% for tumors size between 2.1 and 5.0 cm
- 72% for tumors greater than 5.0 cm

As compared to women, men are more likely to be diagnosed with advanced-stage breast cancer, which can be attributed to delayed detection and decreased awareness. Screening mammography is not recommended for men due to the rarity of the disease.

The majority of women with a strong family history of breast cancer affecting multiple first-degree relatives never develop breast cancer. However, the majority of women who develop breast cancer do not have a family history.

3.3   Breast Imaging Modalities

3.3.1   Mammography

This is a low-dose X-ray method that allows visualisation of the internal structure of the breast.

In screening, this helps in detection of non-palpable mass, calcifications and architectural distortion.

Types of mammography based on technical factors are as follows:

1. *Film screen*: Images are obtained on a film. Though resolution is sharp, the dis-advantage includes higher radiation dose, longer time, cumbersome physical storage, transport of films and multiple retakes.
2. *Digital mammography (2D)*: Film is replaced by a detector plate that enables immediate image processing and viewing on specialised monitors. Post-processing is possible. Digital images can be transferred electronically across locations for comparisons. Radiation dose is lower.
3. *Digital breast tomosynthesis (DBT or 3D)*: This is further modification of digital mammography in which the X-ray tube travels in a predetermined arc. Reconstructed thin images are obtained. The advantages are as below:
   • Overcomes overlapping of tissues so that subtle lesions become sharper.
   • Asymmetries due to overlapping tissue disappear.

This results in lower recall rates and increased invasive cancer detection and involves slightly higher radiation dose but is comparable with 2D with the use of synthesised views.

Screening mammography is recommended as long as women have good overall health with a life expectancy of 10 years or more.

Early cancer detection by screening mammography leads to the following:

• Less-extensive surgery, i.e. breast conservation with axillary sampling is possible.
• In early stages, chemotherapy with fewer side effects can be used.
• In select cases, endocrine therapy will suffice, and chemotherapy can be avoided.

3.3.2   Disadvantages of Screening Mammography

1. False-positive results in initial screening, especially in dense breasts. Leads to additional mammographic views and biopsy where there is no cancer.

2. Overdiagnosis of cancers that remain indolent. However, there is no way of measuring them at present.
3. Radiation exposure: Minimal risk.
4. Limitations of mammography: Not all cancers are screen detected. Some of the screen-detected ones have an aggressive course.

3.3.3 Ultrasound

A dedicated high-resolution, real-time linear array scanner with an adjustable focal zone and having a transducer frequency of 5–18 MHz should be used for breast imaging. Harmonic imaging helps in better visualisation of cystic lesions.

A targeted US is performed for the palpable finding or mammographic abnormality for lesion characterisation. This is the first modality of choice in pregnant and lactating women as they have dense breasts.

Studies have shown that ultrasound along with screening mammography in women with dense breasts detects additional 4 more cancers per 1000 women scanned than mammography alone. Ultrasound screening also detects a lot of indeterminate lesions, leading to an increase in guided biopsy and thereby a false-positive rate of up to 40%. The use of ultrasound instead of mammograms for breast cancer screening is not recommended.

Ultrasound also helps in preoperative staging of the axilla by evaluating the lymph nodes. Initial lesion assessment also helps in planning biopsy that is comfortable under ultrasound guidance. Response assessment is also possible in neoadjuvant setting.

3.3.4 Breast MRI

High-strength magnetic fields with a dedicated breast imaging coil are used to obtain detailed cross-sectional images of the breast. Intravenous contrast is essential to differentiate an enhancing cancer from non-enhancing glandular tissue. Staging breast MRI is very useful in dense breasts when the primary malignancy is in the form of architectural distortion or clusters of calcifications. Exact delineation of the disease extent pre-operatively helps in planning an optimal surgery. Breast MRI should be done at the facilities that should have capability for MRI-guided biopsy or should be able to refer to a facility having the same. Breast MRI can only supplement and not replace screening mammography.

For high-risk women having a lifetime risk of more than 20% of developing breast cancer, annual MRI screening in addition to mammography is recommended beginning at 25 years of age [4]. The indications for high-risk screening have been enumerated in the previous chapter.

3.4   Image-Guided Interventions

Fine needle aspiration cytology (FNAC): 21G needle is preferred.

• Used under ultrasound guidance to remove fluid from a cyst and cellular material from a solid mass.
• Cytological evaluation of non-palpable suspicious lymph nodes.

Image-guided core biopsy: Usually, a 14 G core is preferred.

• Suspicious solid masses or complex cystic lesions under ultrasound guidance.
• Under stereotactic guidance for suspicious calcifications seen only on mammography. Vacuum-assisted biopsy (VAB) with wider cores can be used if available. But, the site of biopsy needs to be marked with a clip inserted immediately after biopsy.
• Vacuum-assisted biopsy can also be used under MRI guidance for assessing suspicious non-mass enhancement.

Wire localisation:

• Once biopsy has confirmed the pathology, for non-palpable lesions, ultrasound, mammography, or MRI-guided wire localisations can be performed.
• Specimen ultrasound or mammography is to be performed to determine adequate margins [5].

3.5   Reporting of Breast Imaging Findings

Breast Imaging Reporting and Data System was established in the early 1990s in order to maintain a uniform quality in breast imaging reporting among radiologists and to enable communications with the non-radiologists who interpret the reports in order to reduce ambiguity. A detailed report has specific components like indication for the study, brief history, breast composition, significant findings in standardised terminology, comparision with previous studies and conclusion to final assessment category. Finally, management recommendations are given with documentation of unexpected findings to the referring clinician or patient. There are seven assessment categories ranging from 0 to 6 (Table 3.1). The fifth edition of BI-RADS has guidelines on reporting and management of mammography, breast ultrasound, and breast MRI. It also includes standardised auditing procedures for all three modalities.

3.6   Approach to Screening-Detected Breast Lesions

A few basic facts need to be revisited before we proceed to breast imaging. Breast is composed of fat and fibroglandular tissue.

Table 3.1 BI-RADS: final assessment categories

	Category	Management	Likelihood of cancer
0	Need additional imaging of prior examinations	Recall for additional imaging and/or await prior examinations	n/a
1	Negative	Routine screening	Essentially 0%
2	Benign	Routine screening	Essentially 0%
3	Probably benign	Short interval follow-up	>0% to ≤2%
4	Suspicious	Tissue diagnosis	4a: (>2% to ≤10%) 4b: >10% to ≤50%) 4c: >50% to <95%)
5	Highly suggestive of malignancy	Tissue diagnosis	≥95%
6	Known biopsy proven	Surgical excision when clinically appropriate	n/a

- In mammography, fat appears lucent and fibroglandular tissue is white. The mass density is compared with fibroglandular tissue.

Non-palpable lesions detected on mammography are masses, calcifications, asymmetry and architectural distortion that are described and characterised using BI-RADS lexicon. This includes the laterality and describing number and location of the lesions in relation to the nipple in a clockwise position.

1. Mass is a 3-dimensional structure and has shape and margins. The density of the mass is also mentioned.
2. Calcifications are of benign and suspicious types on mammography. They may be intralesional or extralesional in location. The suspicious ones are pleomorphic, linear, branching, amorphous and coarse heterogeneous. A linear or focus distribution of suspicious calcifications is more likely to be malignant than regional or segmental distribution.
3. Asymmetry is seen only in one view and does not form mass. Focal asymmetry is seen in both views. Global asymmetry is a benign variant after a proper workup. However developing asymmetry is suspicious of malignancy.
4. Architectural distortion is parenchymal distortion without a mass. This is usually associated with post-operative changes or a radial scar. Tomosynthesis delineates the margins and lucent centre and helps in lesion location.

- In US, subcutaneous tissue is isochoric and fibroglandular tissue is echogenic. Any lesion echogenicity is compared with the subcutaneous tissue.
- Structures identified: Cysts, solids, vascularity

- In breast MRI when contrast is given, it is only the glandular portion that enhances after contrast administration. Therfore, it is easy to differentiate fibrous tissue from active glandular tissue in dense breasts.
- Concerning features: Mass, foci, non-mass enhancement

The following clinical scenarios for suspicious lesions are discussed:

1. Screening mammography-detected lesions (>40 years)
2. Palpable masses (<30 years)
3. Palpable masses (30–40 years)
4. Palpable masses (>40 years)

3.7   Screening Mammography-Detected Lesions on Initial Study

Once suspicious mass, calcifications, asymmetry and architectural distortion are identified, they need to be characterised by targeted ultrasound.
Mass

- If it is a simple cyst on correlative ultrasound, it is characterised as benign with suggestion for no further imaging follow-up. The category will be BI-RADS 2.
- If it is a complicated cyst or a solid mass with probably benign features, a short-term follow-up is recommended for 2 years that is to be performed at 6, 12, and 24 months (BI-RADS 3). If it is stable after two years or regresses before that, downgrade to BI-RADS 2. In the event of lesion progression any time before two years, upgrade it to BI-RADS 4 and proceed with guided biopsy.
- If the mass is suspicious on ultrasound, proceed with ultrasound-guided core biopsy.

Calcificatons (Fig. 3.1)

- Calcifications that are not clearly benign on screening mammography are recalled for additional magnification views and ultrasound examination.
- If suspicious calcifications are seen on ultrasound, proceed with ultrasound-guided core biopsy and specimen mammography.
- If calcifications are not seen on ultrasound, proceed with stereotactic-guided core biopsy. VAB is used when the cluster is <5 mm or calcifications are spread out. Clip is deployed at the biopsy site if VAB is used and check mammography obtained. Specimen mammography of the core samples should demonstrate at least five flecks of calcifications in one core or more than one in three cores [6].

Asymmetry (Fig. 3.2)

- Occurs in 3% of recall mammography. Suspicious if associated with mass, calcifications or architectural distortion.
- Additional mammographic views such as spot compression or rolled overview are to be performed. Tomosynthesis helps to elucidate overlapping fibroglandular tissue that is the most common cause of asymmetry.
- After localisation in 3D view, proceed with diagnostic ultrasound for lesion characterisation. Benign ultrasound correlates are cysts, scar, fat necrosis, hema-

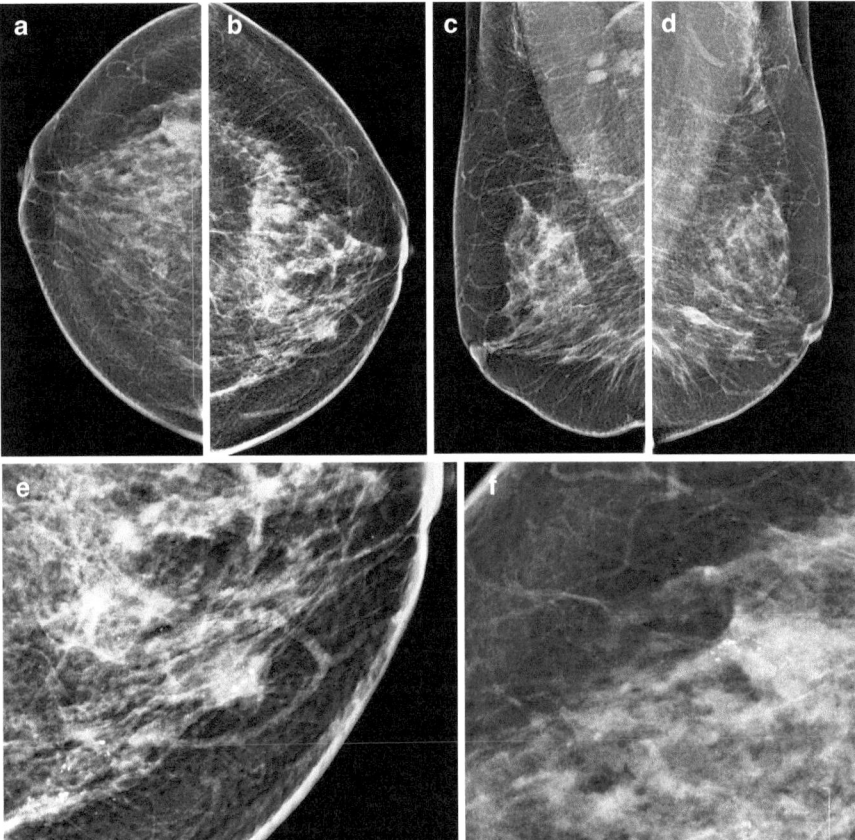

Fig. 3.1 A 49-year-old lady with palpable left breast mass suspicious for neoplasm on FNAC was referred. (**a–d**) Bilateral MG CC and MLO views. Amorphous clusters of calcifications, non-palpable on the right side. (**e**) Palpable left breast mass with focal amorphous clusters calcifications. (**f**) Non-palpable right breast similar to cluster of calcifications. (**g**) US irregular mass in the left breast. Normal axillary lymph nodes. (**h, i**) US irregular mass in the right breast. Abnormal axillary lymph nodes. Bilateral US-guided core biopsy and right axillary lymph node FNAC were performed. The right breast showed invasive mammary carcinoma, grade II, luminal B with metastatic node. The left breast showed invasive mammary carcinoma, grade II, luminal B, Her enriched, negative nodes

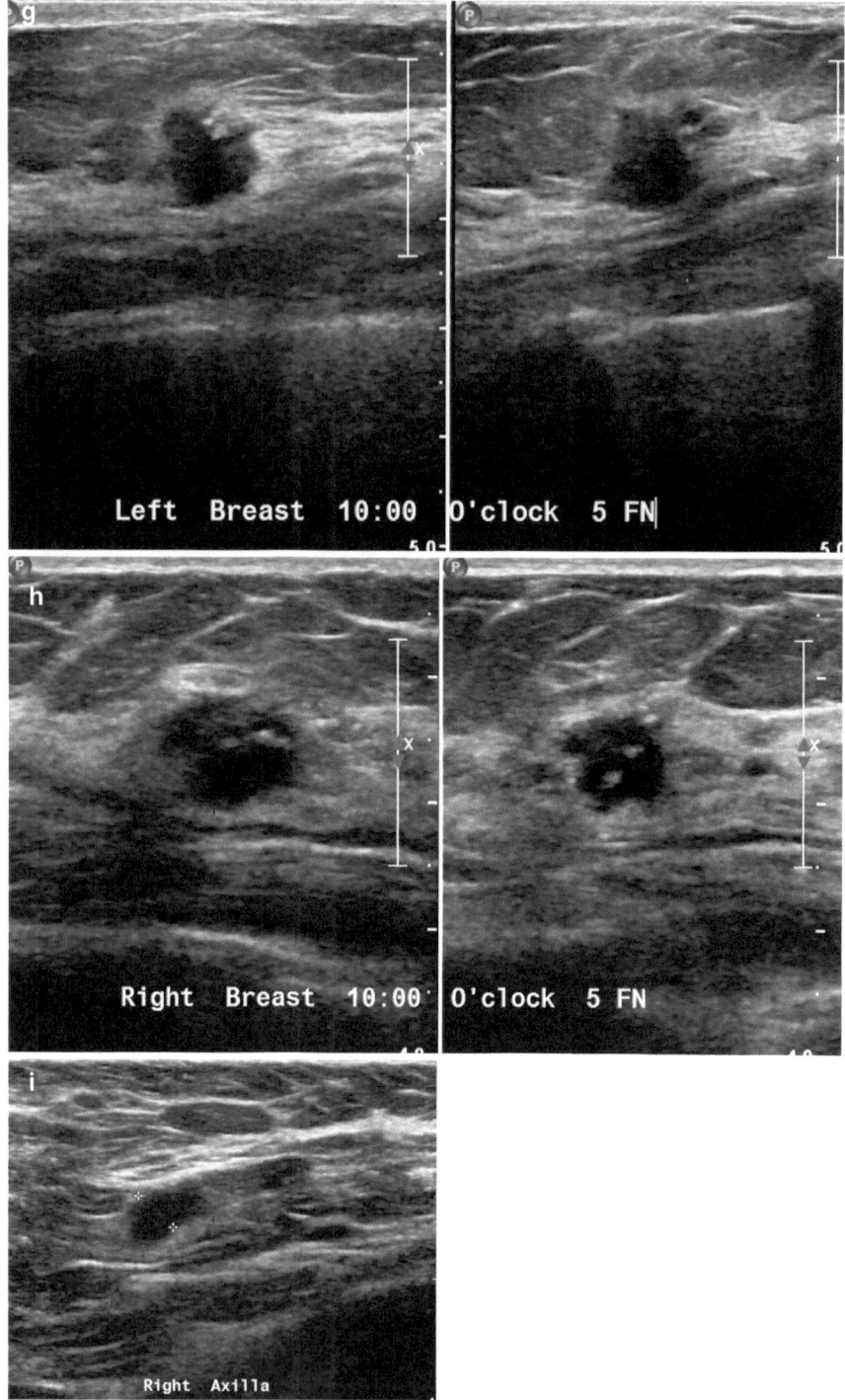

Fig. 3.1 (continued)

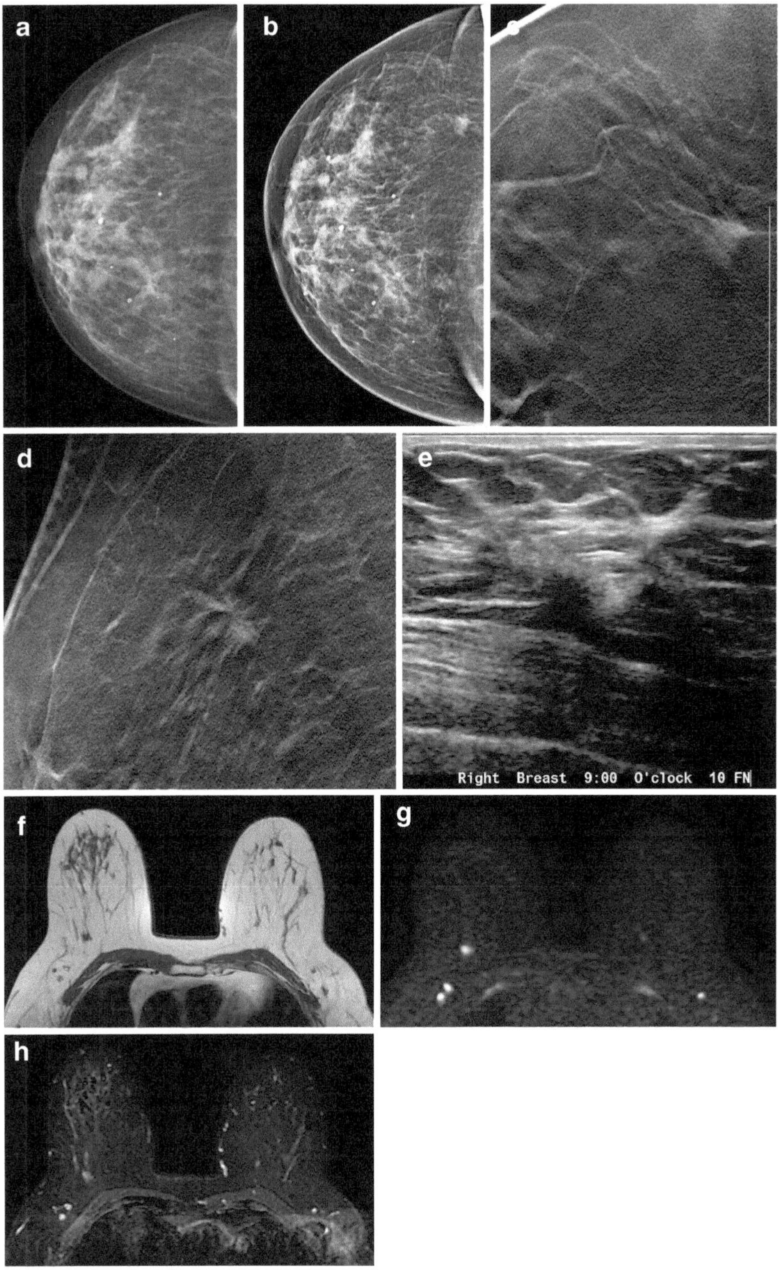

Fig. 3.2 A 68-year-old lady for routine screening mammography. (**a**) Right CC in 2013. (**b**) Developing asymmetry in right breast UOQ in 2015. (**c, d**) Margins appreciated on tomosynthesis. (**e**) Ultrasound showed a 0.8-cm mass. Guided core biopsy showed invasive carcinoma with lobular features. (**f, g**) Breast MRI confirmed unifocality of the mass. T1, DWI b = 1000, post-contrast. Wire localisation with SLNB done. Final HPE showed invasive lobular carcinoma, luminal A, node negative

toma, lymph node and ectopic breast tissue. If there is hypoechoic solid mass with or without posterior shadowing, proceed with ultrasound-guided core biopsy.
- If not seen on ultrasound, proceed with breast MRI. If suspicious on MRI, proceed with mammography or MRI-guided biopsy. If no abnormal imaging features, have a short-term follow-up with mammography for 6 months [7].

Architectural distortion (Fig. 3.3)

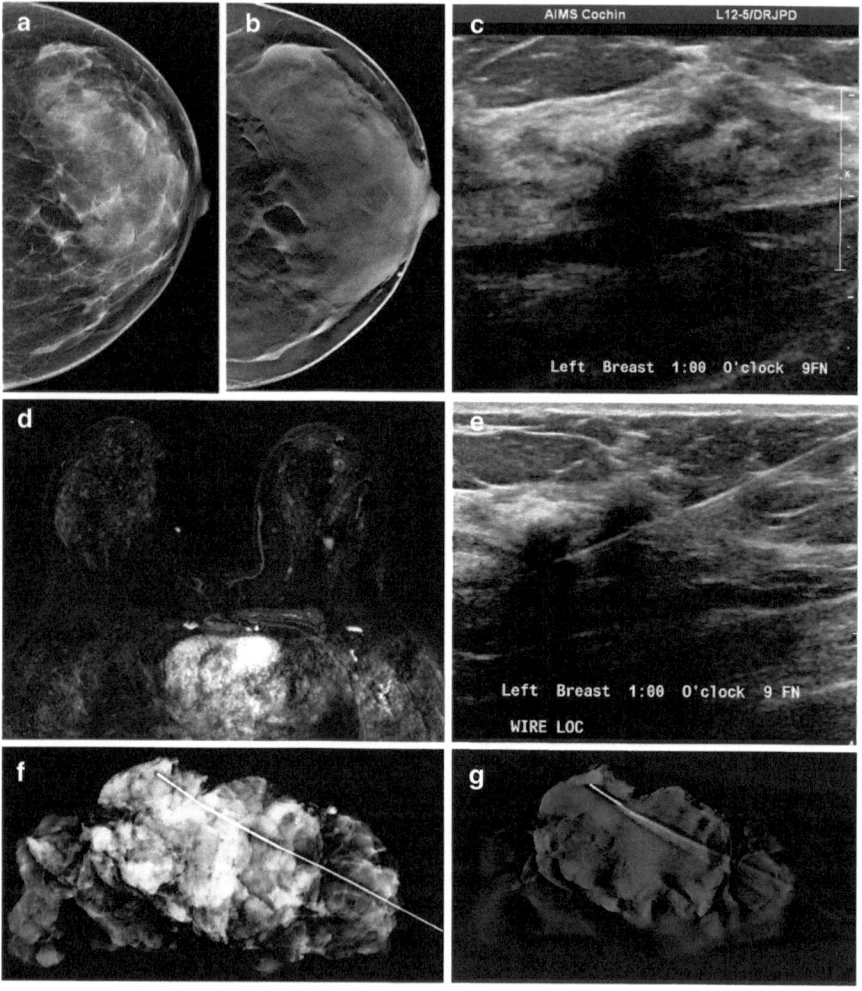

Fig. 3.3 A 51-year-old lady for routine screening mammography. Prior h/o bilateral fibrocystic changes. (**a**) Mammogram showed dense breasts. (**b**) Subtle architectural distortion was seen only in CC tomosynthesis view. (**c**) US showed an irregular mass of 1 cm. US-guided biopsy showed radial scar with a small focus of low-grade carcinoma. (**d**) Unifocality in dense breasts was confirmed by breast MRI. (**e**) US-guided wire localisation. (**f, g**) Specimen tomosynthesis for lesion characterisation. Final HPR was infiltrating mammary carcinoma, grade I arising in a radial scar, luminal A with negative lymph nodes

- Exclude the history of prior surgery at the site.
- If no, additional evaluation with spot compression or tomosynthesis.
- Try to correlate with ultrasound using triangulation between modalities.
- If found on ultrasound, proceed with ultrasound-guided core biopsy.
- If not found on US, proceed with breast MRI. If suspicious, proceed with MR-guided biopsy.
- If seen only on tomosynthesis and not on US and MRI, proceed with tomosynthesis-guided biopsy or wire localisation if available.
- If seen only on one view with no corresponding correlates on US, MRI considering the risk of the patient, a short-term follow-up with tomosynthesis can be opted [8].

3.7.1 Palpable Masses (<30 Years)

Ultrasound is the initial modality to characterise the mass.

- Simple cyst BI-RADS 2.
- Complicated cyst of probably benign solid mass: BI-RADS 3
- If no mass is seen and clinical suspicion is present, proceed with single-view MLO mammography to exclude suspicious calcifications.
- Suspicious mass on ultrasound. Proceed with diagnostic mammography to characterise the mass and exclude multiplicity followed by ultrasound-guided core biopsy (Fig. 3.4).
- Breast MRI is to be performed in high-risk scenario. There is no probably benign category in high-risk cases, and all newly appeared masses have to be biopsied.

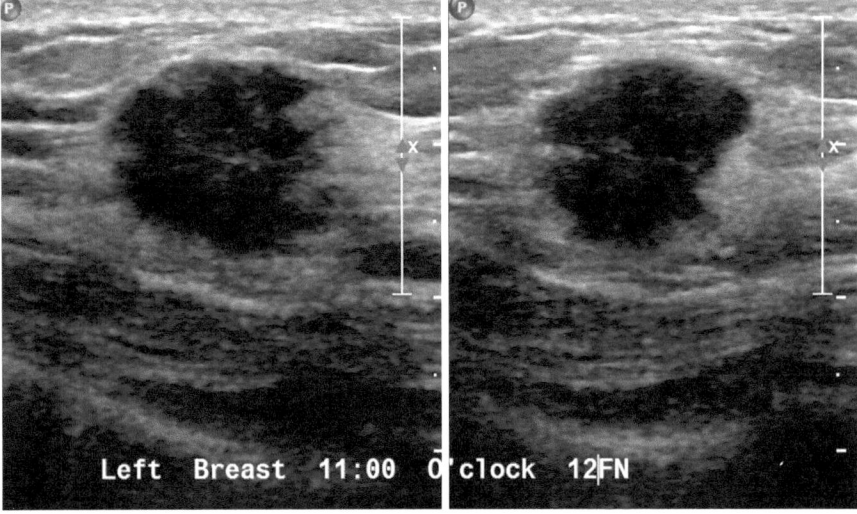

Fig. 3.4 Mass in a 26-year-old pregnant lady. US-guided core biopsy showed invasive mammary carcinoma triple negative

3.7.2 Palpable Masses (30–39 Years)

Both ultrasound and mammography are appropriate and can be used up front.

- If ultrasound is performed initially with negative findings, proceed with mammography to exclude calcifications.
- If ultrasound shows suspicious lesions, proceed with diagnostic mammography and ultrasound-guided biopsy.
- For simple cysts and probably benign lesions, proceed as described above.

3.7.3 Palpable Masses (≥40 Years)

- Initial evaluation is with diagnostic mammography. This can be omitted when a proper prior study performed within 6 months is available for comparison. The opposite side is also to be examined for any abnormalities (Fig. 3.5)
- Proceed with diagnostic ultrasound for lesion characterisation and further recommendations based on lesion morphology as described in above sections.

There is a lot of inconsistency in clinical breast examination. A thorough breast imaging with multiple modalities should be completed before proceeding with biopsy [5, 9].

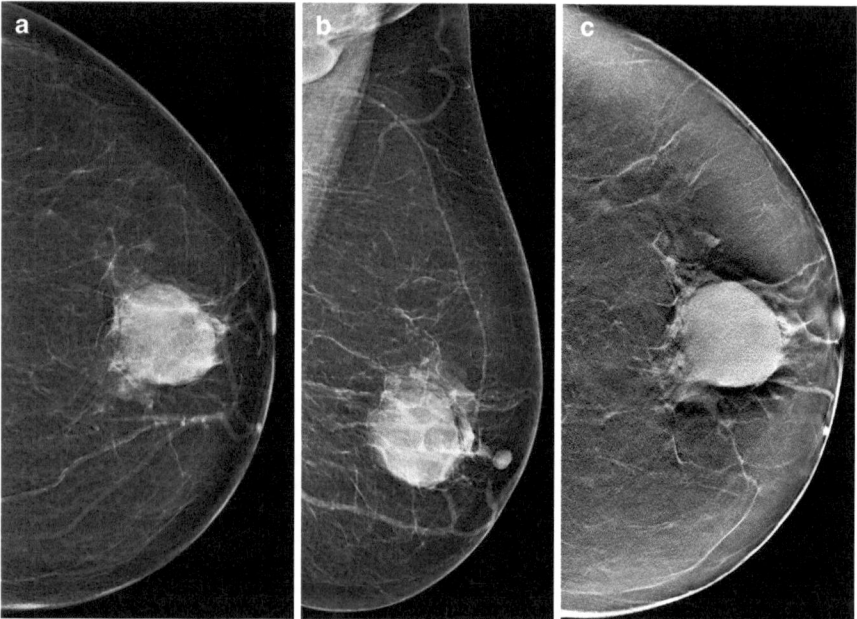

Fig. 3.5 A 69-year-old lady with left breast lump for diagnostic evaluation. (**a, b**) Bilateral mammography performed. Left CC and MLO view show a round high-density mass with circumscribed margins. No calcifications. (**c**) Margins seen on tomosynthesis. (**d, e**) US shows a complex cystic lesion with a vascular solid component. US-guided core biopsy of the solid component after aspiration of bloody cystic aspirate showed invasive mucinous carcinoma with neuroendocrine differentiation, luminal A with negative nodes confirmed on lumpectomy with SLNB

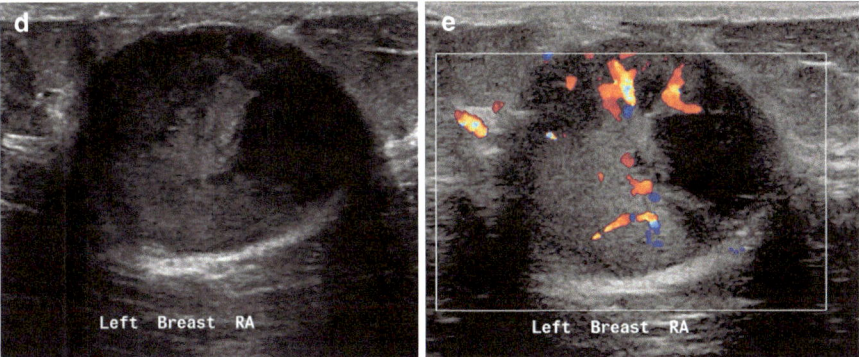

Fig. 3.5 (continued)

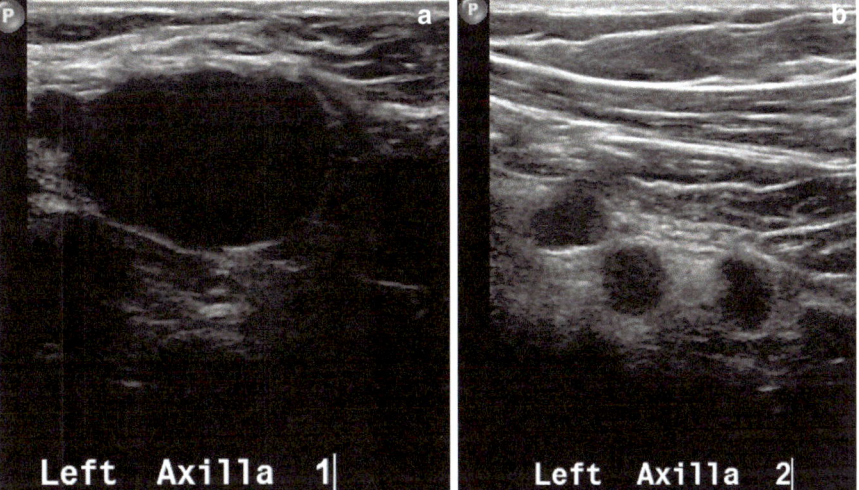

Fig. 3.6 (**a**) Enlarged axillary lymph node with diffuse cortical thickness. (**b**) Level 2 round irregular axillary lymph node

3.8 Evaluation of Axilla (Fig. 3.6)

Involvement of axillary lymph nodes at presentation carries a significant diagnostic and therapeutic implication. All newly diagnosed patients of breast cancer should undergo axillary lymph node staging with ultrasound. The indeterminate or suspicious lymph nodes should be subjected to US-guided FNAC. Sentinel lymph node biopsy will be performed in normal or reactive FNAC lymph nodes. The node-positive patients will be triaged for axillary clearance or neo-adjuvant chemotherapy based on nodal burden, tumour size and immunohistochemistry markers. The false-negative result on cytology is as high as 31% and necessitates axillary clearance even though the nodal burden is low on final histopathology [10].

3.9   Screening Mammography Controversies

Several studies and RCT in North America and Europe in the 1970s and 1980s have shown statistically significant reduction in breast cancer mortality directly attributed to mammographic screening. This is attributed either to early diagnosis due to mammography or to mortality reduction due to better treatment options. Even though many studies have no significant reduction in cancer mortality rates, thereby questioning the validity of mammographic screening, a meta-analysis of the randomised controlled trials by an independent panel in the UK reported a 20% mortality reduction among screened populations.

The main controversies in screening mammography are as below:

- When should screening start in average- and low-risk females?
- How often should it be done?
- Do screening mammography benefits outweigh the harms?
- A false positive on screening involves a recall rate of up to 10%, who needs additional investigation with modified views, ultrasound and sometimes even a biopsy.
- Overdiagnosis range in mammography varies from 1 to 50%. Some of the indolent cancers discovered on screening never become malignant during lifetime. But there is no way of identifying the indolent lesions on imaging.

Additional DBT has led to lesser recall rates and more invasive cancer detection in screening.

According to BI-RADS of ACR, breast is composed of either of four types depending on the degree of fat and fibroglandular tissue and lesion visibility: predominantly fatty in 10%, scattered fibroglandular tissue in 40%, heterogeneously dense in 40% and extremely dense in 10%. Increasing breast density itself is associated with higher cancer incidence, and it can also obscure cancer detection. Carney et al. showed that the sensitivity for screening in women in fatty breasts was 88% and in extremely dense breasts was 62%. There is no enough evidence to suggest that screening ultrasound results in mortality reduction [11].

As compared to the western countries where the cancer peaks between 60 and 70 years of age, in India, the majority of breast cancers peak between 40 and 50 years of age. Many of these cancers are HER2 enriched and hormone negative, or triple negative having a poor prognosis. In India, population-based breast cancer screening is not recommended due to limited resources and the lack of local statistics on mammography and breast cancers. About two-thirds of the patients present with local invasion and 6–25% present with metastases. A significant proportion present with regional T2/T3 tumours and up to one-third of all patients have skin and/or chest wall involvement (T4a-c). A large number of compromises are made at every step right from diagnosis to surgery and multimodality treatment. Preoperative diagnostic tissue biopsy is being performed only in miniscule places. A significant proportion of patients undergo an incomplete or inappropriate surgical excision before being referred to a specialist, making subsequent management challenging [12, 13].

In 1924 address of RSNA, Malvern Clopton, MD, stated that "early breast cancer cannot be diagnosed by palpation or inspection." Breast imaging has come a long way in the past century from direct exposure mammography, xeromammography, film screen mammography with compression of breast and more recently digital breast imaging with tomosynthesis.

To ensure success of mammography screening, high-quality imaging along with accurate interpretation and clear communication of findings and recommendations to referring clinicians was necessary. To ensure this, BI-RADS, the first structured reporting language for imaging, was introduced in 1992. The three important components are the following:

- A lexicon of descriptors
- A reporting structure to include final assessment categories and management
- A framework for data collection and auditing

In 2007, guidelines were issued for breast MRI screening for women with a 20–25% or greater lifetime risk of breast cancer by the American Cancer Society. However, the facility for MRI-guided biopsy is a must as targeted second look ultrasound is able to identify only 46–70% of the lesions [14].

For screening to be effective, there must be a lead time before the mass becomes clinically apparent. Prior to screening programmes, DCIS used to constitute about 2–5% of the cancers. However, now DCIS constitutes about 20–30% of the diagnosed cases. There are a few indolent cases that would have never progressed to invasion during the lifetime of the patient, thereby strengthening the concept of overtreatment. About 37% of DCIS identified at initial screening and about 4% of DCIS during interval screening will not progress. However, there is no way to identify the non-progressive, non-lethal masses from the progressive lethal breast cancers at present [15]. Screening-detected cancers have a more favourable prognosis due to early stage as compared to non-screen-detected cancers. The potential sources of bias towards effectiveness of screening-detected cancers are lead time and length bias [16].

A meta-analysis of RCT showed a 15% reduction in mortality in screening in 40- to 49-year-old women. This however includes a higher rate of recall and false-negative and false-positive results with increased diagnostic interventions [17]. Breast density has a significant effect on sensitivity but not on specificity. Ultrasound in women with dense breasts helps in detecting additional cases of cancer [18].

The screening-detected cancers have a different biology and prognosis, and this has to be kept in mind while tailoring treatment on personalised level [19]. False-negative results of FNAC of axillary lymph nodes are still at 31%, which necessitates preoperative axillary nodal sampling [15].

Neo-adjuvant chemotherapy is initiated after discussion in multidisciplinary tumour board in cases with high tumour volume to breast ratio, lymph node-positive status and younger age with triple negative of HER receptor-enriched tumours [20]. Constant monitoring and assessment is necessary during the course of treatment [16].

Newer modalities such as radiofrequency tumour ablation need further clinical trials after careful selection of cases. Research is also going on in vacuum-assisted biopsy in radiological complete response cases to determine minimal residual disease.

To summarise (Table 3.2):

1. Diagnostic mammography is the initial imaging modality for evaluation of a palpable breast mass in a woman aged 40 or older.
2. Ultrasound is the initial imaging modality for evaluation of a palpable breast mass in a woman younger than the age of 30.
3. For women with palpable mass and aged between 30 and 39 years, either ultrasound or mammography can be used for initial evaluation.
4. Imaging should be able to explain the palpable concern. Any mass suspicious on clinical examination should be biopsied irrespective of imaging findings.
5. Alternatively, any highly suspicious breast mass detected by imaging and not palpable should be biopsied.

To conclude, breast imaging speciality includes screening, diagnostic and surveillance scenarios. With judicious use of available imaging modalities such as mammography, ultrasound and breast MRI with guided interventions, along with triple assessment and concordance, a truly personalised breast care for early breast cancers is possible.

Table 3.2 Algorithm for palpable masses

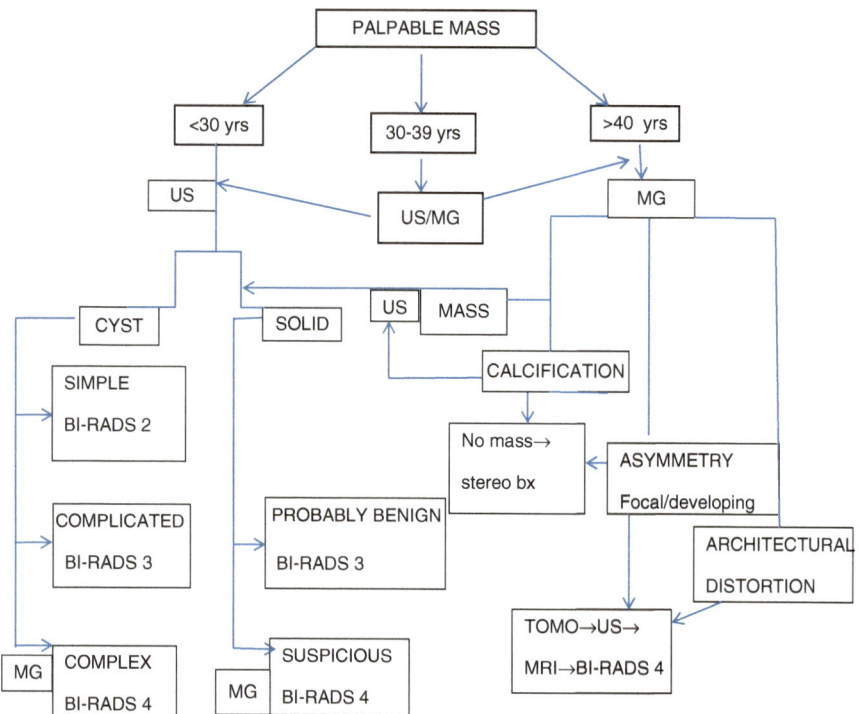

References

1. Ekmektzoglou KA, et al. Breast cancer: from the earliest times through to the end of the 20th century. Eur J Obstet Gynecol Reprod Biol. 2009;145:3–8.
2. Ades F, et al. The past and future of breast cancer treatment—from the papyrus to individualised treatment approaches. Ecancer. 2017;11:746. https://doi.org/10.3332/ecancer.2017.746.
3. India State-Level Disease Burden Initiative Cancer Collaborators. The burden of cancers and their variations across the states of India: the Global Burden of Disease Study 1990–2016. Lancet Oncol. 2018;19:1289–306. Published by Elsevier Ltd. This is an Open Access article under the CC BY 4.0 license.
4. American Cancer Society. Breast cancer facts & figures 2017-2018. Atlanta: American Cancer Society, Inc.; 2017.
5. Harvey JA, Mahoney MC, Newell MS, Bailey L, Barke LD, D'Orsi C, Haffty BG. ACR Appropriateness criteria palpable breast masses. J Am Coll Radiol. 2013;10(10):742–49.e3. https://doi.org/10.1016/j.jacr.2013.06.013.
6. Wilkinson L, Thomas V, Sharma N. Microcalcification on mammography: approaches to interpretation and biopsy. Br J Radiol. 2017;90(1069):20160594.
7. Chesebro AL, et al. Developing asymmetries at mammography: a multimodality approach to assessment and management. Radiographics. 2016;36:322–34.
8. Durand MA, et al. Tomosynthesis-detected architectural distortion: management algorithm with radiologic-pathologic correlation. Radiographics. 2016;36(2):311–21.
9. D'Orsi CJ, Sickles EA, Mendelson EB, Morris EA, et al. ACR BI-RADS® Atlas, Breast Imaging Reporting and Data System. Reston, VA, American College of Radiology; 2013.
10. Kane G, Fleming C, Heneghan H, et al. False-negative rate of ultrasound-guided fine-needle aspiration cytology for identifying axillary lymph node metastasis in breast cancer patients. Breast J. 2019;25(5):848–52.
11. Lee CH. Radiologic screening for breast cancer: current controversies. Curr Radiol Rep. 2014;2:34. Published online: 20 December 2013.
12. Leong SPL, et al. Is breast cancer the same disease in Asian and Western countries? World J Surg. 2010;34:2308–24, 2309. Published online: 7 July 2010.
13. Malvia S, et al. Epidemiology of breast cancer in Indian women. Asia Pac J Clin Oncol. 2017;13:289–95.
14. Joe BN, Sickles EA. The evolution of breast imaging: past to present. Radiology. 2014;273(2 Suppl):S23–44.
15. Kopans DA, et al. Mammographic screening and "overdiagnosis". Radiology. 2011;260(3):616–20. radiology.rsna.org.
16. Cortesi L, et al. Prognosis of screen-detected breast cancers: results of a population based study. BMC Cancer. 2006;6:17. https://doi.org/10.1186/1471-2407-6-17.
17. Suzuki A, et al. Controversies in breast cancer screening for women aged 40–49 years. Jpn J Clin Oncol. 2014;44(7):613–8.
18. Mujagić S, et al. The influence of breast density on the sensitivity and specificity of ultrasound and mammography in breast cancer diagnosis. Acta Med Acad. 2011;40:132–9.
19. Ahmed M, Douek M. The management of screen-detected breast cancer (review). Anticancer Res. 2014;34:1141–6.
20. Cain H, et al. Neoadjuvant therapy in early breast cancer: treatment considerations and common debates in practice. Clin Oncol. 2017;29:642–52.

Pathology of Early Breast Carcinomas

4

Ajith Nambiar

4.1 Introduction

Invasive breast cancer is the most common cancer in women. It accounts for nearly a quarter of all cancers in women. The incidence of breast cancer is increasing in the country. It is also not uncommon to find young females below 30 years to be presenting with breast cancer. In some developed countries, there has been a leveling of or decrease in incidence primarily due to screening and also partly to decreasing use of hormone replacement treatment.

A pathologist role just does not lie in diagnosing breast tumors but also in providing appropriate prognostic variables in each case and finally providing the molecular classification based on immunohistochemistry surrogates into luminal A, luminal B, HER2 overexpressed, and triple-negative categories, which have theranostic relevance.

4.2 Classification

4.2.1 2019 WHO Classification of Tumors of the Breast [1]

- *Epithelial tumors*
- *Invasive breast carcinoma*
  - Infiltrating duct carcinoma (NOS), 8500/3
  - Oncocytic carcinoma, 8290/3
  - Lipid-rich carcinoma, 8314/3
  - Glycogen-rich carcinoma, 8315/3
  - Sebaceous carcinoma, 8410/3

A. Nambiar (✉)
Department of Pathology, Amrita Institute of Medical Sciences, Kochi, Kerala, India
e-mail: ajitn@aims.amrita.edu

© Springer Nature Singapore Pte Ltd. 2021
B. Kunheri, D. K. Vijaykumar (eds.), *Management of Early Stage Breast Cancer*,
https://doi.org/10.1007/978-981-15-6171-9_4

- Lobular carcinoma NOS, 8520/3
- Tubular carcinoma, 8211/3
- Cribriform carcinoma NOS, 8201/3
- Mucinous adenocarcinoma, 8480/3
- Mucinous cystadenocarcinoma NOS, 8480/3
- Invasive micropapillary carcinoma of breast, 8507/3
- Metaplastic carcinoma NOS, 8575/3
- *Rare and salivary gland-type tumors*
  - Secretory carcinoma, 8502/3
  - Acinar cell carcinoma, 8550/3
  - Mucoepidermoid carcinoma, 8430/3
  - Polymorphous adenocarcinoma, 8525/3
  - Adenoid cystic carcinoma, 8200/3
      Classic adenoid cystic carcinoma
      Solid basaloid adenoid cystic carcinoma.
      Adenoid cystic carcinoma with high-grade transformation
  - Tall cell carcinoma with reversed polarity, 8509/3
- *Neuroendocrine neoplasms*
  - Neuroendocrine tumor, NOS, 8240/3
  - Neuroendocrine tumor, grade 1, 8240/3
  - Neuroendocrine tumor, grade 2, 8249/3
  - Neuroendocrine carcinoma NOS, 8246/3
  - Neuroendocrine carcinoma, small cell, 8041/3
  - Neuroendocrine carcinoma, large cell, 8013/3
- *Epithelial–myoepithelial tumors*
  - Pleomorphic adenoma, 8940/0
  - Adenomyoepithelioma NOS, 8983/0
  - Adenomyoepithelioma with carcinoma, 8983/3
  - Epithelial–myoepithelial carcinoma, 8562/3
- *Noninvasive lobular neoplasia*
  - Atypical lobular hyperplasia
  - Lobular carcinoma in situ NOS, 8520/2
      Classic lobular carcinoma in situ
      Florid lobular carcinoma in situ
  - Lobular carcinoma in situ, pleomorphic, 8519/2
- *Ductal carcinoma in situ (DCIS)*
  - Ductal carcinoma, noninfiltrating, NOS, 8500/2
      DCIS of low nuclear grade
      DCIS of intermediate nuclear grade
      DCIS of high nuclear grade
- *Benign epithelial proliferations and precursors*
  - Usual ductal hyperplasia
  - Columnar cell lesions including flat epithelial atypia
  - Atypical ductal hyperplasia

- *Adenosis and benign sclerosing lesions*
  - Sclerosing adenosis
  - Apocrine adenoma, 8401/0
  - Microglandular adenosis
  - Radial scar/complex sclerosing lesion
- *Papillary neoplasms*
  - Intraductal papilloma, 8503/0
  - Ductal carcinoma in situ, papillary, 8503/2
  - Encapsulated papillary carcinoma, 8504/2
  - Encapsulated papillary carcinoma with invasion, 8504/3
  - Solid papillary carcinoma in situ, 8509/2
  - Solid papillary carcinoma with invasion, 8509/3
  - Intraductal papillary adenocarcinoma with invasion, 8503/3
- *Adenomas*
  - Tubular adenoma NOS, 8211/0
  - Lactating adenoma, 8204/0
  - Duct adenoma NOS, 8503/0

- *Mesenchymal tumors*
- Vascular tumors
  - Hemangioma NOS, 9120/0
        Perilobular hemangioma
        Venous hemangioma
        Cavernous hemangioma
        Capillary hemangioma
  - Angiomatosis
  - Atypical vascular lesion, 9126/0
        Lymphatic atypical vascular lesion resembling lymphangioma
        Vascular atypical vascular lesion resembling hemangioma
  - Postradiation angiosarcoma, 9120/3
        Epithelioid angiosarcoma
  - Angiosarcoma, 9120/3
        Epithelioid angiosarcoma
- Fibroblastic and myofibroblastic tumors
  - Nodular fasciitis, 8828/0
  - Myofibroblastoma, 8825/0
  - Desmoid-type fibromatosis, 8821/1
  - Inflammatory myofibroblastic tumor, 8825/1
- Peripheral nerve sheath tumors
  - Schwannoma NOS, 9560/0
  - Neurofibroma NOS, 9540/0
  - Granular cell tumor NOS, 9580/0
  - Granular cell tumor, malignant, 9580/3

- Smooth muscle tumors
  - Leiomyoma NOS, 8890/0
     Cutaneous leiomyoma
     Leiomyoma of the nipple and areola
  - Leiomyosarcoma NOS, 8890/3
- Adipocytic tumors
  - Lipoma NOS, 8850/0
  - Angiolipoma NOS, 8861/0
  - Liposarcoma NOS, 8850/3
- Other mesenchymal tumors and tumorlike conditions
  - Pseudoangiomatous stromal hyperplasia
- *Fibroepithelial tumors*
  - Fibroadenoma NOS, 9010/0
  - Phyllodes tumor NOS, 9020/1
     Periductal stromal tumor
  - Phyllodes tumor, benign, 9020/0
  - Phyllodes tumor, borderline, 9020/1
  - Phyllodes tumor, malignant, 9020/3
  - Hamartoma
- *Tumors of the nipple*
  - Nipple adenoma, 8506/0
  - Syringoma NOS, 8407/0
  - Paget disease of the nipple, 8540/3
- *Malignant lymphoma*
  - Diffuse large B cell lymphoma NOS, 9680/3
  - Burkitt lymphoma NOS/Acute leukemia, Burkitt type, 9687/3
     Endemic Burkitt lymphoma
     Sporadic Burkitt lymphoma
     Immunodeficiency-associated Burkitt lymphoma
  - Breast implant-associated anaplastic large cell lymphoma, 9715/3
  - Mucosa-associated lymphoid tissue lymphoma, 9699/3
  - Follicular lymphoma NOS, 9690/3
- *Metastatic tumors*
- *Tumors of the male breast*
  - Gynaecomastia
  - Carcinoma
     Invasive carcinoma, 8500/3
     In situ carcinoma, 8500/2

4.3   Important Entities

The most common breast cancer comprising about 85% of all carcinomas in breast is the invasive breast carcinoma of no special type (NST). This group comprises all tumors without specific differentiating features which characterize the other categories (special types). The term "ductal" was omitted as it was felt that the term ductal conveys an unproven histogenetic assumption of derivation from the ductal system in 2012. The special types of breast cancer are also frequently associated with ductal carcinoma in situ (DCIS). However, in 2019, it has again found favor in terminology. The rare variants of invasive carcinoma NST include pleomorphic carcinoma and carcinoma with osteoclast-like giant cells.

Invasive lobular carcinomas are composed of noncohesive cells individually dispersed or arranged in a single-file linear pattern, alveolar pattern, or targetoid pattern in a fibrous stroma. These tumors do not characteristically express E cadherin. A pleomorphic variant unlike the above classical variant differs in having pleomorphic cytological characteristics.

Tubular carcinomas are a special type of breast carcinoma with particular favorable prognosis and are composed of round, ovoid, or angulated single-layered tubules, haphazardly distributed in a cellular fibrous or fibroelastotic stroma. Tubular carcinomas usuallycoexist with flat epithelial atypia, low-grade DCIS, and lobular neoplasia.

Cribriform carcinoma is an invasive carcinoma with also a favorable prognosis that grows in a pattern similar to that seen in intraductal cribriform carcinoma; a 50% component of tubular carcinoma may be admixed.

Carcinomas with medullary features include medullary carcinomas (MC), atypical MC, and a subset of invasive carcinomas of no special type (NST). These tumors demonstrate all or some of the following features: a circumscribed or pushing border, a syncytial growth pattern, grade 3 vesicular nuclei with prominent nucleoli, and prominent lymphoid infiltration. The tumors in this group are most often negative for estrogen and progesterone receptors (ER and PR) and HER2 ("triple-negative") and variably express basal markers. Also, these are most frequently associated with BRCA1 gene mutations.

Invasive micropapillary carcinoma is composed of aggregates of cuboidal to columnar neoplastic cells that are devoid of fibrovascular core and lie in empty stromal spaces. The neoplastic cells display reverse polarity such that the apical pole of the cell faces out to the stromal space. These tumors have a propensity for lymphovascular invasion.

Mucinous carcinoma is characterized by nests of cells floating in lakes of mucin partitioned by delicate fibrous septae containing capillary blood vessels. The hypercellular or type B mucinous carcinoma shows frequent neuroendocrine differentiation, as demonstrated by expression of chromogranin and synaptophysin.

Metaplastic carcinomas are a collective term for a group of heterogeneous tumors showing differentiation of malignant epithelium into squamous or mesenchymal elements, e.g., spindle, chondroid, and osseous cells. These tumors may be entirely composed of metaplastic elements or may be a mixture of metaplastic elements and conventional invasive carcinoma NST, including DCIS. Variants of metaplastic carcinoma include squamous cell carcinoma, low-grade adenosquamous carcinoma, fibromatosis-like carcinoma, and spindle cell carcinoma including myoepithelial carcinoma and metaplastic carcinoma with mesenchymal differentiation. Immunohistochemical analysis of metaplastic carcinomas has revealed that >90%

of these cancers are negative for ER, progesterone receptor (PR), and HER2 and express keratins 5/6 and 14 and EGFR. The identification of epithelial differentiation in metaplastic breast carcinomas requires the use of more than one marker. The usual markers are high-molecular-weight keratins, in particular 34betaE12, keratins 5/6 and 14, and AE1/AE3.

4.4 Precancerous Lesions

Duct carcinoma in situ (DCIS) is an intraductal proliferation of malignant epithelial cells. It needs to be distinguished from hyperplastic intraductal proliferations on the one end and from invasive carcinoma by the absence of stromal invasion across the basement membrane. This, if need be, can be confirmed by immunostaining for myoepithelial makers. Despite the name, most DCIS is generally considered to arise from the terminal duct lobular units.

DCIS is mainly associated with invasive malignancy or may be present alone without the invasive component. The DCIS, when present with invasive malignancy in a wide local excision, needs to be quantified. More than 25% of the invasive component, when composed of DCIS, is labeled as extensive intraductal component (EIC). It has implications as the probability of DCIS in the remainder of the breast is high and needs to be addressed either by radiotherapy or mastectomy. In the stand-alone cases, the DCIS needs to be measured. Also importantly, in a wide local excision, the presence or absence of DCIS at the margins of excision needs to be mentioned. The nuclear grade of DCIS needs to be mentioned. The nuclear scoring is done on the same basis as for nuclear scoring on an invasive malignancy, and they can be graded as low-grade, intermediate-grade, or high-grade DCIS. The different morphological categories of a DCIS needs to be mentioned. The various common types include solid, cribriform, comedonecrosis, and papillary. The other types include clear, signet ring, apocrine, neuroendocrine, and cystic hypersecretory type.

DCIS in papilloma: Benign papillomas are sometimes characterized by the presence of a focal population of monotonous cells with the cytological and architectural features of low-grade ductal neoplasia. Myoepithelial cells may be scant or absent from these foci and on immunohistochemistry show the absence of high molecular cytokeratin CK5/6 and diffuse uniform positive staining for estrogen receptor.

Encysted/encapsulated papillary carcinoma is a variant of papillary carcinoma, characterized by fine fibrovascular cores covered by neoplastic epithelial cells of low or intermediate nuclear grade and surrounded by a fibrous capsule. In the majority of cases, there is no myoepithelial cell layer within the papillae or at the periphery of the lesion. These lesions are considered in situ carcinoma. In some cases, there may evidence of frank invasion, when the entity is called encysted/encapsulated papillary carcinoma with invasion.

Paget's disease of nipple is an adenocarcinoma within the epidermis of the nipple. The carcinoma cells are typically high grade and positive for cam 5.2 and HER2. It needs to be reported regardless of whether or not the underlying in situ or invasive carcinoma is identified. The differentials include intraepidermal squamous carcinoma and melanoma, which can be distinguished by immunohistochemistry.

Lobular neoplasia: In view of the subjectivity involved in separating ALH from LCIS and the similar molecular profiles, it has been agreed now to group the two forms together as "lobular neoplasia" (in situ lobular neoplasia). The defining cell type is discohesive, cytologically bland nuclei with occasional small inconspicuous nucleolus. The distension of lobular units may be variable from mild to gross, resulting in either patent lumina or complete obliteration. In difficult cases of differentiating from low-grade DCIS, E cadherin expression on immunohistochemistry can be seen as they are absent to weak in lobular neoplasia.

Microinvasive carcinoma: The entity is typically a dominant, and often extensive, DCIS lesion with one or more clearly separate foci of invasion into the stromal tissue, none of which measures more than 1 mm in diameter. Microinvasive focus is rare in DCIS, except in high-grade ones. In the event of any doubt, DCIS areas can be picked up by organoid architecture and the presence of myoepithelial cells in DCIS with loss in microinvasive foci.

4.5   Grossing

The different specimens received include breast wide local excision and mastectomy.

Wide local excisions: The specimen after receiving is measured in the 3 dimensions and then inked with the same or different colors to represent the different margins. The specimen is oriented based on suture markings (long lateral and short superior tags). The specimen is then breadloafed from one end to the other at a distance of 5 mm. The cut surface shows the tumor, measure the tumor in the 3 dimensions and the distance from all the margins are documented. Smaller tumors less than 3 cm are completely submitted for microscopic examination. In larger tumors, at least one representative bit for each centimeter of the tumor is put. The surgical margins, either shave or radial, are also put.

Mastectomy: The specimen is oriented based on axillary fat, anterior skin, and nipple areola as markers. The neoplasm is palpated and corelated with the clinical and radiology reports as regards the quadrant involvement. The specimen is inked at the base and breadloafed from one end to the other at a distance of at least 5 mm. The tumor is identified along with any other abnormalities. The anterior surface is looked for any peau d'orange, ulceration, or nodule formation. The tumor diameter in three dimensions is recorded. The distance of the tumor from the posterior deep margin is recorded. The axillary tail or dissected nodes are documented for the number, size, and gross involvement by the tumor. Representative sections are taken from the tumor, margins, anterior skin, nipple areola, and the axillary nodes.

Special situations include post-neoadjuvant excisions and nonpalpable excisions. In the post-neoadjuvant excisions, look out for evident gross tumor. In the case of no evident tumor, the area of the original tumor is matched with clinical and radiological findings, and the tumor bed area is sampled completely to look for any microscopic tumor. In nonpalpable tumors, the slices are radiographed, and suspicious areas with calcifications are completely sampled.

4.6   Essentials in a Histopathology Report

- Tumor size
- Tumor type
- Tumor grade (Modified Richardson–Bloom Score)
- Presence of extensive intraductal carcinoma (EIC)*
- Lymphovascular emboli
- Margin status (negative/close/focal positive/gross positive) in wide excision**
- No. of metastatic nodes and total axillary lymph node dissected
- Pathological staging (pTNM)
- Receptor status: ER and PR (by IHC or EIA) and HER2/neu by IHC
- Note:
- *EIC: DCIS in >25% of any low power field within or outside the tumor. It is a strong predictor of local recurrence after BCT, especially if margins are positive.
- **Gross +ve cut margin: Extensive involvement of a cut margin OR > 3 foci of invasive or in situ carcinoma in any inked margin. It requires revision excision or mastectomy.
- **Focal positive cut margin: 3 or less foci of invasive or in situ carcinoma in any inked margin. It requires revision surgery especially if EIC is present.

4.7   Grading

- Modified Richardson–Bloom grading system [2] (Nottingham's modification).
- *Tubule formation*
- Score1 >75%
- Score2 10–75%
- Score3 <10%

4.7.1   Nuclear Grade

Small uniform nuclei, no pleomorphism: 1
    Moderate sized nuclei with pleomorphism: 2
    Marked pleomorphism: 3

4.7.2   Mitosis/10hpf*

0–6: 1
    7–12: 2

>12: 3
*Could vary with microscopes

4.7.3 Final Score

3–5 = Grade I
   6–7 = Grade II
   8–9 = Grade III

4.8 Post-neoadjuvant Chemotherapy Breast Pathology

The needle-core biopsy findings (grade, histological type, necrosis, Ki67 index, hormone-receptor status, and HER2 status) help stratify patients be treated with neoadjuvant therapy. Although neoadjuvant therapy does not provide survival benefit, response to treatment is a strong prognostic factor and is useful for individual patient care.

The residual cancer or tumor bed must be found to assess the tumor response. This is done either by correlating the area with the pretreatment radiological image localization or by placing clips before treatment. If the tumor does not respond or shows minimal response, then the gross dimension of the tumor needs to be recorded. The size of the tumor, the grade of the tumor, and the presence of the viable tumor within the lymph node are powerful predictors of long-term survival. Sometimes, no gross disease may be palpable, and histology may reveal microscopic residual disease. The size and grade of the tumor need to be recorded. In some cases, no microscopic residual viable cancer cells or any viable DCIS remains, and these are recorded as pathological complete response (pCR). What remains in sections from the tumor bed after a complete response may only be a loose edematous, vascularized fibro-elastotic connective tissue with chronic inflammatory cells and macrophages.

Classification of response can be provided as

- R0: complete pathological response
- R1: Microscopic viable tumor
- R2: Macroscopic viable tumor

The AJCC stage before and after treatment also serves as an important additional prognostic information.

4.9 Prognosis and Predictive Factors in Early Breast Cancer

Breast cancer is a heterogeneous group of diseases compounded by tumor heterogeneity within each individual tumor. Following surgery, the patient has a choice of adjuvant hormonal therapy and chemotherapy to reduce the risk of recurrence and death from breast cancer. Adjuvant treatments are aimed to eradicate distant micro-metastasis. Stratifying patients becomes of paramount importance.

The different prognostic and predictive factors in early breast cancers are discussed below. A prognostic factor would determine disease-free or overall survival in a patient. The adjuvant chemotherapy, radiation, and hormonal therapy can alter the natural course and reduce the risk of relapse and therefore alter the natural course of a disease. On the other hand, a predictive factor would address the likelihood of response to a proposed therapy. The assessment of hormone receptors and HER2 status on IHC can be both prognostic and predictive.

Tumor type/grade: Histopathological type have a prognostic significance. Certain special types of breast carcinomas like the tubular, mucinous, and medullary have a more favorable prognosis compared to the usual common infiltrating carcinoma, no special type (NST).

The grading of tumors has prognostic relevance [3]. The modified Bloom–Richardson is the most accepted grading system. Patients with grade 3 have much higher relative risk of recurrence compared to grade 1 tumors. It plays a primary role in decision making in the lymph node-negative cases with borderline tumor size.

Tumor size: An accurate measurement of tumor size is important as it is an important component of the prognostic indices and provides us the T stage. The T4 is a defined criterion with the involvement of chest wall and skin. The skin involvement includes ulceration, nodule, and peau d'orange appearance. The T1 to T3 is based on the size detection of the invasive component. Subdividing the T1 into T1a to T1c is relevant as the probability of metastasis increases with increasing size from less than 5 mm (T1a) to less than or equal to 2 cm (T1c).

A three-dimensional account of the size should be available to then take the largest dimension as the T size. Care should be taken not to take adjacent DCIS areas, and also satellite nodules should not be included in the main mass. If the foci of the tumor are more than 5 mm apart, the chances of satellite deposit representing one mass is considered low and therefore not added to the main mass.

Excision margins: It is recommended that the pathologist mentions the distance between the DCIS and infiltrating duct carcinoma and the inked surgical margin. The presence of DCIS at margins in wide local excision needs to be addressed.

Lymphatic and vascular invasion: The peritumoral lymphatic and vascular invasion (LVI) has prognostic significance for the risk of local and distant recurrence [4]. Criteria for invasion should be strictly adhered in order to avoid false-positive tumor cells floating with lymphatic or vascular channels. The adherence of tumor to the wall or presence of thrombus within the vessel or confirmation of space to be lymphatic or vessel with endothelial markers, if in doubt, confirms LVI. It is primarily used to make decisions for lymph node-negative patients with borderline tumor sizes [5].

Lymph node status: The presence or absence of lymph node involvement is the most significant prognostic indicator in patients with early breast cancer. Also, there is a direct relation between the number of nodes involved and the risk of distant recurrence.

Any nodal involvement needs to be further stratified into macrometastasis or micrometastasis. Micrometastasis is defined as metastatic foci larger than 0.2 mm and/or more than 200 cells, but none larger than 2.0 mm. Macrometastasis is defined as a focus larger than 2 mm.

Isolated tumor cells (ITC) are single tumor cells or small clusters of cells not more than 0.2 mm in greatest extent that can be detected by routine H&E stains or by immunohistochemistry. Also included in the criteria proposed is a cluster of fewer than 200 cells in a single histological cross section. Nodes containing only ITCs are excluded from the total positive node count for purposes of N classification and should be included in the total number of nodes evaluated.

The use of sentinel node (SN) in breast cancer is an established practice. In order to avoid complications of axillary dissection, sentinel node examination becomes relevant. If cancer is not detected in the sentinel node(s), <10% of patients will have other nodes involved. The sentinel nodes are detected by using a blue dye or radiolabeled colloid or a combination to achieve greater detection rates. The optimal pathologic method to assess the SN for involvement remains a question. Serial sectioning of each of the submitted sentinel node increases the sensitivity as does the use of immunohistochemistry (IHC) for histologically negative lymph nodes. The significance, however, of occult micrometastases found by IHC alone remains controversial.

Nottingham Prognostic Index (NPI) is a well-validated prognostic scoring system based on the three established prognostic variables:tumor size, histological grade, and axillary lymph node status [6].

The NPI is calculated using the formula: NPI = Grade (1 to 3) + Node (1 to 3) + [size of invasive carcinoma in cm × 0.2]. Node is the axillary lymph node stage, which is estimated as follows:

- Score 1 = negative nodes
- Score 2 = 1–3 positive axillary nodes or a positive internal mammary node alone (e.g., for medial tumors).
- Score 3 = >3 positive nodes and/or the apical node, or any low axillary node and an internal mammary node together.

Size is the greatest dimension of the invasive tumor, and in multifocal disease, the largest invasive tumor mass is considered. If histological assessment of tumor size or grade is not available, imaging or clinical size or preoperative core biopsy grade can be used.

NPI scores vary from 2.01 to up to >7 and can be subdivided into the following groups:

- <2.4 = excellent prognostic group
- 2.4 – <3.4 = good prognostic group
- 3.4 – <4.4 = moderate 1 prognostic group

- 4.4 – <5.4 = moderate 2 prognostic group
- ≥5.4 = poor prognostic group.

This latter category can be subdivided into poor (≥5.4 to <6.4) and very poor prognostic groups (≥6.4).

The NPI is not applicable to tumors after neoadjuvant therapy, or in locally advanced or metastatic cancers or for recurrent tumors.

Estrogen and progesterone receptors: The presence of estrogen and progesterone receptors in an invasive breast carcinoma is both a prognostic and predictive marker. ER is a nuclear transcription factor that, when activated by the hormone estrogen, stimulates the growth of both normal breast epithelium and even tumor cells. ER regulates the expression of PR, so the presence of PR usually indicates that the estrogen–ER pathway is intact and functional.

The prognostic marker is difficult to assess as it needs to be evaluated in the absence of tamoxifen treatment intervention [7]. The presence of the receptor is a powerful predictive factor for the likelihood of benefit from adjuvant tamoxifen. Tamoxifen binds to ER and blocks estrogen-stimulated growth, resulting in significantly longer disease-free and overall survival in patients with ER-positive invasive breast cancers, compared with those that are ER-negative.

IHC is considered a specific, sensitive, and cheap method to assess the presence of the receptors in formalin-fixed paraffin sections. The IHC scores can be provided as both the percentage of positivity in tumor cells and the intensity of positivity. Even a > 1% weak positive is considered positive for starting treatment. Strict adherence to quality control and accreditations are necessary for predictive markers. The choice of the right clone and the procedure using weak, strong, and negative controls with each test sample is mandatory [8].

HER2 gene: The c-erbB-2 (HER2/*neu*) proto-oncogene is located on chromosome 17q21 and encodes 185,000 transmembrane glycoprotein, which has an intrinsic tyrosine kinase activity. It is amplified and/or overexpressed in approximately 30% of human breast tumors. The overexpression of the human epidermal growth factor receptor 2 (HER2) protein results from the HER2 gene amplification. This is associated with aggressive histological features and also poor prognosis, but anti-HER2-targeted therapy, with trastuzumab, provides substantial survival benefits. The potential side effects of the costly drug and the high response to anti-HER2 drugs emphasize the need for accurate measurement of HER2 status.

HER2 status is primarily determined by immunohistochemistry and, when required, by fluorescence in situ hybridization (FISH) on formalin-fixed parraffin-embedded (FFPE) samples. The scoring on IHC is determined by membrane staining, intensity, completeness, and percentage of tumor cells with the stain [9]. Scoring samples as 3+ are considered unequivocally positive, and those scoring 0/1+ as negative. Borderline scores (2+) are regarded as equivocal and mandate further assessment using FISH.

The FISH analysis using dual probes is used when IHC is equivocal. The most commonly used detection methodology is a dual probe FISH using fluorochrome-labeled probes for (a) the *HER2* locus on the long arm of chromosome 17 and (b) a site near the centromere of chromosome 17 (CEN17 or CEP17). The results are based on the HER2/CEP17 ratio less than or more than 2 and the average HER2 copy number of <4 signals/cell, 4–6 signals/cell, and >6 signals/cell.

Proliferation marker Ki67: Ki67 is a nuclear non-histone protein expressed in proliferating cells and absent in quiescent (G0 phase) cells in the cell cycle. The expression of Ki67 can be provided as the percentage of invasive tumor cell nuclei staining on IHC. It is considered that the Ki67 index can be used as both a prognostic and predictive marker in breast cancers. It is of more value than the mitotic count [10].

The methodology of counting and the choice of the optimal cutoff have been the challenging issues in the evaluation of Ki67 as a prognostic marker. The heterogeneity of Ki67 expression within the tumor and the presence of hot spots raise questions in the counting. As regards optimal cutoff, the values have been revised. The cutoff moved from 14% to 20% in the St Gallen consensus criteria. The 2017 St Gallen meeting has put 20–30% as borderline and high as over 30%.

The predictive relevance in distinguishing between luminal A and luminal B based on high Ki67 may need further validation. The issue of tumor heterogeneity, molecular classification based on needle biopsy, and inter-observer variation have raised questions in a robust evaluation of Ki67. The use of digital pathology may address some of the burning issues in Ki67.

4.10 Molecular Classification

The distribution of breast cancer among routine practice comprised overwhelmingly the invasive mammary carcinoma NST group comprising 80–85%, but all these behaved differently even after matching them for the stage and grade of the tumor. The landmark paper by the Stanford group of Perou and Sorlie et al. using gene expression profiling (GEP) was a game-changer. It classified breast cancers into the luminal A, luminal B, normal breast-like, HER2-enriched, and basal-like subtypes [11]. Each of these subcategories have important prognostic and predictive values, but the application of GEP is neither economical nor practical at most places. With the advent of time, many investigators validated the use of immunohistochemistry as a surrogate marker for the molecular classification of breast cancers [12, 13].

The immunohistochemical markers used included estrogen receptor (ER), progesterone receptor (PR), human epidermal growth factor receptor-2 (HER2), dividing into luminal, HER2, and triple-negative subtypes. The Ki67 proliferation marker further subdivided the luminal into luminal A and luminal B. A further use of more IHC can classify the triple-negative subcategory into basal type, claudin low, and androgen positive.

Luminal A: This group of estrogen-positive tumors predominantly includes invasive breast carcinomas NST along with tubular, cribriform, lobular, mucinous, and neuroendocrine carcinomas. They are negative for HER2 receptors with low Ki67 index below 20%. More recently, a 20% cutoff point of PR to separate luminal A and B subtypes is also considered [14]. They have the best prognosis and also have low recurrence scores in the Oncotype DX test [13].

Luminal B: This group of estrogen-positive tumors has a higher Ki67 index above 20%. They may also be considered with negative PR or low PR less than 20%. Also included is a subgroup that has HER2 positivity apart from the hormonal receptor positivity. This group has higher recurrence scores in the Oncotype DX test.

HER2 positive: Apart from the triple-positive group with hormonal receptors positive, there is also an exclusive group of HER2 enriched with hormonal receptors negative. These are obtained by strong complete membrane positivity in more than 10% of tumor cells. In the event of weak-to-moderate positivity, a borderline score is given with FISH done for confirmation.

Triple-negative tumors: Show lack of the ER, PR, and HER2 IHC markers. This group has a significant overlap with the basal group reported in the initial landmark Stanford work through gene expression profiling. This includes a heterogeneous morphological group including adenoid cystic carcinoma, secretory carcinoma, metaplastic carcinoma, and carcinoma with medullary features apart from the no special type.

4.11 Conclusions

Breast cancer needs a multidisciplinary team approach. The pathologist role is not just as a diagnostician and a prognostician but also as a theranostician. Although infiltrating mammary carcinoma, NOS forms the major cancer prototype in breast cancers, the cancer is a very heterogenous disease. The appropriate diagnosis and the use of validated IHC are of paramount importance at the first stage of diagnosis and molecular classification in the needle biopsy. Further, providing all the prognostic and predictive markers in the radical specimen is of paramount importance in proper stratification and optimal care of patients with breast cancer.

References

1. Lakhani S, et al. WHO classification of tumours of the breast. Lyon: IARC Lyon; 2012.
2. Bloom HJ, Richardson WW. Histological grading and prognosis in breast cancer; a study of 1409 cases of which 359 have been followed for 15 years. Br J Cancer. 1957;1957(11):359–77.
3. Elston CW, Ellis IO. Pathological prognostic factors in breast cancer. I. The value of histological grade in breast cancer: experience from a large study with long-term follow- up. Histopathology. 1991;19:403–10.
4. De Mascarel I, et al. Obvious peritumoral emboli: an elusive prognostic factor reappraised. Multivariate analysis of 1320 node-negative breast cancers. Eur J Cancer. 1998;34:58–65.
5. Lee AH. Prognostic value of lymphovascular invasion in women with lymph node negative invasive breast carcinoma. Eur J Cancer. 2006;42:357–62.
6. Galea MH, Blamey RW, Elston CE, Ellis IO. The Nottingham Prognostic Index in primary breast cancer. Breast Cancer Res Treat. 1992;22:207–19.
7. Schiff R. Clinical aspects of estrogen and progesterone receptors. In: Harris JR, Lippman ME, Morrow M, Osbourne CK, editors. Diseases of the breast. 4th ed. Philadelphia: Wolters Kluwer Lippincott Williams & Wilkins; 2006. p. 408–30.

 8. Hammond ME, et al. American Society of Clinical Oncology/College of American Pathologists guideline recommendations for immunohistochemical testing of estrogen and progesterone receptors in breast cancer. Arch Pathol Lab Med. 2010;134:907–22.
 9. Wolff AC, et al. American Society of Clinical Oncology/College of American Pathologists guideline recommendations for human epidermal growth factor receptor 2 testing in breast cancer. J Clin Oncol. 2007;25:118–45.
10. Goldhirsch A, et al. Thresholds for therapies: highlights of the St Gallen International Expert Consensus on the primary therapy of early breast cancer. Ann Oncol. 2009;20:1319–29.
11. Perou CM, Sorlie T, Eisen MB, et al. Molecular portrait of human breast tumours. Nature. 2000;406(6797):747–52.
12. Tang P, Skinner K, Hicks D. Molecular classification of breast carcinomas by immunohistochemical analysis, are we ready? Diagn Mol Pathol. 2009;18(3):125–32.
13. Goldhirsh A, Winer EP, Coates AS, et al. Personalizing the treatment of women with early breast cancer: highlights of the St. Gallen International Expert Consensus on the primary therapy of early breast cancer 2013. Ann Oncol. 2013;24(9):2206–23.
14. Prat A, Cheang MC, Martin M, et al. Prognostic significance of progesterone receptor–positive tumor cells within immunohistochemically defined luminal A breast cancer. J Clin Oncol. 2013;31(2):203–9.

Molecular Mechanisms of Early Breast Cancer

5

Prasanth Ariyannur and Vijay Kumar Srinivasalu

5.1 Central Molecular Pathophysiology of Cancers

The molecular pathophysiology of three stages of cancer, such as initiation, progression, and metastasis, is dealt with altered molecular signaling pathways that regulate key physiological functions of normal cells such as growth and proliferation, differentiation, stress response, DNA repair, metabolism, and cell survival. Alterations in molecular signaling pathways can also alter the reaction of tumor cells to the adjacent stromal microenvironment, immune cells, tissue macrophages, and vascular endothelial cells. Because of all these changes, carcinogenesis is a dynamic process within a set of distinctive signaling streams/traits which are complementary to each other in the cell. There are about ten of these traits that have been characterized so far [1]. See Fig. 5.1 and legend for more details.

5.2 Molecular Development of Breast

Microscopically, normal breast consists of ducts and glands along with fibrofatty tissues. Ducts are double-layered epithelium consisting of luminal cells and surrounding myoepithelial cells. Luminal cells during development are formed by a combination of ducts and lobules that lead to terminal branching and acinar formation which are the gland units for milk production. During normal development, steroid hormones estrogen and progesterone would act on ER and PR of luminal cells

P. Ariyannur (✉)
Molecular Oncology Laboratory, Department of Biochemistry, Amrita Institute of Medical Sciences, Amrita Vishwa Vidyapeetham, Kochi, Kerala, India
e-mail: prasanthas@aims.amrita.edu

V. K. Srinivasalu
Department of Medical Oncology, Amrita Institute of Medical Sciences, Amrita Vishwa Vidyapeetham, Kochi, Kerala, India

© Springer Nature Singapore Pte Ltd. 2021
B. Kunheri, D. K. Vijaykumar (eds.), *Management of Early Stage Breast Cancer*,
https://doi.org/10.1007/978-981-15-6171-9_5

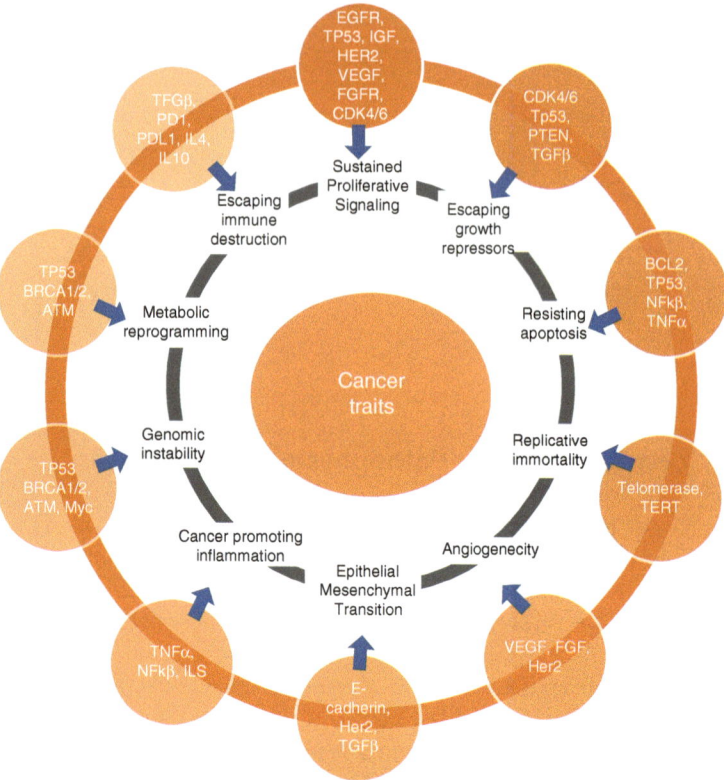

Fig. 5.1 This figure illustrates the key markers associated with respective hallmark traits in the context of breast cancer. (Modified from reference [1].) *Sustained proliferative signaling* by growth factors themselves, overexpression of growth factor receptors, or spontaneous activation of receptor due to altered structure or function of the receptor protein. In breast cancer cells, altered signaling of estrogen receptor (ER), progesterone receptor (PR), and human epidermal growth factor receptor 2 (Her2) are the most common proliferation-inducing traits. In about 70% of breast cancer, proliferation is induced by ERα, which would induce a set of gene regions called estrogen response elements (ERE) and activation of many cell proliferation gene targets [2]. Similarly, Her2 activates a set of receptor tyrosine kinase (RTK) for downstream signaling pathways for proliferation. Downstream signaling pathways consist of mitogen-activated protein kinase (MAPK) and phophatidylionositol-3-kinase (PI3K). Somatic mutations of *PIK3CA*, *BRAF*, *KRAS*, and *EGFR* are involved in breast cancer cells to produce abnormal proliferative downstream signaling in Ras-Raf-MAPK signaling pathways. *Escaping growth suppressors* of both intra- and extracellular tumor microenvironments can be another major trait for the persistence of breast cancer. Retinoblastoma (*RB1*) gene is a gatekeeper and typical tumor suppressor gene having a central role in cell cycle and transducing extracellular growth inhibitory signals [3]. G1 cyclin-dependent kinase (CDK 4/6) inhibitors (such as palbociclib and ribociclib) can hypophosphorylate pRb which leads to cell cycle arrest [4], which are now used in ER-positive Her2-negative breast cancer [5]. TGFβ signaling pathway, which has an anti-proliferative effect by the downregulation of onco-gene cMyc in early breast cancer, is evaded when it is altered by receptor mutation or altered expression of SMAD4 protein which is also involved in TFGβ pathway [6]. *Resisting apoptosis* cell reaction by evading the checkpoint regulator function senses DNA damage by p53 when pathogenic mutations occur on the *TP53* gene in breast cancer tissues. This has been accounted for

to produce cellular response and proliferation. Luminal cells account for 90% of proliferation and most of the hormone receptor-positive cancer [18]. Estrogen acts on nuclear receptors ERα and ERβ, both are transcription factors. ER is expressed normally in all luminal cells, while PR is expressed only in terminal bud cells and induced by estrogen. At the time of puberty and menarche, the ducts enlarge and branch out, and acinar formation occurs [18]. After *menarche*, there is a cyclical proliferation especially during the luteal phase of the menstrual cycle due to the elevated levels of estrogen and progesterone, followed by apoptosis during menstruation. During pregnancy and lactation, massive lobuloalveolar growth occurs due to the proliferation of epithelial cells, followed by apoptosis during the weaning and involution of tubulo-alveolar glands. The ability of mammary gland cells to proliferate and differentiate during each menstrual cycle and pregnancy shows the role of stem cells and their DNA replication and mitosis. Hereditary breast cancer can occur during this period, especially in mammary stem cells, probably due to

←————————————————————

about 37% of breast cancer samples [7]. *Replicative immortality* by upregulating telomerase enzyme was observed in breast cancer tissue (especially ERα induced) [8]. This would add nucleotide repeats and/or maintains the telomere length to provide replicative immortality. Also, this upregulation was found to be associated with poor prognosis with chemotherapy, which was found to be reversed by hormonal (tamoxifen) therapy as well. *Angiogenic* factors such as vascular endothelial growth factor (VEGF) and Her2 were found to have some role initially with breast cancer when clinical trials of anti-VEGF-A antibody (bevacizumab) showed promising results, which was later found to have no progression-free survival (PFS) benefit [9]. *Epithelial-mesenchymal transition* (EMT) [10] and loss of function of E-cadherin causing loss of polarity and promoting EMT are the major traits found in many tumors providing resistance to apoptosis, invasion, and metastasis. *Cancer promoting inflammation* due to immune cell infiltration and expression and secretion of growth and survival factors to the tumor microenvironment causing propagation and invasion of tumors. *Genomic instability* can occur in diverse ways. Mutations in gatekeeper genes (*TP53*, *RB1*, etc.) are significantly higher in cancer cells, and this can cause overall genomic instability which causes clonal evolution and selective growth advantage [11]. Mutations in caretaker genes which are involved in DNA repair (such as *BRCA1*, *BRCA2* in germline cancers) are called *mutator phenotype*, which can give rise to more mutations in other part causing genomic instability in sporadic cancers when the collapse of DNA replication occurs due to oncogene activations [12]. Accordingly, somatic mutations in tumor cells are divided into driver and passenger mutations. Variations in *TP53*, *PIK3CA*, *MAP3K1*, *GATA3*, *CDH1*, *BRCA1*, *PTEN*, *IK3R1*, *AKT1*, and *RB1* are the prominent driver mutations in breast cancer [7]. Passenger mutations are synonymous (without any amino acid change) variation and without any direct role in proliferation. *Metabolic reprogramming* to adapt to cell proliferation and survival is an important change in biochemical physiology. According to the Warburg phenomenon, cancer cells tap cellular energy via anaerobic glycolysis [13]. This is to adapt to the hypoxic microenvironment and mitochondrial dysfunction and ATP depletion [14]. Mutations of certain genes could also trigger this. *PIK3CA* mutations, which are commonly seen in breast cancer, cause abnormal PI3K/Akt signaling pathway stimulating hexokinase and phosphor-fructokinase to drive glycolysis by activation or induction (via mTOR pathway) [15]. *Escaping immune cell destruction* in breast cancer cells has also been identified. Triple (ER, PR, and Her2)-negative breast cancers (TNBC) are associated with FOXP3 (fox head/winged helix) transcription factor which is involved in the development of T-regulatory (Treg) cells, which regulate normal T lymphocytes and NK cell response to make more aggressive tumor [16]. On the other hand, the presence of tumor-infiltrating lymphocytes (TILs) can provide better control over cancer progression and with chemotherapeutic agents [17]

the higher chance of DNA replication errors and damage due to haploinsufficiency and dominant negative effect of mutations in DNA repair genes (see details below). Normal mammary stem cells (NMSC) do not express steroid hormone receptors (ERα, PR) and Her2 [19], which suggest that tumors arising from these cell types form a particular subset of breast cancer. Breast cancer stem cells (CSC) express aldehyde dehydrogenase 1 (ALDH1) [20] and CD44 [21], both have tumorigenic and metastatic potential. Mutations of key regulatory pathways and epigenetic changes can potentially transform NMSC to CSC [22] and clonal evolution during therapeutic response [23].

5.2.1 Molecular Pathogenesis by Estrogen and Progesterone Receptors

The estrogen in breast tissue is acted through ERα and ERβ. Among them, ERα is widely accepted for patient management and treatment decisions. ERα contains three domains, N-terminal activating function-1 (AF-1) domain, DNA binding domain (DBD), hinge domain, and a ligand-binding domain (LBD) or AF-2. This conforms to a common nuclear receptor domain structure where AF-1 is the protein–protein interaction site and AF-2 is the site where enzyme activity is either present intrinsically or coordinated by binding with other protein(s) [24]. As described partially above, classically ERα binds to ERE and coregulators to regulate transcription of target genes involved in many cellular processes. These cellular mechanisms include acetylation, ubiquitination, sumoylation, phosphorylation, ribosylation, RNA splicing, DNA repair, and many other functions. Besides, it can affect transcription indirectly via influencing chromosomal remodeling and post-translational modification. ER can directly affect cell proliferation via cyclin D and activating CDK4 and CDK6. Breast cancer expressing ER is mostly sensitive to endocrine therapy. This includes either competitive (e.g., tamoxifen) [25] or noncompetitive (e.g., fulvestrant) [26] inhibition and inactivation of ER. About 30% of women who undergo anti-hormonal therapy develop resistance due to the evolution of tumor, causing either loss of expression of ERα or mutations in the encoding gene (*ESR1*) [27]. This happens usually in the mutations of the LBD regions [28] or chromosomal translocations where the *ESR1* gene is also involved [29]. In resistant conditions, exemestane (aromatase inhibitor that blocks the peripheral activation of estrogen) and palbociclib (CDK4/6 inhibitor) are found to be effective. Molecular pathogenesis of isolated PR on breast cancer is controversial and emerging. The activation domain (AF3) of PR (like ER) affects several target genes, and PR dimers can bind to PR response elements (PRE) that are supposed to modify transcription of many DNA gene regions.

5.2.2 Her2 Membrane Receptor

Her2 belongs to the EGFR family of tyrosine kinases activating pathways of cell growth differentiation and survival, via its homo-heterodimerization.

Overexpression and/or amplification of Her2 is observed as a driver in 20–30% of early stage breast cancer [30]. Much of the potency of Her2 activity in breast cancer is revealed after the detection of clinical benefits of trastuzumab, aka herceptin [31]. Trastuzumab has shown to inhibit Her2-mediated mitogenic signaling by both ligand-independent and extracellular ligand-dependent dimerization. The dimerization of Her2 and Her3 activates the PI3K signaling pathway, which is also disrupted by trastuzumab [32]. To tap this mechanism for chemotherapeutic use, small molecular inhibitors of Her2, e.g., lapatinib, along with trastuzumab, were found to be effective in advanced stages of Her2-positive breast cancer [33]. Resistance to trastuzumab in the metastatic and recurrent setting has been due to many factors of the tumor microenvironment, such as TGF-β and CD44 receptors. TGFβ via crosstalk between Her2 mediates epithelial–mesenchymal transition of cancer cells via transcriptional regulation of SMAD target genes, activation of PI3K/Akt pathway [34], or induction of a specific long non-coding RNA [35]. A combination of trastuzumab and maytansine (a tubulin inhibitor) was found to be effective in Her2 overexpressing cancer cells resistant to trastuzumab and lapatinib [36].

5.3   Molecular Classification of Breast Cancers

The earlier classification was based on the immunohistochemistry expression levels of ER, PR, Her2, and basal markers (cytokeratin, CK5/6, and EGFR). This classification distinguished breast cancers to their survival as well [37]. But overlapping with the triple-negative breast cancer (TNBC), there was a subtype that has low expression of luminal differentiation markers, high expression of EMT markers, immune-response genes, and stem cell-like features [38]. Due to this and several other studies, comprehensive molecular subtyping was evolved in 2012 identifying the germline, somatic gene variations, copy number variations, epigenetic, and other changes using multiplatform analysis such as mRNA expression, DNA methylation, microRNA sequencing, whole-exome sequencing, and protein expression (reverse phase protein array or RPPA). This comprehensive biological subtyping called The Cancer Genome Atlas (TCGA) adopted most of the earlier classification (given below) and classified breast cancer into four major subtypes: Luminal A, Luminal B, Her2 enriched, and Basal-like [39]. See Table 5.1 for details.

5.3.1   Lehmann's Molecular Classification of Triple-Negative Breast Cancer

Six different molecular subtypes of TNBC have been reported. They are basal-like 1 (BL1), basal-like 2 (BL2), immunomodulatory (IM), mesenchymal (M), mesenchymal stem-like (MSL), and luminal androgen receptor (LAR) [40]. IM subtype has shown better prognosis, whereas the LAR subtype is the worst (hazard ratio of 0.68 vs. 1.47 [41]. About 92% of BL1 subtype contains *TP53* mutation, thus making them highly genomically unstable subtype with a deletion in various genes

Table 5.1 TCGA 2012 molecular subtypes [39]

	Luminal A	Luminal B	Her2-enriched	Basal-like
Receptor status	ER/PR positive Her2 negative	ER/PR positive Her2 variable	High expression of Her2; low in the expression of ER, PR	ER/PR/Her2 negative (TNBC)
RTK-PI3K pathway	High	High	Low	High
P53 pathway	Low	Low	Low	High
RB1 pathway	High	High	Low	High
DNA mutations	*PIK3CA* (49%); *TP53* (12%); *GATA3* (14%); *MAP3K1* (14%)	*TP53* (32%); *PIK3CA* (32%); *MAP3K1* (5%)	*TP53* (84%); *PIK3CA* (7%)	*TP53* (75%); *PIK3CA* (42%); *PIK3R1* (8%)
Protein expression	High estrogen reactive subtype	Low estrogen reactive subtype	High expression of DNA repair proteins	High protein expression of EGFR and HER2
Biological properties	Mostly invasive. Good response to endocrine therapy. Good prognosis	Lesser frequency of invasion, not good better response to endocrine therapy, not as good prognosis Luminal A	Response to trastuzumab (herceptin). Response to anthracycline. Unfavorable prognosis	No response to tamoxifen or herceptin. Sensitive to platinum-based drugs or PARP inhibitors (olaparib) Usually worse prognosis

involved in DNA repair mechanisms such as *BRCA2*, *MDM2*, *PTEN*, and *RB1*. With significantly enriched mutations in *PI3KCA* (55%), *AKT1* (13%), and *CDH1* (13%), a higher number of mutations are seen in LAR tumors. M and MSL subtypes have higher signals of angiogenesis, while IM shows elevated levels of immune signatures and checkpoint inhibitor genes such as *PD1*, *PDL1*, and *CTLA4*. TNBC are mostly represented by invasive ductal carcinomas. LAR and IM subtypes are enriched with invasive lobular and medullary carcinomas, respectively. Similarly, molecular signatures and mutation frequencies are observed in LAR tumors, and IM tumors are also represented in lobular cancers and medullary breast cancers, respectively. MSL tumors are genetically stable, but high expression of *PDGFR* and *VEGFR* makes them more susceptible to antiangiogenic therapy in contrast to the unselected TNBC population. The mesenchymal (M) subtype has upregulated EGFR and Notch signaling pathways by signals such as *EGFR*, *NOTCH1*, and *NOTCH3*. Targeting EGFR and Notch pathways may be a possibility for these tumors. Similar to anti-VEGF inhibitors, EGFR inhibitors did not demonstrate a survival advantage in unselected TNBC.

5.3.2 TCGA Subtypes

The four subtypes of TCGA classification in 2012 featured distinct patterns of molecular pathophysiology [39]. The most common driver mutations are *TP53*, *MAP3K1*, *CDH1*, *PIK3CA*, and *GATA3*. Basal-like and luminal tumors have distinct genes mutated with little overlap. About 80% of *TP53* mutations are found in basal-like cancer subtype (ER-negative), where it is found to be nonsense and frameshift mutations. Same with *PTEN* loss in that subtype. Her2-enriched subtype has Her2 amplification in 80% of cases along with a high frequency of *TP53* mutations. Luminal types have high *PIK3CA* mutations as RTK-PI3K pathway is involved. Luminal/ER+ is the most heterogeneous breast cancer subtype with the highest expression of *ESR1*, *GATA3*, and *FOXA1* and prominent FOXA1/ER signal hub. Luminal A type has intact TP53 and RB1 pathway but inactivated in luminal type B. Relevant molecular details are given in Table 5.1.

5.3.3 Pan-Cancer Atlas Subtypes

After the TCGA in 2012, more comprehensive molecular exploration and analysis were conducted and included more noncoding DNA regions, pathways specific to leukocyte infiltration, and the tumor microenvironment in more than a thousand breast cancer samples called Pan-cancer Pan-Gyn Atlas (PGA). Using 16 molecular features, PGA showed five different prognostic subtypes. PGA also has given a decision tree to classify patients based on clinical laboratory accessible features [42]. While most of the genes which were associated with gynecological tumors in TCGA 2012 were found to be associated with PGA as well, there were additional exclusive genes identified which include mutated (*TP53*, *PIK3CA*, *GATA3*, *CDH1*) and amplified genes (*MYC*, *MCL1*, *ERBB2*, *CCND1*, *KAT6A*, etc.). Many commonalities with the somatic mutational landscape identified earlier by somatic mutation database (COSMIC) were 12 base substitution mutational signatures, 6 rearrangement signatures, and 93 mutated cancer genes [43]. PGA found similar clustering previously identified as characteristic somatic copy number alterations (SCNA) in luminal B, basal-like and Her2+ TCGA types, and mutational signatures in luminal A subtype [44]. Many miRNAs and lncRNA associations from COSMIC were also found to be associated [43]. Gene-lncRNA interaction network of ESR1, DKC1, and lncRNAs TERC, NEAT1, and TUG1 were identified. Identification of association of key lncRNAs (TERC) and their regulator genes (*ESR1*, *DKC1*) has led to prove that ER regulates BRCA expression. In the luminal A subtype, miR-21 targets were positively correlated with TERC. However, many of the identified lncRNAs were not confirmed to be driver mutations in the PGA.

The 16 molecular features included those which are currently used (ER/PR protein expression status, *BRCA1/2* mutation status, *ERBB2* amplification status) or from previous TCGA studies (MSI status, hypermutator type in which DNA contains >10 mutations/million base pair, SCNA load, AR protein expression, leukocyte infiltration (immuno-) score using immune markers and mutation status of

Table 5.2 Pan-cancer Pan-Gyn classification [42]

Cluster No.	SCNA	ER	PR	AR	Hyper-Mut	Immune
C1 (non-hypermutator)	Low	High	High	High	Low	
C2 (hypermutator)	Low	Low	Low	Low	High	
C3 (immune-high)	High	Low	Low	Low		High
C4 (AR/PR low)	High	Low	Low	Low		Low
C5 (AR/PR high)	High	High	High	High		Low

PTEN, *TP53*, *RAS*, *ERBB2*, *PIK3CA*, and *POLE*). Accordingly, for breast cancer, there were five clusters with a decreasing survival score (see Table 5.2). Luminal B and Her2 tissues were found to have higher levels of DNA methylation. Tissues with positive immune markers of Her2 showed a longer survival rate than their immune negative counterparts.

5.4   Hereditary Breast Cancers

An increased incidence of breast or ovarian cancer among multiple close family members with an autosomal dominant inheritance had indicated historically that genetic factors might have a significant contribution at least in a subset of breast and ovarian cancers. Subjects who have had this type of history underwent detailed linkage analysis and were subsequently identified with highly penetrant genes with pathogenic variants. Although pathogenic variants are seen only rarely, estimated to be in about 10% of the total breast and ovarian cancer cases, they might have a significant role in early detection and taking preventive measures to obviate a potentially disastrous occurrence.

In general, many studies have shown that the genetic predisposing factors can be variants of genes that can be divided up into high- and moderate- to low-penetrant genes. High-penetrant genes are associated with most cancer incidences as compared to moderate- and low-penetrant ones. *BRCA1* and *BRCA2* are major examples of high-penetrant genes. Other genres such as *TP53*, *PALB2*, *PTEN*, *CDH1*, and *STK11* are all highly penetrant genes. Moderately penetrant genes are *ATP*, *RAD51*, and *CHEK2*. Each of these genes or combinations of genes might have a definite predilection for a cancer occurrence. A certain cluster of cancer types and/or organ of origin types can be associated with variants of certain genes or one or more genes of a group of genes. Some of these are combined as *syndromes* while others are still *orphan* clusters. For example, variants of the *TP53* gene is associated with a cancer syndrome called *Li-Fraumeni syndrome*, in which there is a high predilection for the association of pre-menopausal breast cancer with brain tumors, leukemia, sarcoma, and adrenocortical carcinoma. Similarly, variants of *BRCA1*, *BRCA2*, *PALB2*, and *RAD51* are all mostly found to be associated with a similar type of cancer predilection.

Some of the frequent questions that arise in this context are:

- When it should be suspected to investigate genetic factors?
- Which are all gene(s) that needs to be selected?
- What type of cluster of cancer disorders should be investigated?
- What are the criteria for genetic testing?
- What are the selection criteria?
- How can a variant be interpreted and assessed further for future cancer predilections?
- How a genetic testing report with clinical interpretation be applied to a patient?
- How to explain subjects about the risk assessment, statistics of predilection, and impact of gene variations?
- How to follow up and manage long term for those who are identified with genetic variants?

Understanding the gene regions and their role in molecular physiology would enable one to better understand and predict the role of the gene and the specific mutations affecting the regions of the gene as well. While many of these questions still cannot be answered completely, we attempt to address them below from each gene scenario.

5.4.1 High-Penetrance Cancer Susceptibility Genes

Most of the occurrences of breast and/or ovarian cancer at an early age of onset, in synchronous or sequential bilateral, in multiple generations with an autosomal dominant pattern of inheritance, either from maternal or paternal lineage could be explained by specific germline pathogenic variation(s) of a particular gene or a set of genes [45–47]. Although a definite estimate is impossible, multiple resources confirmed that high-penetrant germline pathogenic variants occur in about 5–10% of the breast cancers overall [46]. During the last three decades, studies conducted in large families with multiple affected individuals have led to the identification of susceptible genes such as *BRCA1*, *BRCA2*, *TP53*, *PALB2*, *PTEN*, *STK11*, and others. Most of these genes contribute to multiple different pathways converging into some key regulatory components of DNA double-strand break repair mechanisms [48].

5.4.1.1 BRCA1
In the early 1990s, using chromosomal linkage analysis, certain familial breast cancer was identified to be associated with derangements in the long arm of chromosome 17 [49, 50], which subsequently led to the identification of the gene *BRCA1*

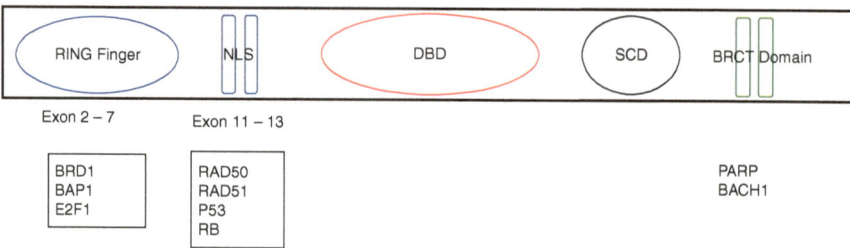

Fig. 5.2 Domains and structure of the *BRCA1* gene. The zinc finger domain, also called the *R*eally *I*nteresting *N*ew *G*ene (RING) domain, holds seven conserved cysteine residues and a histidine residue coordinate with two Zn^{2+} ions to stabilize the structure. It interacts with BRCA1-Associated RING Domain protein 1 (BRD1) to form a heterodimer and interact further with E2 ubiquitin-conjugating enzyme UbcH5 and functions combined as an E3 ubiquitin ligase activity [53]. A large number of cancer-predisposing mutations in the RING domain regions of *BRCA1* and *BRD1* suggest that ubiquitin ligase activity of BRCA1 is central to the tumor suppressor function [54]. BRCA1 E3-ubiquitin ligase activity is to regulate the ubiquitinated degradation of steroid (both estrogen and progesterone) receptors [55], maintain heterochromatic structure via ubiquitylation of histone H2A [56], indirectly assisting DNA double-strand break resection during homologous recombination (HR) by activating a critical intermediate protein called CtIP (carboxy-terminal binding protein-interacting protein) along with ATM, CDK, and MRN proteins as a part of the checkpoint response during G2 and S phases of the cell cycle [57], resulting in DNA repair, condensation, and gene activation. Cells with mutations in the RING domain *BRCA1* were found to be incapable of G2/M phase cell cycle checkpoint function during γ-radiation [58]. The E3 ligase activity of the BRCA1 was inhibited by most of the platinum-based chemotherapeutic agents such as cisplatin, carboplatin, and oxaliplatin [59]. Moreover, the mutations in the RING domain has shown to be partially responsible for the sensitivity of tumors to poly-ADP ribose polymerase (PARP) inhibitor, olaparib [60]

by positional cloning methods [51]. *BRCA1* gene (OMIM[1] #113705) has a size of about 81 kb, 24 exons, and expressing a 190 kDa protein BRCA1 of 1863 amino acids (aa). Three domains in BRCA1 protein are often mutated in cancer. These are (1) an N-terminal cysteine-rich zinc finger domain (exons 2–7), (2) a multifunctional domain spanning exons 11 through 13, and (3) a C-terminal domain (BRCT) [52]. A detailed illustration of the domains is given in Fig. 5.2.

The multifunctional domain spanning four exons (11–13) forms about 65% of the whole sequence of *BRCA1* and contains two nuclear localization signals (NLS). The two NLS (one 501–507 aa, and another 607–614 aa) are required for transport of the BRCA1 protein from the cytoplasm to the nucleus [61]. BRCA1 Exon 11 region binds to retinoblastoma protein (RB), (specifically interacting 304–394 aa) causes suppression of cell cycle progression [62]. Exon 11 region binds to RAD50 and RAD51, both the proteins are involved in DNA double-strand break (DSB) repair. When bound to RAD50, BRCA1 (interacting aa 348–748) protein

---

[1] OMIM: Online Mendelian Inheritance in Man is a comprehensive compendium of human genes and genetic phenotypes that is freely available over the internet at the website omim.org and updated daily. OMIM is authored by McKusick-Nathans Institute of Genetic Medicine and Johns Hopkins University School of Medicine.

is involved in DSB repair by Non-Homologous End Joining (NHEJ) process [63]. With RAD51, BRCA1 (interacting 758–1064 aa) causes DSB repair by HR [64]. The global transcriptional activator c-Myc promotes 15% of the genome [65]. There are two c-Myc binding sites in BRCA1 protein: MB1 in exon 11 between 433 and 511 aa and MB2 in exon 8–11 (175–303 aa). When bound to c-Myc, BRCA1 causes inhibition of the transcriptional activity of c-Myc [66]. Partner and Localizer of BRCA2 (PALB2) protein interact with BRCA1 (at 1364–1437 aa) and BRCA2 to form a trio molecular scaffold to assist HR in DNA repair [67]. A serine cluster domain -SCD- (spans from exon 11 to 13 and aa 1280–1524) holds several serine residues that are phosphorylated by ATM and ATR kinase enzymes to recruit BRCA1 to DSB site. Specifically, serine at positions 1189, 1457, 1524, and 1542 is all known to be critically involved [68].

BRCT domains are a conserved peptide region that are found in a family of proteins that are involved in DNA damage repair and checkpoint. Typically, BRCT domains hold phospho-peptide binding modules, but phosphorylation-independent protein–protein interactions, DNA binding, and poly ADP-ribose (PAR) binding as well. See detailed review in [69]. The consensus sequence identified by the BRCT domain is ^{990}pSer-X-X-Phe^{993}, where X can be any amino acid [69]. BRCT is found to directly bind to DSB [70] or terminal overhangs and adjacent major grooves [71]. BRCT domains can function singly or in multiples. If they interact with each other, there is a 22 aa interacting peptide (BACH1). Mutations in the BRCT domain of the BRCA1 can inhibit the recognition of its phospho-ligands and have been found to affect cancer in breast and ovaries [72]. Since BRCT is a common domain in many proteins, but with different affinities to different phosphoproteins, mutations of BRCT in BRCA1 can change the affinity, compete with other BRCTs, and cause ill-effects of other genes causing cancer as well, e.g., TP53 [73]. Since BRCA1 BRCT mutations affect DSB HR-mediated repair, chemotherapeutic efficiency of single-strand break repair inhibitors such as PARP inhibitors is increased and thus utilized clinically [74].

5.4.1.2 BRCA2

BRCA2 is the second most frequent gene associated with breast cancer is linked to the long arm of chromosome 13 (13q12–13) [75, 76]. The complete gene BRCA2 (OMIM # 600185) consists of 27 exons spanning around 70 kb genomic region expressing a 90 kDa BRCA2 protein containing 3418 aa [77] (Fig. 5.3).

BRCA2 is involved in several processes such as maintaining genome stability, including DNA replication, telomere homeostasis, chromosome segregation during mitosis, and cell cycle progression. See the recent review in [80] for more details. Owing to the multifaceted roles, BRCA2 pathogenic variations not only lead to DNA replication stalling, secondary replication fork stability, and stress but also causes (1) aneuploidy due to centromere duplication defects [81], (2) defect in cytokinesis [82] and (3) defect in spindle assembly checkpoint during M-phase of the cell cycle [83]. More active research is currently underway to understand many of the nuclear and cytoplasmic roles of BRCA2.

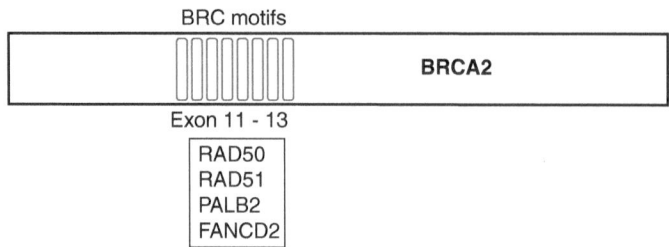

Fig. 5.3 BRCA2 structure. Apart from the NLS in the C-terminal region, there is only one functional domain identified in the protein. This is from exon 11 genomic region expressing eight copies of 39 aa motif repeats spanned across a middle 1000 residues of BRCA2 (aa 638–2280) called BRC motif. This region is conserved for binding RAD51 protein and positioning RAD51 to the DNA DSB repair sites [78]. BRC region is followed by a COOH-terminal region containing specific oligonucleotide binding and helix-turn-helix motif which binds to a protein named DSS1 and attaches to ssDNA and assist RAD51-mediated HR method of DSB DNA repair [79]. Furthermore, BRCA2 acts as a hub to several regulatory proteins such as RAD51, PALB2, and FANCD2 in DSB repair by HR

Tumor Suppressor Effects by BRCA Proteins

Both *BRCA1* and *BRCA2* are tumor suppressor genes. Germline pathogenic variation in one allele of either gene, with the acquired loss of the second allele during a lifetime, can confer a predisposition to breast and ovarian cancer. The autosomal dominant pattern of inheritance of breast cancer cannot be entirely addressed by haploinsufficiency or a trans-dominant negative effect by a single mutant allele. One large collaborative study had shown that *BRCA1* variant carriers have more ER-negative and PR-positive tumors than *BRCA2* variant carriers [84]. However, this opposes the ubiquitylation and degradation of ER and PR by E3 ubiquitin ligase activity of the BRCA1 RING domain. The propensity of *BRCA1* pathogenic variants in ER-positive or TNBC cannot be explained by the current knowledge [85]. Since BRCA1 and BRCA2 are the hub of many different proteins and have a central role in DNA DSB error-free repair by HR, there could be a greater dependency on the gene dose at least during the initial induction of tumors. Though more direct evidence is required in this mechanism, the recent finding of a large increase in skewed X-inactivation and activation of many X-linked genes as a protective in *BRCA1/2* mutation carriers [86] suggests a wider effect of BRCA1/2 dose in the breast and ovarian cells where X-linked gene expressions can be critical. In summary, the *BRCA1/2* pathogenic variants cannot explain the complete pathogenesis of breast cancer.

5.4.1.3 TP53

Germline variants of the *TP53* gene (OMIM #191170) on chromosome 17p have been known to be associated with early onset breast cancer, especially when it is associated with the familial occurrence of adrenocortical carcinoma, brain tumors, childhood sarcomas, or leukemias (see Table 5.3). These conditions were consolidated

Table 5.3 2015 Chompret Criteria for LFS [93]

Familial presentation	A proband with tumor belonging to LFS tumor spectrum (According to 2015 criteria, LFS tumor spectrum includes premenopausal breast cancer, soft tissue sarcoma, osteosarcoma, central nervous system (CNS) tumor, and adrenocortical carcinoma) before age 46 years At least one first/second-degree relative with LFS tumor before 56 years or with multiple tumors
Multiple primitive tumors	A proband with multiple tumors (except multiple breast tumors), two of which belong to the LFS tumor spectrum and the first of which occurred before age 46 years
Rare tumors	A patient with adrenocortical carcinoma, choroid plexus tumor, or rhabdomyosarcoma of embryonal anaplastic subtype, irrespective of family history
Early onset breast cancer	Breast cancer before the age of 31 years

clinically into Li-Fraumeni syndrome (LFS) (OMIM #151623) (Table 5.5) [87, 88]. While occurrences of somatic pathogenic variants of *TP53* are quite common in most of the tumors [89], inherited germline mutations causing breast cancer is only less than 1% [90]. Because of the rare confluence of some or all of these tumor types in one family, certain clinical criteria (called Chompret criteria) were developed to help decide whether genetic testing of the *TP53* gene to be done [91, 92]. This has recently been updated as given in Table 5.3 [93]. However, the cumulative cancer incidence by the age of 70 years in *TP53* variant-positive patients is 100% and is about 54% for female breast cancer [94].

5.4.1.4 Molecular Pathogenesis of TP53

TP53 is a tumor suppressor gene of 20 kb and 11 exons. The protein product of the gene called cellular tumor antigen protein-53 (p53) has two main functions upon sensing DNA damage: (1) acts as a transcriptional trans-activator of a set of genes (e.g., *CDKN1A*, *MDM2*, *GADD45A*, *Bax*, *IGFBP1*, cyclin G1, cyclin G2) to repair damaged DNA or (2) inducing apoptosis of the cell. Because of these two functions, the *TP53* gene is known as the "guardian of the human genome." To do these functions, p53 protein can arrest the cell cycle by the proper activation of the retinoblastoma (RB) pathway and can directly involve in the DNA repair process [95]. The protein p53 contains five conserved domains. Domain-I (start to codon 62) has the transactivation properties. Rest of the domains make up DNA-binding core, which contains DNA-binding domain (DBD) (codon 94–292) and tetramerization domain (TET) (codons 325–356). Most of the mutations of *TP53* were identified in DBD and TET regions. In a normal unstressed cell, p53 is inactivated by a ligase enzyme (*MDM2* gene function). Upon stress, it gets activated and induces cell cycle arrest, apoptosis, senescence, DNA repair, and change in metabolism. Mutated p53 cannot bind to either proper gene regions of the DNA repair and apoptosis (dominant-negative effect) [96] or trans-activate inappropriate target genes involved in the cell cycle [97].

5.4.2 Other High-Penetrant Genes

5.4.2.1 PTEN

PTEN hamartoma tumor syndrome is a spectrum of disorders that are linked to mutations of a tumor suppressor gene called phosphatase and tensin homolog (*PTEN*) gene. This includes Cowden syndrome (OMIM # 158350), Bannayan-Ripley-Ruvalcaba syndrome (BRRS), adult Lhermitte-Duclos disease (LDD), and autism spectrum disorders associated with macrocephaly [98] (see Table 5.6). This syndrome is highly associated with both benign and malignant breast cancer between the ages of 38 and 50 years, and the cumulative cancer risk for subjects having PTEN mutation is about 85% [99]. According to the latest clinical criteria, breast cancer is one of the major criteria for the diagnosis of these syndromes [98]. PTEN protein is a phosphatase enzyme that dephosphorylates phosphatidylinositol (3,4,5) trisphosphate regulating cell growth, survival, and migration. It also acts as a protein phosphatase enzyme regulating cell cycle [100], contributing a central role in tumorigenesis.

5.4.2.2 CDH1

Another high-penetrant gene is *CDH1*, which was found to have a lifetime risk of about 50% for invasive breast cancer with predominant lobular histology [101], and a higher association with diffuse gastric cancer [102]. *CDH1* is located on chromosome 16q22.1 and encodes the E-cadherin, a calcium-dependent adhesion molecule that plays a key role in cellular adhesion, polarity, orientation, and maintenance of cellular differentiation and tissue morphology by binding to β-catenin, plakoglobin, and actin filaments by driving subsequent Wnt cell signaling [101, 103]. Association of these two cancers in one person can be a hereditary syndrome called hereditary diffuse gastric cancer syndrome (HDGC) (OMIM #137215) [102].

5.4.2.3 STK11

Germline pathogenic variants of the *STK11* gene were identified in many subjects who fall under the clinical criteria of Peutz–Jeghers syndrome (PJS) (OMIM #175200), an autosomal dominant hamartomatous polyposis syndrome [104, 105]. Though gastrointestinal cancers are common in PJS, the cumulative risk of breast cancers with pathogenic mutations of *STK11* gene is 30–50% [106]. The gene *STK11*, located on chromosome 19p13.3, encodes an enzyme called serine/threonine kinase 11 or liver kinase b1 (LKB1). This enzyme is required for assessing the energy requirement of cells by activating 14 other kinases and regulates cell growth and proliferation when energy levels are low. By activating adenosine monophosphate-activated protein kinase (AMPK)-related kinases, it regulates cell polarity and inhibits abnormal expansion of tumor cells. Studies have shown that estradiol upon dose-dependent binding to the estrogen receptor (ERα) affects the promoter region of *STK11* and reduces kinase expression, thus reducing AMPK activity as well [107]. This suggests a mechanism of STK11-related tumorigenicity in ER-positive breast cancers. Furthermore, *STK11* is identified as a tumor suppressor gene, a haploinsufficiency itself can induce cancers, and an associated somatic *TP53* mutation can accelerate the occurrence as well [108].

5.4.2.4 PALB2

Many genetic studies conducted in families and probands of breast cancer suggested the occurrence of mutations of partner and localizer of BRCA2 or *PALB2* gene [109, 110]. Though large group studies on breast cancer patients showed less than 5% incidence of *PALB2* mutation [111], 70-year breast cancer risk for those having *PALB2* variation was found to be ranging from 30 to 50% [110, 112]. As described earlier, PALB2 interacts with BRCA2 and other proteins and involves in several central cell growth and apoptosis by facilitating DNA repair via HR mechanisms. Among *PALB2* carriers, a cut-off value of 2 cm for the tumor size seems to affect 10-year survival outcomes (32.4% in tumors >2 cm vs. 82.4% in tumors <2 cm). Approximately, one-third of those with a *PALB2* pathogenic variant had triple-negative breast cancer, and the average age at breast cancer diagnosis was around 53 years. In about 3–4% of pancreatic cancers, *PALB2* pathogenic variation was identified [113, 114], which warrants genetic testing of *PALB2* in breast cancer patients with family history pancreatic cancer.

5.4.3   ACMG Criteria for Genetic Testing

Owing to the association of many high-penetrance genes, the American College of Medical Genetics and Genomics (ACMG) recommended practice guidelines (2014) laid out criteria for breast cancer (see Tables 5.4, 5.5 and 5.6) [115].

5.4.4   Moderate- to Low-Penetrant Cancer Susceptibility Genes

Genes described above would comprise only less than 25% of the familial breast cancer. For genes that showed a life-time risk of breast cancer of less than 50% in

Table 5.4 Tumors that warrant genetic testing for breast cancer predisposition [115]

When to refer to genetic counseling	What syndromes to consider
• Breast cancer age of diagnosis ≤50 years. • Triple-negative breast cancer dx at age ≤ 60 years. • ≥2 primary breast cancers in the same person • Ashkenazi Jewish ancestry and breast cancer at any age. • ≥3 cases of breast, ovarian, pancreatic, and/or aggressive prostate cancer in close relatives, including the patient • Breast cancer and one added LFS tumor (Tables 5.3 and 5.5) in the same person or two relatives, one dx at age ≤ 45 years.	HBOC (OMIM #604370, #612555) LFS (OMIM #151623)
• Breast cancer and ≥1 PJ polyp.	PJS (OMIM #175200)
• Lobular breast cancer and diffuse gastric cancer in the same person. • Lobular breast cancer in one relative and diffuse gastric cancer in another, one dx at age < 50 years.	HDGC (OMIM #137215)
• Breast cancer and two added Cowden syndrome criteria (Table 5.6) in the same person.	Cowden (OMIM #158350)

Table 5.5 Tumors associated with Li-Fraumeni syndrome [87, 115]

- Soft tissue sarcoma.
- Osteosarcoma.
- Brain tumor.
- Breast cancer (often early onset).
- Adrenocortical tumor.
- Leukemia.
- Bronchoalveolar cancer.
- Colorectal cancer.

Table 5.6 Cowden syndrome criteria (NCCN 2013) [98, 99, 115]

Major criteria
- Breast cancer.
- Endometrial cancer (epithelial).
- Thyroid cancer (follicular).
- Gastrointestinal hamartomas (including ganglioneuromas; excluding hyperplastic polyps; ≥3).
- Lhermitte–Duclos disease (adult).
- Macrocephaly (≥97th percentile: 58 cm for adult women, 60 cm for adult men).
- Macular pigmentation of the glans penis.
- Multiple mucocutaneous lesions (any of the following):
  - Multiple trichilemmomas (≥3, at least 1 proven by biopsy).
  - Acral keratoses (≥3 palmoplantar keratotic pits and/or acral hyperkeratotic papules).
  - Mucocutaneous neuromas (≥3).
  - Oral papilloma (particularly on tongue and gingival), multiple (≥3).
  - OR biopsy-proven OR dermatologist diagnosed.

Minor criteria
- Autism spectrum disorder.
- Colon cancer.
- Esophageal glycogenic acanthosis (≥3).
- Lipomas (≥3).
- Intellectual disability (i.e., intelligence quotient ≤75).
- Renal cell carcinoma.
- Testicular lipomatosis.
- Thyroid cancer (a papillary or follicular variant of papillary).
- Thyroid structural lesions (e.g., adenoma, multinodular goiter).
- Vascular anomalies (including multiple intracranial developmental venous anomalies).

various studies, a separate group is created, which comprises the largest number of studies and literature on the genetic and genomic associations and breast cancer risk. A few of them are only of major interest as they have been replicated in later studies. As the list is exhaustive, only selected ones from public curated databases and robust metanalysis have been included in the list. Many of them are now included in the popular multi-gene panel. The clinical utility of these genomic regions is not clear from these studies. This may be due to the lower impact of variations of these genes to mount a gross tissue level clinical response.

5.4.5 Fanconi Anemia (FA) Genes

FA is a syndrome characterized by bone marrow failure, physical abnormalities, and increased the risk of many types of malignancy. It can be caused either by an autosomal recessive biallelic pathogenic variants of any of the 19 known genes that occur or as an autosomal dominant inheritance of heterozygous variant of *RAD51* gene or a hemizygous variant of *FANCB* when it is called X-lined FA [116]. Out of the 19 genes, *FANCA* is attributed to 60–70% pathogenic variants, followed by *FANCC* and *FANCG*, accounting for about 24%, and the rest of the genes, each accounting for 3% or lower. FA genes with breast cancer risk of high penetrance are *BRCA1*, *BRCA2*, and *PALB2*. Lower penetrance FA genes are *BRIP1*, *FANCD2*, and *RAD51C*. FA genes are involved in the repair of DNA damage caused by interstrand crosslinking defects. Genetic testing of FA genes of married partners might be more important when it comes to making decisions on reproduction as pathogenic variants of these genes can cause serious childhood-onset disease if parents are carriers of pathogenic variants.

A helicase enzyme that interacts with BRCT, *BRIP1*, is involved in DNA repair and cell cycle checkpoint function [117]. Pathogenic variants of *BRIP1* can cause breast cancer similar to that of *BRCA2* [118]. Many large population studies have shown that *CHEK2* pathogenic variants, especially 1100delC, is associated with familial breast cancer. The breast cancer risk by the age of 70 years was found to be as high as 42% in a certain population [119] and associated with ER positivity [120]. CHK2 (OMIM #604373) is a protein kinase that is activated in response to DNA damage and involved in cell cycle arrest. Ataxia Telangiectasia Mutated gene (*ATM*) was found to be associated in large epidemiologic studies with a relative risk of >2 and a cumulative risk of 33% at the age of 80 years [121]. Ataxia Telangiectasia (OMIM #208900) is an autosomal recessive disorder characterized by neurological derangement, telangiectasias, immunodeficiency states, and hypersensitivity to ionizing radiation caused by more than 300 types of variations in the *ATM* gene. However, there is less evidence to recommend against radiation therapy in heterozygous carriers of the *ATM* pathogenic variant. *RAD51*-related genes (*RAD51* paralogs) encode proteins, by their interaction with many proteins including BRCA1 and BRCA2, involved in DNA damage repair via HR [122]. There is substantial evidence for the association between germline variants of *RAD51C* and HBOC, similarly the association of *RAD51* 135G>C and homozygous CC genotypes and breast cancer in *BRCA2* variant carriers [123, 124]. A vast number of other genes have been studied with moderate to low risk (odds ratio of <1.5). But these genes were found to have a lesser impact to improve models for individualized risk assessment, and models that included these variants did not produce a significant improvement in clinical utility assessment.

5.5 Conclusion

Understanding molecular mechanisms help in better prognostication and risk stratification in early breast cancer. In this chapter, we have attempted to summarize the vast advances that occurred in the current molecular pathologies of early breast cancer along with its deficiencies and the need for more knowledge in certain highly demanding areas as well. Luminal A tumors have the best prognosis compared to luminal B or other subgroups due to significantly high responses with endocrine therapy. Despite many past and ongoing clinical trials investigating therapeutic targets in TNBC, chemotherapy is still the only standard treatment possibility available in this subset. However, the molecular pathologies of TNBC are found to have more overlaps with hormone-positive tumors. Similarly, DSB and HR abnormalities seen in somatic as well as hereditary breast cancers cannot be explained entirely by the abnormalities of *BRCA* genes as they are interacting with many other proteins of vital importance to the cell function. We have summarized the current knowledge and practical clinical approach to hereditary breast cancers. A clinician needs to know the functional domains and cellular functions of high-penetrant genes to make right clinical decisions on ordering, interpreting, understanding, and explaining genetic associations to breast cancer patients and caretakers.

References

1. Hanahan D, Weinberg RA. Hallmarks of cancer: the next generation. Cell. 2011;144(5): 646–74. https://doi.org/10.1016/j.cell.2011.02.013.
2. Yue W, Yager JD, Wang JP, Jupe ER, Santen RJ. Estrogen receptor-dependent and independent mechanisms of breast cancer carcinogenesis. Steroids. 2013;78(2):161–70. https://doi.org/10.1016/j.steroids.2012.11.001.
3. Burkhart DL, Sage J. Cellular mechanisms of tumour suppression by the retinoblastoma gene. Nat Rev Cancer. 2008;8(9):671–82. https://doi.org/10.1038/nrc2399.
4. Finn RS, Dering J, Conklin D, Kalous O, Cohen DJ, Desai AJ, et al. PD 0332991, a selective cyclin D kinase 4/6 inhibitor, preferentially inhibits proliferation of luminal estrogen receptor-positive human breast cancer cell lines in vitro. Breast Cancer Res. 2009;11(5):R77. https://doi.org/10.1186/bcr2419.
5. Sherr CJ, Beach D, Shapiro GI. Targeting CDK4 and CDK6: from discovery to therapy. Cancer Discov. 2016;6(4):353–67. https://doi.org/10.1158/2159-8290.CD-15-0894.
6. Drabsch Y, ten Dijke P. TGF-beta signalling and its role in cancer progression and metastasis. Cancer Metastasis Rev. 2012;31(3–4):553–68. https://doi.org/10.1007/s10555-012-9375-7.
7. Cancer Genome Atlas Research N, Weinstein JN, Collisson EA, Mills GB, Shaw KR, Ozenberger BA, et al. The cancer genome atlas Pan-Cancer analysis project. Nat Genet. 2013;45(10):1113–20. https://doi.org/10.1038/ng.2764.
8. Lu L, Zhang C, Zhu G, Irwin M, Risch H, Menato G, et al. Telomerase expression and telomere length in breast cancer and their associations with adjuvant treatment and disease outcome. Breast Cancer Res. 2011;13(3):R56. https://doi.org/10.1186/bcr2893.
9. Cella D, Wang M, Wagner L, Miller K. Survival-adjusted health-related quality of life (HRQL) among patients with metastatic breast cancer receiving paclitaxel plus bevacizumab versus paclitaxel alone: results from Eastern Cooperative Oncology Group Study 2100 (E2100). Breast Cancer Res Treat. 2011;130(3):855–61. https://doi.org/10.1007/s10549-011-1725-6.

10. Polyak K, Weinberg RA. Transitions between epithelial and mesenchymal states: acquisition of malignant and stem cell traits. Nat Rev Cancer. 2009;9(4):265–73. https://doi.org/10.1038/nrc2620.
11. Greaves M, Maley CC. Clonal evolution in cancer. Nature. 2012;481(7381):306–13. https://doi.org/10.1038/nature10762.
12. Negrini S, Gorgoulis VG, Halazonetis TD. Genomic instability—an evolving hallmark of cancer. Nat Rev Mol Cell Biol. 2010;11(3):220–8. https://doi.org/10.1038/nrm2858.
13. Warburg O, Wind F, Negelein E. The metabolism of tumors in the body. J Gen Physiol. 1927;8(6):519–30. https://doi.org/10.1085/jgp.8.6.519.
14. Pelicano H, Martin DS, Xu RH, Huang P. Glycolysis inhibition for anticancer treatment. Oncogene. 2006;25(34):4633–46. https://doi.org/10.1038/sj.onc.1209597.
15. Jones RG, Thompson CB. Tumor suppressors and cell metabolism: a recipe for cancer growth. Genes Dev. 2009;23(5):537–48. https://doi.org/10.1101/gad.1756509.
16. Bohling SD, Allison KH. Immunosuppressive regulatory T cells are associated with aggressive breast cancer phenotypes: a potential therapeutic target. Mod Pathol. 2008;21(12):1527–32. https://doi.org/10.1038/modpathol.2008.160.
17. Denkert C, von Minckwitz G, Brase JC, Sinn BV, Gade S, Kronenwett R, et al. Tumor-infiltrating lymphocytes and response to neoadjuvant chemotherapy with or without carboplatin in human epidermal growth factor receptor 2-positive and triple-negative primary breast cancers. J Clin Oncol. 2015;33(9):983–91. https://doi.org/10.1200/JCO.2014.58.1967.
18. Anderson E, Clarke RB, Howell A. Estrogen responsiveness and control of normal human breast proliferation. J Mammary Gland Biol Neoplasia. 1998;3(1):23–35. https://doi.org/10.1023/a:1018718117113.
19. Asselin-Labat ML, Shackleton M, Stingl J, Vaillant F, Forrest NC, Eaves CJ, et al. Steroid hormone receptor status of mouse mammary stem cells. J Natl Cancer Inst. 2006;98(14):1011–4. https://doi.org/10.1093/jnci/djj267.
20. Ginestier C, Hur MH, Charafe-Jauffret E, Monville F, Dutcher J, Brown M, et al. ALDH1 is a marker of normal and malignant human mammary stem cells and a predictor of poor clinical outcome. Cell Stem Cell. 2007;1(5):555–67. https://doi.org/10.1016/j.stem.2007.08.014.
21. Al-Hajj M, Wicha MS, Benito-Hernandez A, Morrison SJ, Clarke MF. Prospective identification of tumorigenic breast cancer cells. Proc Natl Acad Sci U S A. 2003;100(7):3983–8. https://doi.org/10.1073/pnas.0530291100.
22. Shah M, Allegrucci C. Stem cell plasticity in development and cancer: epigenetic origin of cancer stem cells. Subcell Biochem. 2013;61:545–65. https://doi.org/10.1007/978-94-007-4525-4_24.
23. Shackleton M, Quintana E, Fearon ER, Morrison SJ. Heterogeneity in cancer: cancer stem cells versus clonal evolution. Cell. 2009;138(5):822–9. https://doi.org/10.1016/j.cell.2009.08.017.
24. Jordan VC, O'Malley BW. Selective estrogen-receptor modulators and antihormonal resistance in breast cancer. J Clin Oncol. 2007;25(36):5815–24. https://doi.org/10.1200/JCO.2007.11.3886.
25. Shiau AK, Barstad D, Loria PM, Cheng L, Kushner PJ, Agard DA, et al. The structural basis of estrogen receptor/coactivator recognition and the antagonism of this interaction by tamoxifen. Cell. 1998;95(7):927–37. https://doi.org/10.1016/s0092-8674(00)81717-1.
26. Wakeling AE, Dukes M, Bowler J. A potent specific pure antiestrogen with clinical potential. Cancer Res. 1991;51(15):3867–73.
27. Robinson DR, Wu YM, Vats P, Su F, Lonigro RJ, Cao X, et al. Activating ESR1 mutations in hormone-resistant metastatic breast cancer. Nat Genet. 2013;45(12):1446–51. https://doi.org/10.1038/ng.2823.
28. Toy W, Shen Y, Won H, Green B, Sakr RA, Will M, et al. ESR1 ligand-binding domain mutations in hormone-resistant breast cancer. Nat Genet. 2013;45(12):1439–45. https://doi.org/10.1038/ng.2822.
29. Ma CX, Reinert T, Chmielewska I, Ellis MJ. Mechanisms of aromatase inhibitor resistance. Nat Rev Cancer. 2015;15(5):261–75. https://doi.org/10.1038/nrc3920.

30. Latta EK, Tjan S, Parkes RK, O'Malley FP. The role of HER2/neu overexpression/amplifica-
    tion in the progression of ductal carcinoma in situ to invasive carcinoma of the breast. Mod
    Pathol. 2002;15(12):1318–25. https://doi.org/10.1097/01.MP.0000038462.62634.B1.
31. Piccart-Gebhart MJ, Procter M, Leyland-Jones B, Goldhirsch A, Untch M, Smith I, et al.
    Trastuzumab after adjuvant chemotherapy in HER2-positive breast cancer. N Engl J Med.
    2005;353(16):1659–72. https://doi.org/10.1056/NEJMoa052306.
32. Junttila TT, Akita RW, Parsons K, Fields C, Lewis Phillips GD, Friedman LS, et al. Ligand-
    independent HER2/HER3/PI3K complex is disrupted by trastuzumab and is effectively
    inhibited by the PI3K inhibitor GDC-0941. Cancer Cell. 2009;15(5):429–40. https://doi.
    org/10.1016/j.ccr.2009.03.020.
33. Geyer CE, Forster J, Lindquist D, Chan S, Romieu CG, Pienkowski T, et al. Lapatinib plus
    capecitabine for HER2-positive advanced breast cancer. N Engl J Med. 2006;355(26):2733–43.
    https://doi.org/10.1056/NEJMoa064320.
34. Wang SE. The functional crosstalk between HER2 tyrosine kinase and TGF-beta signal-
    ing in breast cancer malignancy. J Signal Transduct. 2011;2011:804236. https://doi.
    org/10.1155/2011/804236.
35. Shi SJ, Wang LJ, Yu B, Li YH, Jin Y, Bai XZ. LncRNA-ATB promotes trastuzumab resistance
    and invasion-metastasis cascade in breast cancer. Oncotarget. 2015;6(13):11652–63. https://
    doi.org/10.18632/oncotarget.3457.
36. Verma S, Miles D, Gianni L, Krop IE, Welslau M, Baselga J, et al. Trastuzumab emtansine
    for HER2-positive advanced breast cancer. N Engl J Med. 2012;367(19):1783–91. https://
    doi.org/10.1056/NEJMoa1209124.
37. Blows FM, Driver KE, Schmidt MK, Broeks A, van Leeuwen FE, Wesseling J, et al. Subtyping
    of breast cancer by immunohistochemistry to investigate a relationship between subtype and
    short and long term survival: a collaborative analysis of data for 10,159 cases from 12 studies.
    PLoS Med. 2010;7(5):e1000279. https://doi.org/10.1371/journal.pmed.1000279.
38. Prat A, Parker JS, Karginova O, Fan C, Livasy C, Herschkowitz JI, et al. Phenotypic and
    molecular characterization of the claudin-low intrinsic subtype of breast cancer. Breast
    Cancer Res. 2010;12(5):R68. https://doi.org/10.1186/bcr2635.
39. Cancer Genome Atlas N. Comprehensive molecular portraits of human breast tumours.
    Nature. 2012;490(7418):61–70. https://doi.org/10.1038/nature11412.
40. Lehmann BD, Bauer JA, Chen X, Sanders ME, Chakravarthy AB, Shyr Y, et al. Identification
    of human triple-negative breast cancer subtypes and preclinical models for selection of tar-
    geted therapies. J Clin Invest. 2011;121(7):2750–67. https://doi.org/10.1172/JCI45014.
41. Bareche Y, Venet D, Ignatiadis M, Aftimos P, Piccart M, Rothe F, et al. Unravelling triple-
    negative breast cancer molecular heterogeneity using an integrative multiomic analysis. Ann
    Oncol. 2018;29(4):895–902. https://doi.org/10.1093/annonc/mdy024.
42. Berger AC, Korkut A, Kanchi RS, Hegde AM, Lenoir W, Liu W, et al. A comprehensive pan-
    cancer molecular study of gynecologic and breast cancers. Cancer Cell. 2018;33(4):690–705.
    e9. https://doi.org/10.1016/j.ccell.2018.03.014.
43. Nik-Zainal S, Davies H, Staaf J, Ramakrishna M, Glodzik D, Zou X, et al. Landscape of somatic
    mutations in 560 breast cancer whole-genome sequences. Nature. 2016;534(7605):47–54.
    https://doi.org/10.1038/nature17676.
44. Ciriello G, Miller ML, Aksoy BA, Senbabaoglu Y, Schultz N, Sander C. Emerging landscape
    of oncogenic signatures across human cancers. Nat Genet. 2013;45(10):1127–33. https://doi.
    org/10.1038/ng.2762.
45. Newman B, Austin MA, Lee M, King MC. Inheritance of human breast cancer: evi-
    dence for autosomal dominant transmission in high-risk families. Proc Natl Acad Sci U S
    A. 1988;85(9):3044–8. https://doi.org/10.1073/pnas.85.9.3044.
46. Phipps RF, Perry PM. Familial breast cancer. Postgrad Med J. 1988;64(757):847–9. https://
    doi.org/10.1136/pgmj.64.757.847.
47. Sellers TA, Potter JD, Rich SS, Drinkard CR, Bostick RM, Kushi LH, et al. Familial cluster-
    ing of breast and prostate cancers and risk of postmenopausal breast cancer. J Natl Cancer
    Inst. 1994;86(24):1860–5. https://doi.org/10.1093/jnci/86.24.1860.

48. Walsh T, King MC. Ten genes for inherited breast cancer. Cancer Cell. 2007;11(2):103–5. https://doi.org/10.1016/j.ccr.2007.01.010.
49. Hall JM, Lee MK, Newman B, Morrow JE, Anderson LA, Huey B, et al. Linkage of early-onset familial breast cancer to chromosome 17q21. Science. 1990;250(4988):1684–9. https://doi.org/10.1126/science.2270482.
50. Lenoir G. Familial breast-ovarian cancer locus on chromosome 17q12-q23. Lancet. 1991;338(8759):82–3. https://doi.org/10.1016/0140-6736(91)90076-2.
51. Miki Y, Swensen J, Shattuck-Eidens D, Futreal PA, Harshman K, Tavtigian S, et al. A strong candidate for the breast and ovarian cancer susceptibility gene BRCA1. Science. 1994;266(5182):66–71. https://doi.org/10.1126/science.7545954.
52. Clark SL, Rodriguez AM, Snyder RR, Hankins GD, Boehning D. Structure-function of the tumor suppressor BRCA1. Comput Struct Biotechnol J. 2012;1(1):e201204005. https://doi.org/10.5936/csbj.201204005.
53. Brzovic PS, Keeffe JR, Nishikawa H, Miyamoto K, Fox D 3rd, Fukuda M, et al. Binding and recognition in the assembly of an active BRCA1/BARD1 ubiquitin-ligase complex. Proc Natl Acad Sci U S A. 2003;100(10):5646–51. https://doi.org/10.1073/pnas.0836054100.
54. Greenberg RA. Cancer. BRCA1, everything but the RING? Science. 2011;334(6055):459–60. https://doi.org/10.1126/science.1214057.
55. Heine GF, Parvin JD. BRCA1 control of steroid receptor ubiquitination. Sci STKE. 2007;2007(391):pe34. https://doi.org/10.1126/stke.3912007pe34.
56. Zhu Q, Pao GM, Huynh AM, Suh H, Tonnu N, Nederlof PM, et al. BRCA1 tumour suppression occurs via heterochromatin-mediated silencing. Nature. 2011;477(7363):179–84. https://doi.org/10.1038/nature10371.
57. You Z, Bailis JM. DNA damage and decisions: CtIP coordinates DNA repair and cell cycle checkpoints. Trends Cell Biol. 2010;20(7):402–9. https://doi.org/10.1016/j.tcb.2010.04.002.
58. Ruffner H, Joazeiro CA, Hemmati D, Hunter T, Verma IM. Cancer-predisposing mutations within the RING domain of BRCA1: loss of ubiquitin protein ligase activity and protection from radiation hypersensitivity. Proc Natl Acad Sci U S A. 2001;98(9):5134–9. https://doi.org/10.1073/pnas.081068398.
59. Atipairin A, Canyuk B, Ratanaphan A. The RING heterodimer BRCA1-BARD1 is a ubiquitin ligase inactivated by the platinum-based anticancer drugs. Breast Cancer Res Treat. 2011;126(1):203–9. https://doi.org/10.1007/s10549-010-1182-7.
60. Drost R, Bouwman P, Rottenberg S, Boon U, Schut E, Klarenbeek S, et al. BRCA1 RING function is essential for tumor suppression but dispensable for therapy resistance. Cancer Cell. 2011;20(6):797–809. https://doi.org/10.1016/j.ccr.2011.11.014.
61. Chen CF, Li S, Chen Y, Chen PL, Sharp ZD, Lee WH. The nuclear localization sequences of the BRCA1 protein interact with the importin-alpha subunit of the nuclear transport signal receptor. J Biol Chem. 1996;271(51):32863–8. https://doi.org/10.1074/jbc.271.51.32863.
62. Aprelikova ON, Fang BS, Meissner EG, Cotter S, Campbell M, Kuthiala A, et al. BRCA1-associated growth arrest is RB-dependent. Proc Natl Acad Sci U S A. 1999;96(21):11866–71. https://doi.org/10.1073/pnas.96.21.11866.
63. Zhong Q, Chen CF, Li S, Chen Y, Wang CC, Xiao J, et al. Association of BRCA1 with the hRad50-hMre11-p95 complex and the DNA damage response. Science. 1999;285(5428):747–50. https://doi.org/10.1126/science.285.5428.747.
64. Scully R, Chen J, Plug A, Xiao Y, Weaver D, Feunteun J, et al. Association of BRCA1 with Rad51 in mitotic and meiotic cells. Cell. 1997;88(2):265–75. https://doi.org/10.1016/s0092-8674(00)81847-4.
65. Zeller KI, Zhao X, Lee CW, Chiu KP, Yao F, Yustein JT, et al. Global mapping of c-Myc binding sites and target gene networks in human B cells. Proc Natl Acad Sci U S A. 2006;103(47):17834–9. https://doi.org/10.1073/pnas.0604129103.
66. Wang Q, Zhang H, Kajino K, Greene MI. BRCA1 binds c-Myc and inhibits its transcriptional and transforming activity in cells. Oncogene. 1998;17(15):1939–48. https://doi.org/10.1038/sj.onc.1202403.

67. Sy SM, Huen MS, Chen J. PALB2 is an integral component of the BRCA complex required for homologous recombination repair. Proc Natl Acad Sci U S A. 2009;106(17):7155–60. https://doi.org/10.1073/pnas.0811159106.

68. Cortez D, Wang Y, Qin J, Elledge SJ. Requirement of ATM-dependent phosphorylation of brca1 in the DNA damage response to double-strand breaks. Science. 1999;286(5442):1162–6. https://doi.org/10.1126/science.286.5442.1162.

69. Leung CC, Glover JN. BRCT domains: easy as one, two, three. Cell Cycle. 2011;10(15):2461–70. https://doi.org/10.4161/cc.10.15.16312.

70. Yamane K, Katayama E, Tsuruo T. The BRCT regions of tumor suppressor BRCA1 and of XRCC1 show DNA end binding activity with a multimerizing feature. Biochem Biophys Res Commun. 2000;279(2):678–84. https://doi.org/10.1006/bbrc.2000.3983.

71. Kobayashi M, Ab E, Bonvin AM, Siegal G. Structure of the DNA-bound BRCA1 C-terminal region from human replication factor C p140 and model of the protein-DNA complex. J Biol Chem. 2010;285(13):10087–97. https://doi.org/10.1074/jbc.M109.054106.

72. Castilla LH, Couch FJ, Erdos MR, Hoskins KF, Calzone K, Garber JE, et al. Mutations in the BRCA1 gene in families with early-onset breast and ovarian cancer. Nat Genet. 1994;8(4):387–91. https://doi.org/10.1038/ng1294-387.

73. Liu J, Pan Y, Ma B, Nussinov R. "Similarity trap" in protein-protein interactions could be carcinogenic: simulations of p53 core domain complexed with 53BP1 and BRCA1 BRCT domains. Structure. 2006;14(12):1811–21. https://doi.org/10.1016/j.str.2006.10.009.

74. Javle M, Curtin NJ. The role of PARP in DNA repair and its therapeutic exploitation. Br J Cancer. 2011;105(8):1114–22. https://doi.org/10.1038/bjc.2011.382.

75. Wooster R, Neuhausen SL, Mangion J, Quirk Y, Ford D, Collins N, et al. Localization of a breast cancer susceptibility gene, BRCA2, to chromosome 13q12-13. Science. 1994;265(5181):2088–90. https://doi.org/10.1126/science.8091231.

76. Gayther SA, Mangion J, Russell P, Seal S, Barfoot R, Ponder BA, et al. Variation of risks of breast and ovarian cancer associated with different germline mutations of the BRCA2 gene. Nat Genet. 1997;15(1):103–5. https://doi.org/10.1038/ng0197-103.

77. Tavtigian SV, Simard J, Rommens J, Couch F, Shattuck-Eidens D, Neuhausen S, et al. The complete BRCA2 gene and mutations in chromosome 13q-linked kindreds. Nat Genet. 1996;12(3):333–7. https://doi.org/10.1038/ng0396-333.

78. Wong AK, Pero R, Ormonde PA, Tavtigian SV, Bartel PL. RAD51 interacts with the evolutionarily conserved BRC motifs in the human breast cancer susceptibility gene brca2. J Biol Chem. 1997;272(51):31941–4. https://doi.org/10.1074/jbc.272.51.31941.

79. Yang H, Jeffrey PD, Miller J, Kinnucan E, Sun Y, Thoma NH, et al. BRCA2 function in DNA binding and recombination from a BRCA2-DSS1-ssDNA structure. Science. 2002;297(5588):1837–48. https://doi.org/10.1126/science.297.5588.1837.

80. Fradet-Turcotte A, Sitz J, Grapton D, Orthwein A. BRCA2 functions: from DNA repair to replication fork stabilization. Endocr Relat Cancer. 2016;23(10):T1–T17. https://doi.org/10.1530/ERC-16-0297.

81. Schlacher K, Wu H, Jasin M. A distinct replication fork protection pathway connects Fanconi anemia tumor suppressors to RAD51-BRCA1/2. Cancer Cell. 2012;22(1):106–16. https://doi.org/10.1016/j.ccr.2012.05.015.

82. Mondal G, Rowley M, Guidugli L, Wu J, Pankratz VS, Couch FJ. BRCA2 localization to the midbody by Filamin A regulates cep55 signaling and completion of cytokinesis. Dev Cell. 2012;23(1):137–52. https://doi.org/10.1016/j.devcel.2012.05.008.

83. Choi E, Park PG, Lee HO, Lee YK, Kang GH, Lee JW, et al. BRCA2 fine-tunes the spindle assembly checkpoint through reinforcement of BubR1 acetylation. Dev Cell. 2012;22(2):295–308. https://doi.org/10.1016/j.devcel.2012.01.009.

84. Mavaddat N, Barrowdale D, Andrulis IL, Domchek SM, Eccles D, Nevanlinna H, et al. Pathology of breast and ovarian cancers among BRCA1 and BRCA2 mutation carriers: results from the Consortium of Investigators of Modifiers of BRCA1/2 (CIMBA). Cancer Epidemiol Biomark Prev. 2012;21(1):134–47. https://doi.org/10.1158/1055-9965.EPI-11-0775.

85. Silver DP, Livingston DM. Mechanisms of BRCA1 tumor suppression. Cancer Discov. 2012;2(8):679–84. https://doi.org/10.1158/2159-8290.CD-12-0221.
86. Lose F, Duffy DL, Kay GF, Kedda MA, Spurdle AB, Kathleen Cuningham Foundation Consortium for Research into Familial Breast C, et al. Skewed X chromosome inactivation and breast and ovarian cancer status: evidence for X-linked modifiers of BRCA1. J Natl Cancer Inst. 2008;100(21):1519–1529. https://doi.org/10.1093/jnci/djn345
87. Schneider K, Zelley K, Nichols KE, Garber J. Li-Fraumeni syndrome. In: Adam MP, Ardinger HH, Pagon RA, Wallace SE, LJH B, Stephens K, et al., editors. GeneReviews((R)). Seattle, WA: University of Washington, Seattle; 1993. GeneReviews is a registered trademark of the University of Washington, Seattle. All rights reserved.
88. Malkin D. Li-Fraumeni syndrome. Genes Cancer. 2011;2(4):475–84. https://doi.org/10.1177/1947601911413466.
89. Tomkova K, Tomka M, Zajac V. Contribution of p53, p63, and p73 to the developmental diseases and cancer. Neoplasma. 2008;55(3):177–81.
90. Sidransky D, Tokino T, Helzlsouer K, Zehnbauer B, Rausch G, Shelton B, et al. Inherited p53 gene mutations in breast cancer. Cancer Res. 1992;52(10):2984–6.
91. Chompret A, Abel A, Stoppa-Lyonnet D, Brugieres L, Pages S, Feunteun J, et al. Sensitivity and predictive value of criteria for p53 germline mutation screening. J Med Genet. 2001;38(1):43–7. https://doi.org/10.1136/jmg.38.1.43.
92. Gonzalez KD, Noltner KA, Buzin CH, Gu D, Wen-Fong CY, Nguyen VQ, et al. Beyond Li Fraumeni syndrome: clinical characteristics of families with p53 germline mutations. J Clin Oncol. 2009;27(8):1250–6. https://doi.org/10.1200/JCO.2008.16.6959.
93. Bougeard G, Renaux-Petel M, Flaman JM, Charbonnier C, Fermey P, Belotti M, et al. Revisiting Li-Fraumeni syndrome from TP53 mutation carriers. J Clin Oncol. 2015;33(21):2345–52. https://doi.org/10.1200/JCO.2014.59.5728.
94. Mai PL, Best AF, Peters JA, DeCastro RM, Khincha PP, Loud JT, et al. Risks of first and subsequent cancers among TP53 mutation carriers in the National Cancer Institute Li-Fraumeni syndrome cohort. Cancer. 2016;122(23):3673–81. https://doi.org/10.1002/cncr.30248.
95. Varley JM, Evans DG, Birch JM. Li-Fraumeni syndrome–a molecular and clinical review. Br J Cancer. 1997;76(1):1–14. https://doi.org/10.1038/bjc.1997.328.
96. Willis A, Jung EJ, Wakefield T, Chen X. Mutant p53 exerts a dominant negative effect by preventing wild-type p53 from binding to the promoter of its target genes. Oncogene. 2004;23(13):2330–8. https://doi.org/10.1038/sj.onc.1207396.
97. Weisz L, Zalcenstein A, Stambolsky P, Cohen Y, Goldfinger N, Oren M, et al. Transactivation of the EGR1 gene contributes to mutant p53 gain of function. Cancer Res. 2004;64(22):8318–27. https://doi.org/10.1158/0008-5472.CAN-04-1145.
98. Pilarski R, Burt R, Kohlman W, Pho L, Shannon KM, Swisher E. Cowden syndrome and the PTEN hamartoma tumor syndrome: systematic review and revised diagnostic criteria. J Natl Cancer Inst. 2013;105(21):1607–16. https://doi.org/10.1093/jnci/djt277.
99. Bubien V, Bonnet F, Brouste V, Hoppe S, Barouk-Simonet E, David A, et al. High cumulative risks of cancer in patients with PTEN hamartoma tumour syndrome. J Med Genet. 2013;50(4):255–63. https://doi.org/10.1136/jmedgenet-2012-101339.
100. Chu EC, Tarnawski AS. PTEN regulatory functions in tumor suppression and cell biology. Med Sci Monitor. 2004;10(10):RA235–41.
101. McVeigh TP, Choi JK, Miller NM, Green AJ, Kerin MJ. Lobular breast cancer in a CDH1 splice site mutation carrier: case report and review of the literature. Clin Breast Cancer. 2014;14(2):e47–51. https://doi.org/10.1016/j.clbc.2013.10.007.
102. Benusiglio PR, Malka D, Rouleau E, De Pauw A, Buecher B, Nogues C, et al. CDH1 germline mutations and the hereditary diffuse gastric and lobular breast cancer syndrome: a multicentre study. J Med Genet. 2013;50(7):486–9. https://doi.org/10.1136/jmedgenet-2012-101472.
103. Beeghly-Fadiel A, Lu W, Gao YT, Long J, Deming SL, Cai Q, et al. E-cadherin polymorphisms and breast cancer susceptibility: a report from the Shanghai Breast Cancer study. Breast Cancer Res Treat. 2010;121(2):445–52. https://doi.org/10.1007/s10549-009-0579-7.

104. Jenne DE, Reimann H, Nezu J, Friedel W, Loff S, Jeschke R, et al. Peutz-Jeghers syndrome is caused by mutations in a novel serine threonine kinase. Nat Genet. 1998;18(1):38–43. https://doi.org/10.1038/ng0198-38.
105. Aretz S, Stienen D, Uhlhaas S, Loff S, Back W, Pagenstecher C, et al. High proportion of large genomic STK11 deletions in Peutz-Jeghers syndrome. Hum Mutat. 2005;26(6):513–9. https://doi.org/10.1002/humu.20253.
106. Hearle N, Schumacher V, Menko FH, Olschwang S, Boardman LA, Gille JJ, et al. Frequency and spectrum of cancers in the Peutz-Jeghers syndrome. Clin Cancer Res. 2006;12(10):3209–15. https://doi.org/10.1158/1078-0432.CCR-06-0083.
107. Brown KA, McInnes KJ, Takagi K, Ono K, Hunger NI, Wang L, et al. LKB1 expression is inhibited by estradiol-17beta in MCF-7 cells. J Steroid Biochem Mol Biol. 2011;127(3–5):439–43. https://doi.org/10.1016/j.jsbmb.2011.06.005.
108. Takeda H, Miyoshi H, Kojima Y, Oshima M, Taketo MM. Accelerated onsets of gastric hamartomas and hepatic adenomas/carcinomas in Lkb1+/−p53−/− compound mutant mice. Oncogene. 2006;25(12):1816–20. https://doi.org/10.1038/sj.onc.1209207.
109. Rahman N, Seal S, Thompson D, Kelly P, Renwick A, Elliott A, et al. PALB2, which encodes a BRCA2-interacting protein, is a breast cancer susceptibility gene. Nat Genet. 2007;39(2):165–7. https://doi.org/10.1038/ng1959.
110. Antoniou AC, Casadei S, Heikkinen T, Barrowdale D, Pylkas K, Roberts J, et al. Breast-cancer risk in families with mutations in PALB2. N Engl J Med. 2014;371(6):497–506. https://doi.org/10.1056/NEJMoa1400382.
111. Cybulski C, Kluzniak W, Huzarski T, Wokolorczyk D, Kashyap A, Jakubowska A, et al. Clinical outcomes in women with breast cancer and a PALB2 mutation: a prospective cohort analysis. Lancet Oncol. 2015;16(6):638–44. https://doi.org/10.1016/S1470-2045(15)70142-7.
112. Heikkinen T, Karkkainen H, Aaltonen K, Milne RL, Heikkila P, Aittomaki K, et al. The breast cancer susceptibility mutation PALB2 1592delT is associated with an aggressive tumor phenotype. Clin Cancer Res. 2009;15(9):3214–22. https://doi.org/10.1158/1078-0432.CCR-08-3128.
113. Hofstatter EW, Domchek SM, Miron A, Garber J, Wang M, Componeschi K, et al. PALB2 mutations in familial breast and pancreatic cancer. Familial Cancer. 2011;10(2):225–31. https://doi.org/10.1007/s10689-011-9426-1.
114. Jones S, Hruban RH, Kamiyama M, Borges M, Zhang X, Parsons DW, et al. Exomic sequencing identifies PALB2 as a pancreatic cancer susceptibility gene. Science. 2009;324(5924):217. https://doi.org/10.1126/science.1171202.
115. Hampel H, Bennett RL, Buchanan A, Pearlman R, Wiesner GL, Guideline Development Group ACoMG, et al. A practice guideline from the American College of Medical Genetics and Genomics and the National Society of Genetic Counselors: referral indications for cancer predisposition assessment. Genet Med. 2015;17(1):70–87. https://doi.org/10.1038/gim.2014.147.
116. Mehta PA, Tolar J. Fanconi anemia. In: Adam MP, Ardinger HH, Pagon RA, Wallace SE, LJH B, Stephens K, et al., editors. GeneReviews((R)). Seattle, WA: University of Washington, Seattle; 1993. p. 1993–2018.
117. Levitus M, Waisfisz Q, Godthelp BC, de Vries Y, Hussain S, Wiegant WW, et al. The DNA helicase BRIP1 is defective in Fanconi anemia complementation group. J Nat Genet. 2005;37(9):934–5. https://doi.org/10.1038/ng1625.
118. Seal S, Thompson D, Renwick A, Elliott A, Kelly P, Barfoot R, et al. Truncating mutations in the Fanconi anemia J gene BRIP1 are low-penetrance breast cancer susceptibility alleles. Nat Genet. 2006;38(11):1239–41. https://doi.org/10.1038/ng1902.
119. Weischer M, Bojesen SE, Tybjaerg-Hansen A, Axelsson CK, Nordestgaard BG. Increased risk of breast cancer associated with CHEK2*1100delC. J Clin Oncol. 2007;25(1):57–63. https://doi.org/10.1200/JCO.2005.05.5160.
120. Cybulski C, Huzarski T, Byrski T, Gronwald J, Debniak T, Jakubowska A, et al. Estrogen receptor status in CHEK2-positive breast cancers: implications for chemoprevention. Clin Genet. 2009;75(1):72–8. https://doi.org/10.1111/j.1399-0004.2008.01111.x.

121. Marabelli M, Cheng SC, Parmigiani G. Penetrance of ATM gene mutations in breast cancer: a meta-analysis of different measures of risk. Genet Epidemiol. 2016;40(5):425–31. https://doi.org/10.1002/gepi.21971.
122. Suwaki N, Klare K, Tarsounas M. RAD51 paralogs: roles in DNA damage signalling, recombinational repair and tumorigenesis. Semin Cell Dev Biol. 2011;22(8):898–905. https://doi.org/10.1016/j.semcdb.2011.07.019.
123. Wang Z, Dong H, Fu Y, Ding H. RAD51 135G>C polymorphism contributes to breast cancer susceptibility: a meta-analysis involving 26,444 subjects. Breast Cancer Res Treat. 2010;124(3):765–9. https://doi.org/10.1007/s10549-010-0885-0.
124. Zhou GW, Hu J, Peng XD, Li Q. RAD51 135G>C polymorphism and breast cancer risk: a meta-analysis. Breast Cancer Res Treat. 2011;125(2):529–35. https://doi.org/10.1007/s10549-010-1031-8.

Surgical Management of Early Breast Cancer

6

Misha J. C. Babu

6.1 Introduction

By definition, early breast cancer is defined as breast cancer that has not spread beyond the breast or the axillary lymph nodes. This includes ductal carcinoma in situ and stage I, stage IIA, stage IIB and stage IIIA breast cancers. Early-stage breast cancers are potentially curable and always include surgical removal of breast tumour and axillary nodes. Surgery alone will result in long-term survival for a select group of patients, depending on cancer biology and the tumour stage.

6.2 Evolution of Surgical Treatment of Early Breast Cancer

- For nearly 60 years, starting from the 1890s, surgical treatment of breast cancer was based on the 'Halstedian Paradigm', in which a tumour was considered to invade local tissue and spread in a sequential centrifugal manner and came to be known as Halsted's radical mastectomy (1890–1891) [12]. In 1954 and 1967, an alternative theory was formulated and was put forward in a definitive form by Dr Bernard Fisher in a lecture in 1980. The paradigm of 'biological predeterminism', by Fisher paved the way for conservative approaches in surgical treatment of breast cancer and more emphasis on the use of adjuvant chemotherapy and endocrine therapy [12]. As per the theory of biological predeterminism, breast cancer is considered to be largely a systemic disease from the outset as a consequence of cancer cells entering the bloodstream in an early stage in tumour development. The haematogenous dissemination is not conditional upon lymph node involvement.

M. J. C. Babu (✉)
Department of General Surgery and Breast Clinic, Amrita Institute of Medical Sciences, Kochi, Kerala, India

© Springer Nature Singapore Pte Ltd. 2021
B. Kunheri, D. K. Vijaykumar (eds.), *Management of Early Stage Breast Cancer*,
https://doi.org/10.1007/978-981-15-6171-9_6

Between Halsted and the modern era of breast surgery, there have been attempts at more radical surgical procedures like supraradical mastectomies with significant morbidity and little therapeutic benefit. With the evolution of less radical techniques, modified radical mastectomy was popularised by Patey and Dyson in 1948 as an acceptable therapeutic option to the Halsted procedure. Conservative mastectomies were popularised by Scanlon [6] and Auchincloss as well. The current standard in modified radical mastectomy was established by John Madden in 1972, which involves making an elliptical incision circumscribing the breast and including the nipple-areola complex keeping the tumour as the central landmark.

6.3   Breast Conservation Therapy

Breast conservation therapy (BCT) involves complete removal of tumour with a surrounding margin of healthy breast tissue and followed by radiotherapy to breast [1]. Surgical evaluation of axilla is a part of BCT. The technique of breast conservation was pioneered by Umberto Veronesi of Italy. The effectiveness of quadrantectomy, radiotherapy and axillary dissection in the treatment of small breast cancers (<2 cm) was proved by large-scale clinical trials conducted by Veronesi et al. in Milan in the 1970s and 1980s [14]. Also, in a randomised clinical trial involving 701 patients with early breast cancer, patients were grouped into Halsted's mastectomy and Quadrectomy, Radiotherapy, Axillary Treatment (QUART), and there was no difference in overall survival between the two groups [13]. BCT and mastectomy offer equivalent long-term survival in selected patients.

As per the 2019 ESMO guidelines, Breast Conservation Surgery (BCS) has been considered as primary surgery for suitable patients with breast cancer [10]. Greater emphasis is now placed on acceptable cosmesis after wide local excision, and surgeons are trained to undertake oncoplastic procedures whenever possible [10].

Breast conservation therapy may be contraindicated in the following situations [10]:

- Tumour size (relative to the breast)
- Tumour multicentricity
- Inability to achieve negative surgical margins after multiple resections
- Prior radiation to chest wall/breast, or other contraindications to RT
- Unsuitability for oncoplastic breast conservation
- Patient's wishes

Pregnancy is considered an absolute contraindication to external-beam RT. A relative contraindication for whole breast RT is a history of mantle field radiation for lymphoma. A personal history of scleroderma, systemic or discoid lupus erythematosus or dermatomyositis is also considered a relative contraindication for RT. Rheumatoid arthritis was not considered a contraindication [11].

6.4   Surgical Techniques in BCS

6.4.1   Primary Lesion

Wide excision of the primary lesion is crucial. Clear margins around the tumour must be achieved even if additional procedures are required. Currently, a majority of women with T1 and small T2 (<3 cm) are amenable for breast conservation. Oncoplastic techniques may be needed for larger tumour excisions for acceptable cosmesis.

6.4.2   Tumour Margins

Adequate surgical margins have been an area of debate. The current accepted margin width required is no tumour at the inked margin for invasive cancer and 2 mm for in situ cancer [2, 3]. The technique of shave margin or cavity excision after wide excision is also acceptable, as this ensures a minimum of 10 mm wide margin. The presence of lobular carcinoma in situ, atypical ductal hyperplasia or atypical lobular hyperplasia at the margin does not warrant re-excision [11]. Marking the boundaries of the tumour with radiopaque clips is advocated by most radiation oncologists.

6.4.3   Non-palpable Lesions

Non-palpable lesions can be localised by either wire localisation or ROLL (radioguided occult lesion localisation). Whatever be the technique used, satisfactory identification of the lesion, proof of excision and attaining clear margins define appropriateness of excision.

Assessment of Margin

1. Frozen section analysis: Frozen section is the most widely used test for intraoperative analysis of breast tumours. However, the quality of diagnosis can be influenced by freezing artefacts common in fatty tissue. Some lesions like low-grade Ductal carcinoma insitu (DCIS) and Atypical Ductal Hyperplasia (ADH) can be difficult to differentiate microscopically [9].
2. Touch prep/imprint cytology: Here, tumour cells stick to clean glass surface, and fat cells do not adhere to the glass slide. The cells are then stained with H&E. The procedure takes only 2–3 min. The diagnostic accuracy with Frozen section analysis (FSA) was comparable in many studies (Klinberg et al.) Since drying and surface cautery can affect the accuracy, this technique is not in widespread use.
3. Imaging: Intraoperative ultrasound and intraoperative specimen radiographs can be used to yield negative margins and to guide initial surgery.

6.4.4 Axilla

Regional lymph node status is one of the most important predictors of prognosis of breast cancer. Sentinel node biopsy, rather than axillary dissection, is the standard of care in node-negative early breast cancer [10]. Further axillary surgery following positive Sentinel Lymph Node Biopsy (SLNB) is not required in case of low axillary disease burden (micrometastases or 1–2 Sentinel Lymph Node (SLNs) containing metastases) [10].

6.4.5 BCT in Special Situations

6.4.5.1 Multicentric Cancers
Multicentricity is the occurrence of twoseparate cancers in different quadrants of the same breast. They may not be excisable through a single incision. BCT could still be used if the two cancers could be excised as a single specimen, with clear margins and acceptable cosmesis [10].

6.4.5.2 Pregnancy
Breast conservation is possible in pregnancy-associated breast cancer as well. However, this needs to be coordinated with a high-risk obstetric specialist, because delivery might be induced at an earlier than usual gestational age. Surgery could be performed and radiation therapy could be started after delivery, and a delay of up to 3 months is not considered harmful [10].

6.4.5.3 Earlier Breast Augmentation
The presence of a silicone or saline implant does not affect the decision to do BCT. The implant need not be removed if clear margins of excision can be obtained. With the use of RT, capsular contracture and fibrosis can occur, and the patient needs to be educated about this.

6.5 Mastectomy for Early Breast Cancer

Mastectomy is a better option for decreasing the chance of local clearance [8] in the following situations:

- Multicentric tumours
- In the presence of extensive microcalcification
- In situations where external-beam RT is contraindicated, which precludes breast conservation surgery
- In advanced disease as a palliative procedure
- Inflammatory breast cancer
- In recurrent disease following initial lumpectomy

Many patients also choose mastectomy because of the wish to avoid radiotherapy and a desire for rapid treatment. When done along with immediate reconstruction, mastectomy gives acceptable cosmetic result along with good locoregional control. The introduction of skin-sparing and nipple-sparing mastectomies has further widened the scope of mastectomy in terms of cosmetic appeal, and the improved aesthetic outcome has a positive impact on patients.

The hypothesis on the futility of extensive resections in Halsted's mastectomy was confirmed by the first prospective study comparing Halsted's mastectomy with Patey's modification of radical mastectomy, by Bernard Fisher in 1971. In Patey's modification, pectoralis major muscle was preserved, sacrificing only pectoralis minor, with better functional and cosmetic outcome and comparable survival results.

Various modifications were further proposed to the Patey's modification of mastectomy, with a view to preserve the function of pectoralis minor muscle, which is important in the innervation of pectoralis major muscle as well as in the prevention of lymphedema. In 1975, Scanlon et al. published a paper in which he described a technique to preserve the function of minor muscle [6]. This involves division of the lower lateral fibres of pectoralis major and detaching the origins of pectoralis minor. This manoeuvre provides sufficient exposure of the axilla without traction injury to the neurovascular bundle supplying the muscle.

Before this in 1965, Hugh Auchincloss [5] published a paper, in which both the pectoral muscles were preserved to gain access to axilla and the nodes in the axilla were removed in continuity with the breast and overlying skin.

The current standard in mastectomy has been devised by Madden in 1972 [4, 7]. In this, both the pectoral muscles are preserved. The tumour is kept as the centre of skin incision encompassing the breast and nipple-areolar complex. Axillary lymph node clearance is part of any radical mastectomy. The levels of nodes cleared are brachial lymph node group (lateral), pectoral lymph node groups (anterior), subscapular lymph node groups (posterior), central nodal group, and apical lymph node group (medial or subclavicular). The interpectoral or Rotter's nodes are also excised. Additionally, in clinically N0 axilla, sentinel node biopsy is the standard.

6.5.1 Skin-Sparing Mastectomy

The increase in indications of mastectomy coincided with the increased availability of immediate reconstruction to reduce the sequelae of mastectomy. Skin-sparing mastectomy (SSM) was introduced to optimise the cosmetic outcomes of smaller incisions and to preserve breast anatomy. In June 1991, Toth and Lappert first used the term 'skin-sparing mastectomy' for immediate reconstruction [15]. This operation consists of removal of all breast tissue and nipple-areola complex through an elliptical incision, with the removal of skin overlying the tumour, if required. The rest of the breast skin was left to facilitate reconstruction.

6.5.2 Nipple-Sparing Mastectomy

Nipple-sparing mastectomy was developed to preserve all breast glandular tissue with total preservation of skin and Nipple Aereolar Complex (NAC) [15]. The cosmetic results are superior, with the look of a virtually unchanged breast. Nipple-sparing mastectomy has become more popular due to the increased detection rate of early breast cancer and has become more popular for prophylactic mastectomy in high-risk carriers of BRCA 1 and BRCA 2 mutations.

Contraindications to nipple-sparing mastectomy include the following:

- Carcinoma involving the skin and/NAC (defined as cancer <2 cm of NAC)
- Pathologic discharge from the nipple
- Paget's disease of the breast
- Previous radiotherapy
- Smoking
- Obesity (BMI >30 kg/sq m)
- Large breast and grade 3 to grade 4 ptosis, due to the chance of nipple necrosis due to poor vascularity

6.6 Conclusion

Apart from the Halstedian and Fisher's concept, we now know that 'breast cancer is a heterogeneous disease, thought of as a spectrum of proclivities extending from a disease that remains local throughout its course to one that is systemic when first detectable,' said Dr Hellman, in 1994 Karnofsky Memorial Lecture [16]. Even though new systemic and targeted treatment modalities are evolving, surgical extirpation of tumours for locoregional control will remain the mainstay of the management of breast cancer for many years to come.

References

1. Goldhirsch A, Wood WC, Coates AS, Gelber RD, Thurlimann B, Senn H-J, Panel. Strategies for subtypes—dealing with the diversity of breast cancer: highlights of the St Gallen International Expert Consensus on the Primary Therapy of Early Breast Cancer 2011. Ann Oncol. 2011;22(8):1736–47.
2. Hortobagyi G, Connolly JL, D'Orsi CJ, et al. Breast. In: Amin MB, Edge S, Greene F, et al (eds). AJCC Cancer Staging Manual, 8th Ed. Chicago, IL: Springer; 2017. Google Scholar. https://doi.org/10.1007/978-3-319-40618-3_48.
3. Breast cancer | Topic | NICEwww.nice.org.uk > guidance > conditions-and-diseases > breast-cancer.
4. Plesca M, Bordea C, El Houcheimi B, Ichim E, Blidaru A. Evolution of radical mastectomy for breast cancer. J Med Life. 2016;9(2):183–6. ISSN 1844-3117.
5. Rube JW, Pickren J, Auchincloss H Jr. Modification of conventional radical mastectomy; a detailed study of lymph node involvement and follow-up information to show its practicality. Cancer. 1965;18:942–9.

6. Scanlon EF, Caprini JA. Modified radical mastectomy. Cancer. 1975;35(3):710–3.
7. Plesca M, Bordea C, El Houcheimi B, Ichim Blidaru A. Evolution of radical mastectomy for breast cancer. 2nd Department of Oncological Surgery, Oncological Institute, Bucharest, Romania.
8. Freeman MD, Gopman JM, Salzberg CA. The evolution of mastectomy surgical technique: from mutilation to medicine. Gland Surg. 2018;7(3):308–15. https://doi.org/10.21037/gs.2017.09.07.
9. Singletary SE. Surgical margins in patients with early-stage breast cancer, treated with breast conservation therapy. Am J Surg. 2002;184(5):383–93. Review.
10. Cardoso F, Kyriakides S, Ohno S, Penault-Llorca F, Poortmans P, Rubio IT, Zackrisson S, Senkus E, ESMO Guidelines Committee. Early breast cancer: ESMO, Clinical Practice Guidelines for diagnosis, treatment and follow-up. Ann Oncol. 2019;30(10):1674. https://doi.org/10.1093/annonc/mdz189.
11. Schwartz GF, Veronesi U, Clough KB, Dixon JM, Fentiman IS, Heywang-Köbrunner SH, Holland R, Hughes KS, Mansel RE, Margolese R, Mendelson EB, Olivotto IA, Palazzo JP, Solin LJ, Consensus Conference Committee. Consensus conference on breast conservation, Milan, Italy, April 28-May 1, 2005. Breast J. 2006;12(4):398–407.
12. Fisher B. From Halsted to prevention and beyond: advances in the management of breast cancer during the twentieth century. Eur J Cancer. 1999;35(14):1963–73. Review.
13. Veronesi U, Saccozzi R, Del Vecchio M, Banfi A, Clemente C, De Lena M, Gallus G, Greco M, Luini A, Marubini E, Muscolino G, Rilke F, Salvadori B, Zecchini A, Zucali R. Comparing radical mastectomy with quadrantectomy, axillary dissection, and radiotherapy in patients with small cancers of the breast. N Engl J Med. 1981;305(1):6–11.
14. Zurrida S, et al. The Veronesi quadrantectomy: an established procedure for conservative treatment of early breast cancer. Int J Surg Investig. 2001;2(6):423–31.
15. González EG, Rancati AO. Skin-sparing mastectomy. Gland Surg. 2015;4(6):541–53.
16. Hellman S. Karnofsky memorial lecture. Natural history of small breast cancers. J Clin Oncol. 1994;12(10):2229–34. Review.

Sentinel Lymph Node in Early Breast Cancer: Evidence, Techniques, and Controversies

7

Sheikh Zahoor Ahmad and D. K. Vijaykumar

Outline

- History of sentinel node biopsy.
- Evidence for SLN biopsy in breast cancer (randomized study results).
- Techniques of SLN biopsy and validation (including complications and morbidity).
- Pathology of sentinel node (macro/micro/ITC, serial sectioning, IHC, role of OSNA).
- Special circumstances (pregnancy, post-surgery, recurrent case, post-NACT, internal mammary node, etc.)
- What after sentinel node biopsy (status of completion ALND/no surgery/RT only) in SLNB-positive cases.

7.1 Introduction

The lymphatic system has historically been established as a network of vessels that works complementary to the cardiovascular system by draining the extravasated fluid from the interstitium [1]. In tumors, the lymphatics act as a conduit for transport of tumor cells to regional nodes, which in turn might facilitate systemic seeding [2]. The biological understanding of breast cancer has progressed from a purely "mechanistic model" (forming the basis of Halstedian radical resections) to Fisher's "systemic model" (forming the basis of systemic therapy in breast cancer), and

S. Z. Ahmad
Department of Surgical Oncology, Sher-i-Kashmir Institute of Medical Sciences, Srinagar, Jammu and Kashmir, India

D. K. Vijaykumar (✉)
Department of Breast and Gynecological Oncology, Amrita Institute of Medical Sciences, Amrita Vishwa Vidyapeetham University, Kochi, Kerala, India
e-mail: dkvijaykumar@aims.amrita.edu

© Springer Nature Singapore Pte Ltd. 2021   93
B. Kunheri, D. K. Vijaykumar (eds.), *Management of Early Stage Breast Cancer*,
https://doi.org/10.1007/978-981-15-6171-9_7

finally to "spectrum model" [3, 4]. With the evolution of evidence, the surgical management of breast cancer has been tailored from radical/supra-radical surgeries to ultra-conservative approaches. Regional management of breast cancer has also evolved with sentinel lymph node biopsy (SLNB) becoming the "evidence-based standard" in clinically appropriate settings. In this chapter, we will trace the evolution and incorporation of SLNB in early breast cancer.

7.2   Biological Significance of Nodal Metastases in Breast Cancer

Involvement of regional nodes in breast cancer is an established poor prognostic factor, with the 5-year survival decreasing by approximately 28–40% [5, 6]. Axillary lymph node dissection (ALND) was the cornerstone of locoregional treatment in breast cancer, established way back in Halstedian times. However, Bernard Fisher shook the very basis of the axillary treatment in breast cancer when he reported the provocative results of the National Surgical Adjuvant Breast and Bowel Project (NSABP) B-04 trial (Fig. 7.1) [7]. This trial demonstrated a lack of benefit of axillary treatment in clinically negative axilla (cN0). Even after 25 years of follow-up,

Fig. 7.1 Schema of NSABP B-04 trial (numbers in brackets depict the number of patients)

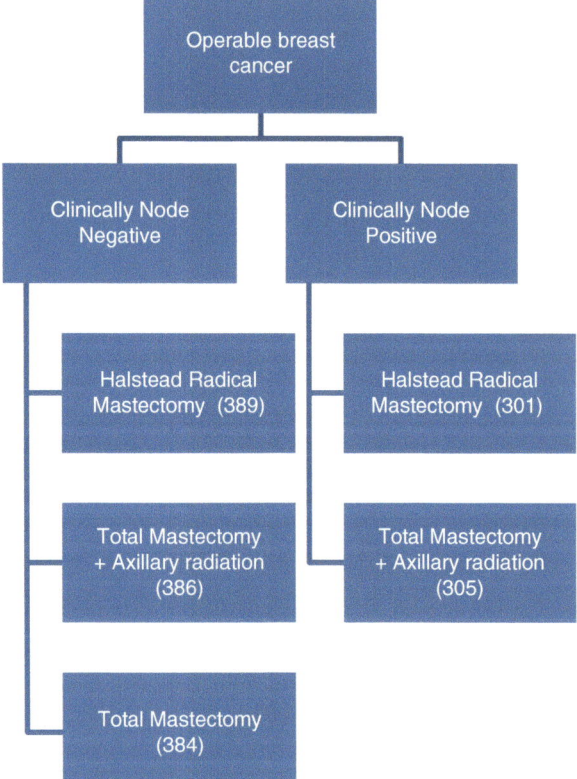

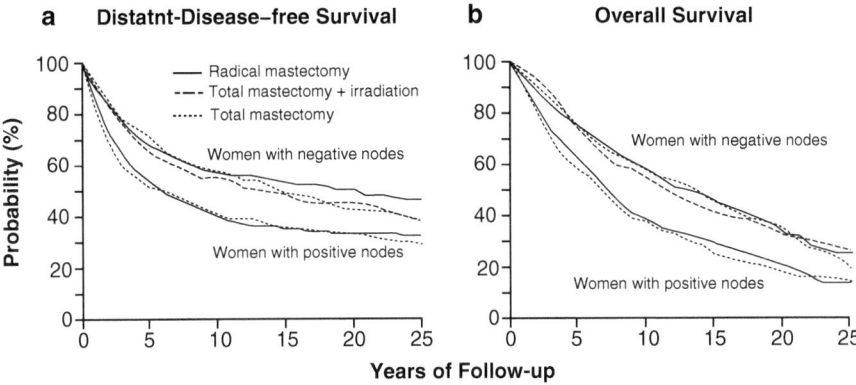

Fig. 7.2 Survival curves depicting distant-disease-free survival (**a**) and overall survival (**b**) during 25 years of follow-up after surgery among patients enrolled in NSABP B-04 trial (Ref. 8)

no beneficial effect on survival (Fig. 7.2) was noted in patients who underwent axillary treatment of any form (ALND or radiotherapy) [8]. Furthermore, patients with clinically positive nodes (cN+) fared worse than those with cN0 disease even after axillary treatment. These results were confirmed by another multicentric trial conducted in Europe [9]. However, both these trials observed increased axillary recurrences in the patients enrolled in the observation group, albeit with no deleterious effects on survival. Thus, these studies proved that axillary nodal involvement is a marker of "unfavourable "biology rather than a reflection of the chronological age of the tumor as hypothesized by Halstead.

The question of the biological significance of axillary nodes has been addressed in many studies, where they have tried to draw an association between the surrogates of tumor chronology (tumor size) and tumor biology (grade, ER/PR,HER2-neu, lymphovascular invasion, etc.) with nodal metastases. The results are conflicting with studies pointing toward the nodal metastases being the function of either tumor chronology [6, 10] or tumor biology [11, 12], or both [13, 14].

7.3   Need for Axillary Staging in Breast Cancer

Although the true biological nature of axillary nodal metastases is still debated [2], the status of axilla is still an important prognostic variable [5, 6] and a pivotal factor in the planning of systemic therapy in breast cancer. Furthermore, the removal of pathologically positive nodes (pN+) in a cN0 axilla does improve the regional recurrence rate as demonstrated even by the NSABP B-04 trial [8]. Hence, the National Institutes of Health (NIH) consensus conference in 1990 concluded that ALND should be part of treatment for potentially curable breast cancer [15]. In fact, a meta-analysis (which was published in subsequent years) including over 3000 patients, which compared ALND vs no ALND, demonstrated an absolute improvement of survival by 4.5% at 10 years [16].

7.4   Methods of Axillary Assessment in Breast Cancer

Most of the contemporary studies have reported about 20–30% pathological nodal positivity in patients with cN0 axilla [32]. Clinical examination is inaccurate in pre-operatively assessing the status of axilla, even if performed by an expert clinician. It suffers from poor sensitivity (~45%) and low overall accuracy [17, 18]. Various imaging modalities (ultrasonography, mammography, computed tomography, magnetic resonance imaging, and positron emission tomography) also perform poorly in the setting of cN0 axilla [19–21]. Axillary lymphadenectomy is the historical gold standard of axillary staging in breast cancer with accuracy approaching 100%. However, it is associated with significant morbidity (seroma, lymphedema, axillary paraesthesia, and shoulder dysfunction) [22], and given the fact that 70–80% of patients ultimately will have pathologically uninvolved nodes (pN0 axilla), it seems to be an overtreatment in the majority of the cases. Hence, there was a need for an equally effective and less morbid procedure for staging axilla in breast cancer, the idea being to do ALND in only those patients who have pathologically involved axillary nodes, based on the findings of this staging procedure. The sentinel lymph node biopsy (SLNB) was developed as a procedure in order to achieve these objectives.

7.5   Evolution of Concept of SLNB

The sentinel lymph node (SLN) is the primary draining node/s that receive/s the lymph from a specific organ, which can later on drain into other nodes in the regional basin (non-SLNs) (Fig. 7.3). The scientific basis of sentinel node concept was laid down by the seminal works of Gilchrist [23] and Zeidman and Buss [24] in the 1940s, when they demonstrated that lymph flows in the regional lymphatic basin in an orderly and reproducible manner. The feasibility of SLNB in the clinical setting was successfully demonstrated by Gould [25], Cabanas [26], and Morton [27] in parotid cancer, penile cancer, and melanoma, respectively. The sentinel node concept in the breast was validated through the works of Kett et al. [28] and Krag et al. [29].

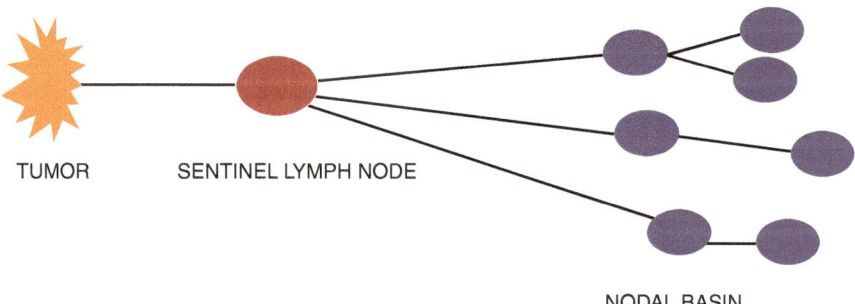

TUMOR   SENTINEL LYMPH NODE

NODAL BASIN

Fig. 7.3 Diagram depicting the concept of SLN

Guiliano et al. in his landmark paper in 1994 described the feasibility of SLNB in breast cancer with intraoperative mapping using isosulfan blue vital dye [30]. They successfully identified the sentinel node in 65.5% procedures. The sentinel node was able to accurately predict the status of the rest of the axilla in 95.6% of cases in their study, and they reported a low false-negative rate of only 4.3%, thus paving way for subsequent work, which established efficacy of SLNB as a significantly less morbid option for axillary assessment in breast cancer.

Thus, the rationale for sentinel node biopsy is established on the assumption of an orderly and foreseeable pattern of spread of cancer cells to the regional lymph nodes and the functioning of the first lymph node as an effective filter. The concept can fit into the explanation of the Halstedian theory of stepwise spread and therefore of locoregional control. It also fits the explanation of the spectrum and systemic theory that propounded that lymph node involvement is an indicator of systemic disease, and hence, SLNB serves as a staging tool to select patients for systemic therapy.

7.6   Evidence for SLNB in Early Breast Cancer

7.6.1   SLNB in Pathologically Negative Axilla (cN0/pN0)

From 1994 onward, there have been many small and large observational studies, which assessed SLNB+ALND in breast cancer, using either blue dyes or radioisotopes or their combination with fairly consistent good identification rates (IR) and acceptably low false-negative rates (FNR). Most of these studies yielded IR of approximately 74–94% and FNR up to 13% [31]. Kim et al. in a meta-analysis of 69 such studies showed IR of $\geq$90% in more than half of them and an overall FNR of 8.4% [32]. The American College of Surgeons Oncology Group (ACOSOG) conducted a multicenter study (ACOSOG Z-0010), which reported very low regional recurrence rates in patients with pathologically negative (pN0) sentinel nodes and not undergoing completion ALND [33].

The noninferiority of SLNB vs SLNB+ALND in patients with pathologically negative sentinel nodes (pN0) has been evaluated in multiple randomized controlled trials (RCTs). These trials compared survival rates (disease-free and overall survival), axillary failure rates, morbidity, and quality of life (QOL) between these two approaches in this patient population (pN0). Most of these studies reported IR $\geq$95%, and FNR less than 10% [34–39] (Table 7.1) [40]. In these trials, SLNB was associated with significantly less incidence of arm edema, numbness, shoulder movement deficits, and wound seroma compared to ALND [34, 35, 37, 41–43] (Table 7.2) [40]. All these trials confirmed the noninferiority of SLNB only vs SLNB+ALND in patients with pathologically negative sentinel nodes. The regional recurrence rates, disease-free survival (DFS), and overall survival (OS) were not negatively affected by leaving the rest of the axilla unaddressed [35, 39–41, 44, 45] (Table 7.3). The findings of these RCTs were confirmed by two recent meta-analyses, which included all major trials addressing this question [46, 47]. The

Table 7.1 Accuracy of SLNB in early breast cancer (Ref. 40)

Trial/author	Year	SLN identification	Sensitivity	False negativity
Veronesi et al. [34]	2003	98.5%	91.2%	8.8%
ALMANAC [35]	2006	98%	93.3%	6.7%
Sentinella-GIVOM [36]	2007	95%	83.3%	16.7%
SNAC [37]	2009	94%	94.5%	5.5%
NSABP B-32 [38]	2010	97.3%	90.2%	9.8%
Canavese et al. [39]	2009	98.6%	77.1%	9.1%

Table 7.2 Comparison of morbidity outcomes (SLNB vs. ALND) (Ref. 40)

Trial/author	No. of patients	Arm lymphedema (%)	Axillary numbness (%)	Abduction deficit (%)	Seroma (%)
Veronesi et al. [34]					
SLNB	259	7	1	0	NR
ALND	257	75	68	21	
ALMANAC [35]					
SLNB	478	5	11	Significantly impaired in ALND group	NR
ALND	476	13	31		
SNAC [37]					
SLNB	544	2.8	NR	2.5	17
ALND	539	4.2		4.4	36
Sentinella-GIVOM [41]					
SLNB	345	Odds ratio (OR)	OR = 0.51	OR = 0.55	NR
ALND	352	0.48 ($p = 0.01$)	($p < 0.0001$)	($p = 0.02$)	
Purushotham et al. [42]					
SLNB	143	OR = 0.30	66	No significant change	14
ALND	155	($p = 0.004$)	84		21
NSABP B-32 [43]					
SLNB	2697	8	8.1	13	NR
ALND	2619	14	31.1	19	

SLNB sentinel lymph node biopsy, *ALND* axillary lymph node dissection, *NR* not reported, *OR* odds ratio

American Society of Clinical Oncology (ASCO) on the basis of high level of available evidence has recommended against routine ALND in early breast cancer (cT1/T2) with clinically negative axilla (cN0) [48].

7.6.2 SLNB in Limited Axillary Disease (cN0/pN+)

After the efficacy of SLNB was proven through RCTs, the paradigm established for treatment of cN0 axilla in breast cancer was to perform SLNB and do completion ALND only in patients with pathologically positive sentinel nodes, the aim being to improve locoregional control and accurately stage the axilla (as the number of pathologically involved axillary nodes is the most powerful prognosticator in breast

Table 7.3 Comparison of survival outcomes (ALND vs. SLNB) (Ref. 40)

Trial/author	Axillary recurrences (ALND vs SLNB)	Disease-free survival (ALND vs SLNB)	Overall survival (ALND vs SLNB)
ALMANAC [35]	0.84% vs 0.2% (at 1 year)	NR	NR
Canavese et al. [39]	0.87% vs 0%	89.8% vs 94.5% (p = 0.715)	97.2% vs 97.2% (p = 0.697)
Sentinella-GIVOM [41]	0.05% vs 0.01%	89.9% vs 87.6%	95.5% vs 94.8%
Veronesi et al. [44]	0% vs 0.01%	88.8% vs 89.9% (10 years) (p = 0.52)	89.7% vs 93.5% (10 years) (p = 0.15)
NSABP B-32 [45]	0.1% vs 0.3%	82.4% vs 81.5% (8 years)	91.8% vs 90.3% (8 years)

ALND axillary lymph node dissection, *SLNB* sentinel lymph node biopsy, *NR* not reported

cancer). However, many studies have reported the rate of involvement of nonsentinel nodes in patients with positive SLNs as low as 15% [49]. A review of 69 studies revealed an incidence of metastases of upto 50% in nonsentinel nodes in patients with positive sentinel nodes [32]. Furthermore, it is noted from other studies that this risk decreases further if SLNs harbor micrometastases (20%) or isolated tumor cells (12%) [50, 51]. A number of clinicopathological factors have been associated with increased risk of non-SLN involvement, which include (although not exclusively) tumor diameter, grade, lymphovascular invasion, estrogen-receptor status, multifocality, size of SLN metastasis, proportion of SLNs involved, etc. [52]. Utilizing these risk factors, a number of predictive nomograms have been developed to predict the status of non-SLNs in patients with positive SLNs [53, 54]. These developments laid the foundation for the trend of foregoing ALND in a subset of patients having very low likelihood of harboring disease in non-SLNs, even in the presence of positive SLNs. Two large retrospective studies (analyzing huge datasets from Surveillance, Epidemiology, and End Results database and National Cancer Data Base) captured this trend by reporting a rate of 16% and 20.8% of omitting completion ALND in patients with positive SLNs, without any negative consequences on their axillary failure rates and OS [55, 56]. Both these studies noted that trend was more common in patients with micrometastases or ITCs in SLNs. However, with time the tendency increased even among patients with macrometastases. In both these studies, patients who underwent SLNB alone were older, had smaller and low-grade tumors, and mostly underwent breast-conserving surgeries.

Atleast three RCTs have tried to assess the therapeutic efficacy of observation versus completion ALND in patients with positive SLNs. The first of these ACOSOG Z0011 was a noninferiority trial conducted in patients with early breast cancer with ≤2 positive SLNs (macrometastases), undergoing breast-conserving surgery (BCS) and was aimed to examine whether ALND can be safely omitted in these patients (Fig. 7.4). All patients were planned to receive postoperative whole breast radiation through two defined tangential fields without axillary radiation. This study recruited only 891 patients against a planned accrual of 1900 patients and was closed early

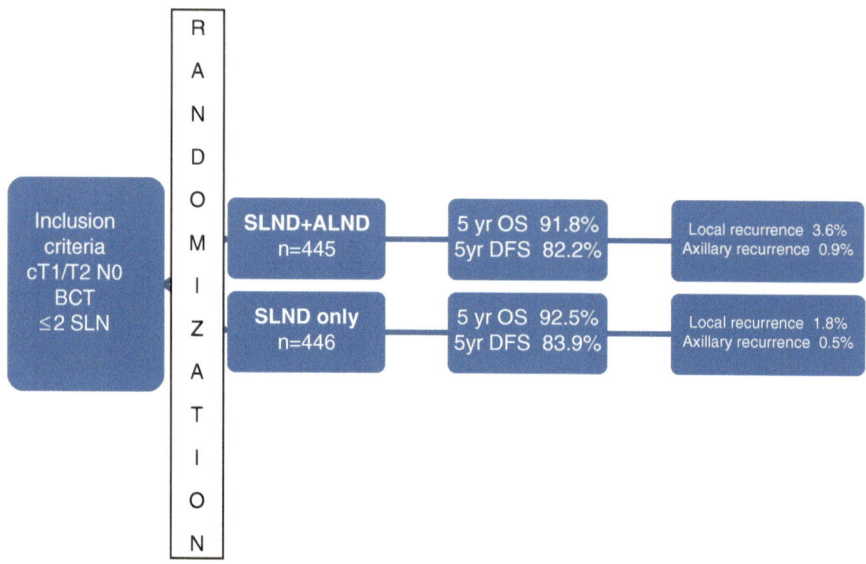

Fig. 7.4 Schema of ACOSOG Z0011 trial (Ref. 57)

due to slow accrual and very low event rate. Most of the patients (>95%) in each group received adjuvant systemic therapy (chemotherapy ± hormone therapy). In the SLNB+ALND group, 27% of patients had additional nodal metastases. After a median follow-up of 6.3 years, the 5-year OS was 91.8% in the ALND arm and 92.5% in the observation arm ($p = 0.008$ for noninferiority), and the corresponding 5-year DFS was 82.2% and 83.9%, respectively. The regional recurrences were also comparable in both the groups (0.5% in ALND and 0.9% in SLNB alone) [57]. Older age, estrogen-receptor status, and lack of adjuvant systemic therapy were the only factors associated with worse overall survival in multivariate analysis. Although this trial has been criticized for various reasons, queries related to this trial have been answered in subsequent publications [52]. Two other trials (International Breast Cancer Study Group—IBCSG 23-01 and AATRM 048) with a similar design (as that of ACOSOG Z0011) asked the same question in patients in whom the SLNs harbored micrometastases [58, 59]. Both these trials corroborated the findings of ACOSOG Z0011 and showed that ALND is unnecessary in patients with micrometastatic disease in SLNs. Recent 10-year follow-up updates of ACOSOG Z0011 [60] and IBCSG 23-01 [61] corroborate their results obtained at initial analysis.

The findings of the ACOSOG Z0011 trial basically reinforced the Fisher's hypothesis that axillary lymph node metastases in breast cancer are a surrogate of unfavorable biology rather than a mere progression of disease, hence precluding the need for local treatment of axilla. These observations were not unlike those of NSABP B-04 conducted decades ago; however, the impact ACOSOG Z0011 had on clinical practice was much more significant. Post-Z0011 era has shown a notable decrease in the use of completion ALND in patients fulfilling the ACOSOG Z0011 criteria [62–66]. Two trials are presently underway to assess the validity of Z0011 results in an expanded patient cohort. The SENOMAC trial is a noninferiority trial that includes patients with T3 disease as well as those who have undergone mastectomy [67]. The SERC trial is a French noninferiority trial, which accrues patients with positive sentinel nodes, but unlike the Z0011 trial, it does not have any upper limit for the number of positive SLNs [68].

7.7   SLNB After Neoadjuvant Chemotherapy

Neoadjuvant chemotherapy (NACT) was inducted in the treatment landscape of breast cancer in the 1970s, in locally advanced (inoperable) stage, to convert it into operable disease [69]. NACT was later extended in the setting of early breast cancer also, mainly to allow breast conservation and also with the possible hypothetical benefit of tackling micrometastatic disease at the earliest, and it also might mitigate the stimulatory effect of surgery on occult metastases. In addition, it allows in vivo testing of chemosensitivity of tumors to various chemotherapy regimens [70]. NACT helps in downstaging the disease, resulting in complete pathological response in 20–50% of patients, which can be increased up to 60% with the use of anti-human epidermal growth factor receptor 2 (anti-HER2) therapies [40]. Although historically ALND has been the standard after NACT in breast cancer, it might be an overtreatment in a significant number of patients. Although there have been concerns regarding poor identification and high FNR (up to 30% in some studies) in patients undergoing SLNB after NACT [40], a number of studies have allayed these fears by demonstrating that the SLN identification rate and FNR are comparable before and after NACT in patients with cN0 axilla [71].

7.7.1   SLNB in Clinically Negative Axilla (cN0)

The timing of SLNB in patients with cN0 axilla planned for NACT is debatable. Although each approach has its own advantages [40], the most relevant advantage of upfront SLNB is its ability to assess the pathological status of axilla beforehand, which can have implications on locoregional treatment options to be used later on during treatment. The main theoretical concern regarding SLNB post-NACT is possible nonidentification and high FNR due to differential effects of chemotherapy on diseased sentinel and nonsentinel nodes, with the possibility of persistent residual disease in non-SLNs in the presence of complete eradication of tumor in SLNs [40].

The earliest evidence for the feasibility of SLNB in the setting of NACT was provided by a retrospective analysis of the NSABP-27 trial. In this, a subset of 428 patients underwent SLNB+ALND after NACT. The SLN identification rate was reported to be 85%, with an FNR of 11%, with the FNR being lower with radioisotopes (8%) than with blue dyes (14%). Although this study included patients with pre-NACT cN0 and cN+ axilla, the FNR was not significantly different between these two groups (12.4% vs. 7%, respectively, $p = 0.51$) [72]. The French prospective multicenter Ganglion Sentinelle et Chimiotherapie Neoadjuvante (GANEA) trial enrolled 195 patients with cT0-3N0-1 breast cancer for SLNB after NACT using a dual mapping method (99mTc-labeled sulfide colloids + patent blue). Among the 130 patients with cN0 disease, the SLN identification rate was 95%, with an FNR of 9% [73]. In a combined analysis of these two studies, overall identification rate was reported as 86.5% (lesser than that reported in upfront setting), and overall FNR 10.9% (comparable with that in upfront SLNB) [74]. A number of systematic reviews and meta-analyses of studies of SLNB post-NACT in patients with cN0 axilla (pre-NACT) have revealed identification rates of 94–96% and FNR of 6–11.4% [75–77].

The issue of SLNB before and after NACT has been assessed in a number of observational studies. Van der Heiden-van der Loo et al., in a population-based study, compared SLNB in patients with clinically negative axilla before ($n = 980$) and after ($n = 203$) NACT. They observed higher identification rate in the pre-NACT group (98% vs 95%, $p = 0.032$). Furthermore, they noted significantly less chance of SLN being positive for disease in post-NACT group; consequently, the need for additional axillary treatment was significantly less in this group (33% vs 45%, $p = 0.006$), despite the fact that higher proportion of patients had T1/T2 tumors in the pre-NACT group (81% vs 68%) [78]. However, this study did not report any data on morbidity, locoregional recurrence, or survival, thus leaving many questions unanswered. In another retrospective study reported from MD Anderson Cancer Centre (MDACC) comparing SLNB before ($n = 3171$) and after ($n = 575$) NACT, identification rates (98.7% and 97.4%, respectively) and FNR (4.1% vs 5.9%, respectively) were similar. Adjusting for clinical stage revealed no differences in locoregional recurrences, disease-free survival, or overall survival between groups [79]. GANEA2 was a prospective study designed to assess the accuracy and safety of SLNB after NACT in breast cancer patients. In this, the patients with cytologically proven nodal metastases were allocated to the pN1 group ($n = 351$) and others to the cN0 group ($n = 606$). Patients in the pN1 group underwent SLNB and ALND after NACT. Patients allocated to the cN0 group underwent SLNB and subsequent completion ALND only in cases of mapping failure or SLN involvement. Among the 419 patients from the cN0 group, which underwent SLNB alone, only one regional recurrence (0.2%) was noted on follow-up. The 3-year DFS was 94.8% (95%CI 91–97.1%) and OS 97.8% (95%CI 94.9–99.1%) [80].

Collectively, these results point toward the feasibility of SLNB after NACT in patients with cN0 axilla and suggest dispensability of additional axillary treatment in those with negative SLN (ypN0). Consequent to this, even in the absence of RCTs, ASCO, on the basis of available evidence, recommends that SLNB may be offered in early breast cancer (with cN0) after NACT [48].

7.7.2   SLNB in Pre-NACT Clinically Positive Axilla (cN+/ycN0)

The role of SLNB in those who present initially with cN+ axilla and attain complete clinical response (ycN0) post-NACT is most contentious. These patients have the potential to avoid the morbidity of ALND if proven to be pN0 by SLNB. The controversy revolves around high FNR and the biological significance of residual disease (post-NACT) in axilla, detected only after applying molecular techniques (immunohistochemistry and polymerase chain reaction) [81]. Although initial studies have reported unacceptably high FNR (>25%) in this setting [82, 83], a recent meta-analysis of 1395 patients with cN1 axilla reported post-NACT SLN identification rate of 92.3% (90.8–93.7%) and FNR of 15.1% [84].

The feasibility of SLNB in these patients has been assessed recently in three large prospective studies (ACOSOG Z1071, SENTINA, and SN FNAC) [85–87]. These studies assessed SLNB in patients with cN+ axilla who achieved ycN0 status (Table 7.4). The lessons learnt from these studies to optimize SLNB after NACT can be summed up as below:

1. Utilization of dual tracer lymphatic mapping for identification of SLNs.
2. Identification and retrieval of >2 SLNs.
3. Use of IHC for detection of disease in SLNs.
4. Performance of completion ALND in pN(i+) disease.

A recent meta-analysis of 3398 patients (from 19 studies) with cN+ axilla reported a pooled SLN identification rate of 90.9% and FNR of 13%, corroborating the above findings [88]. As mentioned above, false negativity is the main area of concern in these patients. In addition to measures enumerated above, other methods

Table 7.4 Summary of prospective studies of sentinel node biopsy after NACT in cN+ axilla (Ref. 40)

	ACOSOG Z1071 [85]	SENTINA [86]	SN FNAC [87]
Design	Single arm	4 arm	Single arm
Number of patients	756	Arm C (592)	153
Patient population	T0-4, N1-2, M0	N1-2, M0	T0-3, N1-2
SLN identification rate	92.9%	80.1%	87.6%
False-negative rate	12.6%	14.2%	9.6%
• 2 SLNs	21.1%	18.5%	4.9% (≥2 SLNs)
• 3 SLNs	9.1%	7.3%	–
• Dual tracer technique.	10.8%	8.6%	5.2%
• Inclusion of ypN0(i+)	8.7%	–	8.4%

have been proposed to decrease FNR of SLNB post-NACT in this set of patients. ACOSOG Z1071 assessed the utility of post-NACT axillary ultrasound (AUS) in a subset of patients and classified patients into AUS-suspicious patients ($n = 181$) and AUS-normal ($n = 430$) before surgery. The investigators observed that FNR decreased from 12.6% (in the whole cohort) to 9.8% in AUS-normal patients, thus suggesting that AUS enables selection of patients with the highest probability of complete axillary response, in whom ALND can be omitted if SLNs are negative [89]. Clipping the positive node before NACT and removing it at the time of SLNB is the other method that has been shown to decrease the FNR significantly [90]. Researchers from MDACC refined this method further to develop the technique of "targeted axillary dissection" (TAD). In this, the biopsy-proven axillary node is clipped before NACT and after completion of chemotherapy I^{125} is inserted into it for intraoperative localization. TAD involves SLNB and selective removal of the clipped node. They observed FNR of only 2% in patients undergoing TAD followed by ALND [91]. The Dutch developed a similar technique using I^{125} seeds (Marking Axillary Lymph Nodes with Radioactive Iodine ^{125}I Seeds – MARI). In this, the pre-NACT-marked positive node is selectively removed (after completion of chemotherapy) without SLNB. False-negative rates of 7% were reported with this technique [92].

Taken together, the studies discussed above tried to evaluate the feasibility and improve the accuracy of SLNB after NACT in patients with a cN+/ycN0 setting. However, at present, no clinically relevant data are available regarding the therapeutic efficacy of SLNB in these patients, and hence, ALND is still considered the standard in these patients. Furthermore, the role of radiotherapy after NACT in these patients is also not clear. Two ongoing trials will try to answer these questions. NSABP B51 trial will try to assess the role of regional nodal radiation in patients with pN+/ypN0 axilla (assessed by post-NACT SLNB ± ALND or ALND) by randomizing patients to two groups—regional RT and no regional RT. The primary endpoint of this trial is invasive breast cancer recurrence-free interval (IBC-RFI). The safety of the omission of ALND in this setting will also be assessed [93]. The second trial (Alliance A11202) is looking at patients with cT1-3N1 breast cancer, with biopsy-proven nodal disease. Patients who are converted to ycN0 will undergo SLNB, and those with positive SLNs are eligible and will be registered to axillary dissection (levels I + II ± III) + nodal RT (undissected axilla, supraclavicular nodes, and internal mammary nodes in the first 3 intercostal spaces) or axillary RT + nodal RT. The primary endpoint is the 5-year invasive breast cancer recurrence-free interval [94].

7.8   Other Indications of SLNB

Sentinel lymph node biopsy has also been used in clinical situations other than those discussed above.

7.8.1   Ductal Carcinoma In Situ

Ductal carcinoma in situ (DCIS) can comprise up to one-fifth of the newly diag-nosed breast cancers, especially in populations undergoing screening mammogra-phy [40, 95]. Theoretically, DCIS is a preinvasive lesion and is not supposed to metastasize via a hemo-lymphatic route. However, up to 14% of patients with a preoperative diagnosis of DCIS are found to harbor metastases in axillary nodes, which is because of an invasive or microinvasive component present in the breast lump which was not revealed on initial biopsy [40]. Even in patients with a defini-tive postoperative diagnosis of DCIS, up to 3.7% will reveal occult metastases in axillary nodes [96]. Because of this, associations, such as the National Comprehensive Cancer Network (NCCN) and ASCO, endorse its selective use in certain situations, like in those undergoing mastectomy, or when the lesion is located at a site that precludes future SLNB, or when the lesion is palpable on examination, or when imaging is highly suggestive of an invasive lesion, and when the area of DCIS is greater than 5 cm [40].

7.8.2   Prophylactic Mastectomy

Patients with an increased lifetime risk for the development of breast cancer (germ-line mutation carriers, strong family history, etc.) are offered prophylactic mastec-tomy (PM) as a risk-reducing measure. An extensive pathological examination of these specimens has revealed up to 5% incidence of occult cancer [97, 98]. A few retrospective studies have reported very low incidence of SLN positivity in these groups of patients. In a meta-analysis of six retrospective studies comprising 1343 prophylactic mastectomies, occult cancer was found in 1.7% specimens ($n = 21$) and a positive SLN was detected in 1.9% patients ($n = 23$). Interestingly, among these 23 patients, approximately half had locally advanced malignancy in the oppo-site breast [99]. These findings were corroborated in another meta-analysis of 14 studies, wherein occult malignancy was reported in 1.8% and positive SLN in 1.3% prophylactic mastectomy specimens [100]. Thus, although routine use of SLNB during PM cannot be advocated, as it would incur unnecessary morbidity and costs, its selective use may be considered in those with a high risk of harboring an occult malignancy [101].

7.8.3   Multicentric Lesions

There is a theoretical concern regarding multicentric lesions (which can be present in up to 10% of newly diagnosed breast cancers) that different lesions might drain into different SLNs. However, observational studies related to this issue have yielded identification rates (>95%) and false-negative rates (<9%) comparable to those in unicentric lesions. Furthermore, the axillary recurrence rates are also similar to those in unicentric lesions [40]. Thus, SLNB is feasible and can be offered in multicentric early breast cancer.

7.8.4 Previous Axillary or Breast Surgery

The improvement in treatment of breast cancer has led to a large number of long-term survivors, who may develop local recurrences in residual breast or chest wall [40]. Although most of these patients are treated with re-excision or salvage mastectomy with ALND (if treated with SLNB alone previously), only one-fourth of these patients will be harboring occult metastases in axilla [102, 103]. Hence, SLNB can potentially avoid unnecessary axillary surgery in these patients. However, there is a theoretical concern regarding the disruption of normal lymphatic drainage (due to previous surgery/RT) leading to aberrant pathways, potentially compromising the safety and accuracy of this procedure. There are no large studies reporting on the feasibility and safety of SLNB in this setting. The investigators from Memorial Sloan-Kettering Cancer Centre (MSKCC) have published their experience with 117 patients undergoing re-SLNB after previous SLNB or/ and ALND. The overall identification rate was 55% and was higher after previous SLNB (74%) than ALND (38%). They noted aberrant location of SLN in 30% ($n = 19$) of patients. Furthermore, they did not report any regional recurrence in these patients on short-term follow-up [104]. A recent meta-analysis of 692 patients (from 25 studies) reported aberrant drainage in up to 43.2% patients, which was noted more frequently in those with the previous history of ALND than SLNB (69.2% vs. 17.4%, $p < 0.0001$). The SLN identification rate was also better in those with previous SLNB (81.0% vs. 52.2%, $p < 0.0001$) [103]. A more recent meta-analysis of seven studies (1053 patients) reporting on lymphatic mapping in recurrent breast cancer revealed an SLN identification rate of 59.6%, which was significantly higher in those with prior SLNB than ALND (odds ratio, 2.97; 95% CI, 1.66–5.32). Aberrant drainage was noted in about 25.7% (23%–28%), which was again higher in those with initial ALND. Occult metastasis was noted in 10.4% of patients (8.6–12.3%) and was usually located within ipsilateral axilla [105].

These observations reveal the feasibility of SLNB (preferably by dual mapping technique) in recurrent breast cancer, which can potentially help us in avoiding ALND in >50% of patients. In fact, it can potentially facilitate the identification of regional nodes outside the ipsilateral axillary basin. However, larger studies with longer follow-up, reporting on the recurrence and survival rates, are needed.

7.9   Contraindications

There is very limited evidence available for the feasibility of SLNB in advanced tumors (T4) and inflammatory breast cancer [48]. In patients with palpable axillary nodes with cytologically or biopsy-proven metastasis, SLNB is futile and does not serve its purpose of staging the axilla and hence is not recommended [48]. In view of the lack of a high level of evidence, ASCO weakly recommends against the use of SLNB in pregnancy [48]. However, data from nonrandomized studies have proven the safety of SLNB using technetium^{99}-based radiocolloid in pregnancy. These studies have demonstrated low radioactivity with negligible systemic diffusion and absorption by the fetus [106, 107]. Due to its potential to cause anaphylactic maternal reactions (1%), blue dye injection is not recommended in pregnancy [48].

7.10   Techniques of SLNB

Technically, SLNB involves injection of a tracer in the target location and subsequent identification of the nodes labeled by it. Krag et al. [29]. was the first to employ ^{99m}technetium-labeled sulfur colloid, and Guiliano et al. [40] pioneered the use of blue dye, whereas Albertini et al. [108] used combination of both for localization of the sentinel nodes in breast cancer. Different variations in the SLNB technique have evolved on the basis of the type of tracer used and its site of injection (peritumoral vs periareolar, subcutaneous vs intradermal vs intraparenchymal). Although initial studies have revealed higher identification rates and low false-negative rates using combination methods [109], later studies have revealed no significant difference between either of the single-agent methods used (blue dyes or radioisotopes) when compared to the combination method [110, 111]. These studies have revealed the surgeon's experience as a significant predictor of success. In addition to the surgeon's inexperience, previous biopsy, obesity, advanced patient age, and location of tumor in upper outer quadrant are associated with poor results in SLNB [112]. However, lymphoscintigraphy has the potential to identify nonaxillary SLNs, for example, in the internal mammary chain.

The ideal site of injection of the tracer was shrouded in controversy initially, with studies favoring intraparenchymal and peritumoral routes [112]. Later studies showed that parenchyma and skin of breast act as a single biological unit [113] and that lymph drains to the same node irrespective of the location of the tumor within the breast [112]. Most of the surgeons prefer periareolar route (subdermal or intradermal) as it facilitates rapid uptake via subareolar plexus and it can obviate use of image guidance in nonpalpable tumors, and it potentially avoids the problem of a shine-through phenomenon in outer quadrant tumors and has a rapid learning curve [112].

The use of the sentinel node technique has reached a plateau with about 60% of patients in developed countries having access to this procedure, whereas in China, only 5% of patients are offered this and this figure is even lower in rest of the world [114]. One of the main reasons for this is the constraints associated with the present techniques. The blue dyes (isosulfan blue, methylene blue, and patent blue) are associated with anaphylaxis (0.7–1.1%), skin necrosis, pain, skin pigmentation, pulmonary edema, and rarely serotonin syndrome in patients taking serotonergic medications [115]. The most commonly used radioisotope is ^{99m}technetium (^{99m}Tc), in the form of sulfur colloid (USA) or nanocolloid human serum albumin (Europe). Newer tracers have been developed using ^{99m}Tc (^{99m}Tc-tilmanocept, ^{99m}Tc-rituximab, and ^{99m}Tc-isosulfan blue) to improve its pharmacokinetics and sentinel node localization [115]. Although lymphoscintigraphy is convenient, effective, safe, and comfortable for the patient, it poses logistical challenges for hospitals, which includes the handling and disposal of radioisotopes, training of staff, and legislative requirements. Furthermore, 6-h half-life of the radioisotope puts limits on the scheduling of surgery as the radiotracer injection is administered by the nuclear medicine department [115]. These limitations in conventional methods have ushered in the development of new SLNB techniques.

7.11 New Techniques in SLNB

A number of new techniques have been developed in recent years to overcome the limitations posed by blue dye and radioisotope methods. These techniques utilize novel tracers such as indocyanine green (ICG), microbubbles, and superparamagnetic iron oxide (SPIO). Each of these techniques has their respective advantages and disadvantages (Table 7.5) and have shown promising results.

7.11.1 Indocyanine Green (ICG)

Indocyanine green is an FDA-approved low-molecular-weight fluorophore, which fluoresces when exposed to light in the near infra-red (NIR) spectrum (absorption 765 nm, emission 840 nm) and thus provides a very high signal-to-background ratio [71]. In essence, it involves injection of tracer in breast and subsequently tracing the movement of dye through the lymphatics (lymphography) into the sentinel lymph node/s with the help of an optical imaging camera system, of which several have been tested in clinical studies [115]. ICG has been compared with blue dyes, radioisotopes, and combination methods in various clinical studies. The identification and false-negative rates of ICG have been reported to be better or comparable to these conventional techniques in most of these studies, with no severe adverse effects related directly to it [71, 114, 115]. However, lack of standardization in the administration of ICG was noted in these studies, although 5 mg/ml (range 0.0625–25 mg) was the most common concentration used in these studies [114].

Table 7.5 Advantages and disadvantages of new SLNB techniques (Ref. 115)

Technique	Advantages	Disadvantages
Indocyanine green (ICG)	• Real-time visualization. • Cheap. • Quick. • *No nuclear medicine department needed.* • *No severe allergic reactions reported.*	• Low molecular weight. • ICG leaking out after SLN is excised. • Difficult to be detected at a depth of more than 1 cm. • Cannot be used in patients with iodine allergy.
Superparamagnetic iron oxide (SPIO)	• Short preparation time. • Comfortable timeframe. • Appropriate molecular weight. • Several years shelf-life. • Fast learning curve. • Brown color helps during axillary dissection. • Does not require any special storage. • *No nuclear medicine department needed.* • *No severe allergic reactions reported.*	• Large diameter of the magnetometer. • Regular re-balancing of the probe during usage. • Possible interference of the surgical instrumentation with the ferromagnetic signaling. • Magnetometer does not reach the same depth as a gamma probe. • Intra-mammary persistence which can create void MRI artifacts. • Cannot be used in patients with hypersensitivity to iron or dextran compounds and those with pacemakers or metal implants.
Contrast-enhanced ultrasound (CEUS) with microbubbles	• Real-time visualization. • Cheap. • Requires only an US apparatus and a contrast agent. • *No nuclear medicine department needed.* • *No severe allergic reactions reported.*	• Long learning curve. • Not so quick as the others. • Operator dependent.

Nonetheless, European Society of Medical Oncology endorsed the use of ICG in early breast cancer in its 2015 breast cancer guidelines [71].

7.11.2 Superparamagnetic Iron Oxide (SPIO)

Superparamagnetic iron oxide, which has been used as a contrast in magnetic resonance imaging, can be injected into the breast and later traced in the sentinel nodes using a handheld magnetometer. SPIO travels into the SLNs within minutes after injection and is trapped within the sinuses and macrophages of the uninvolved areas of the node. It colors the node brown or black in the process, thus aiding in its visual localization in addition to its magnetic detection [115]. A number of trials and their meta-analyses have revealed noninferiority of SPIO to conventional SLNB techniques [71, 114, 115]. The SPIO method offers a number of advantages over the conventional methods (Table 7.5), and it has been standardized in the published studies making it a technique easier to learn [71]. However, before being applied in clinical practice, it needs to be evaluated in properly planned randomized controlled trials.

7.11.3 Contrast-Enhanced Ultrasound (CEUS) with Microbubbles

In this novel technique, microbubbles formed by dispersion of sulfur hexafluoride gas is used as a contrast, detected by ultrasonography. The contrast after periareolar intradermal injection is traced and followed until it enters the SLNs (which usually takes less than a minute). These nodes are marked by guidewires and then dissected out [115]. CEUS is a cheap and noninvasive technique, which allows real-time visualization of SLNs, without the use of any radioisotopes or iodine-containing tracers. However, the studies comparing the standard methods (of SLNB) with CEUS have not proven its noninferiority convincingly [114, 115]. Furthermore, it has got a long learning curve and is highly operator dependent.

7.12 Biological Significance of Micrometastases and Isolated Tumor Cells in SLNs

With incorporation of SLNB in the surgical practice of breast cancer, upstaging of nodal status has been observed in up to almost one-third of patients [49]. This has largely been attributed to intense pathological interrogation of the nodal samples, using methods such as serial sectioning, immunohistochemistry (IHC), and molecular techniques, such as polymerase chain reaction (PCR), one-step nucleic acid amplification (OSNA), fluorescent in situ hybridization (FISH), etc. This has led to the detection of minute metastatic deposits, which were otherwise not picked-up on routine histopathological examination using hematoxylin and eosin (H&E) staining. The American Joint Committee on Cancer has categorized these nodal deposits into three groups based on their size: (1) isolated tumor cells (ITCs): when no deposit is >0.2 mm, pN0 [i+]; (2) micrometastasis: deposit/s 0.2–2.0 mm, pN1mi; and (3) macrometastasis: deposit/s >2.0 mm [116]. As expected, the biological import of these additional pathological findings (micrometastasis and ITCs) has been a topic of intense debate.

Two large retrospective studies (Dutch MIRROR study and International "Ludwig" Breast Cancer Study) reported a negative prognostic impact of micrometastases and ITCs on DFS and OS of these patients as compared to those with "true" pN0 disease [117, 118]. In another large retrospective analysis of 209,720 patients retrieved from the Surveillance, Epidemiology and End Results (SEER) database, nodal micrometastases were shown to be a significant poor prognostic factor with a hazard ratio of 1.35 compared to pN0 disease and 0.82 when compared to pN1 disease ($p < 0.0001$) [119]. Two large prospective studies (ACOSOG Z0010 and NSABP-32) have looked into the impact of ITCs and micrometastases on outcome in early breast cancer. The NSABP-B32 trial, which is the largest trial conducted to date to assess the efficacy of SLNB in early breast cancer, revealed occult metastases in 16% (of 3887) patients (using IHC) who had otherwise pN0 nodes on routine HPE. The observed differences (occult metastases vs no occult metastases) in OS (1.2%; $p = .03$) and DFS (2.8%; $p = .02$), although statistically significant, were small and clinically not significant [120]. In the ACOSOG Z0010 trial, occult metastases were noted in an additional 10.5% of 3326 patients (pN0) re-examined by IHC. The presence of occult metastases did not translate into worse survival in patients with cT1/T2N0M0 disease, thus corroborating the findings of NSABP-32 [121]. Thus, these findings do not favor routine use of enhanced pathological techniques in the evaluation of SLNs, and this view is endorsed by ASCO and NationalComprehensive Cancer Network (NCCN) guidelines [122]. However, this approach might not be valid in patients who undergo SLNB after NACT, as the occult metastases detected by IHC or molecular techniques represent chemoresistant residual disease with a different biological potential [71].

7.13   Conclusion and Future Trends: Omission of Axillary Surgery in Early Breast Cancer

Axillary surgery in early breast cancer has come a long way from being an indispensable therapeutic tool to an ideal staging modality, which aids in decision making for adjuvant treatment. The decision about adjuvant treatment is increasingly being driven by the biomarker profile of the primary tumor, undermining the role of axillary surgery as a key staging tool. Consequent to this, there is growing interest to omit SLNB in patients who have a low likelihood of SLN involvement. Three RCTs are presently accruing patients to assess the safety and efficacy of omission of SLNB in patients with low risk of axillary lymph nodal metastases (Table 7.6) [71]. The data emanating from these studies will probably be the next big step toward de-escalating axillary surgery in early breast cancer.

Table 7.6 Ongoing randomized clinical trials evaluating safety and efficacy of SLNB omission in patients with early breast cancer

Study	Sample size	Study arms	Inclusion criteria	Primary end points
INSEMA (Intergroup-Sentinel-Mamma)	7095	Experimental: no axillary surgery Standard: SLNB ± ALND	• T1-2 cN0. • Negative AUS. • BCS + whole breast RT.	Invasive DFS
Sentinel Node vs Observation After Axillary Ultra-souND (SOUND)	1560	Experimental: no axillary surgery Standard: SLNB ± ALND	• T < 2 cm. • Negative AUS. • BCS + whole breast RT.	Distant-disease-free survival
NCT01821768	460	Experimental: no axillary surgery Standard: SLNB + standard of care	• T1-2 cN0. • Negative AUS.	Regional (axillary) recurrence

AUS axillary ultrasound, *DFS* disease-free survival, *RT* radiotherapy, *SLNB* sentinel lymph node biopsy, *ALND* axillary lymph node dissection, *BCS* breast-conserving surgery

References

1. Natale G, Bocci G, Ribatti D. Scholars and scientists in the history of the lymphatic system. J Anat. 2017;231(3):417–29.
2. Sleeman J, Schmid A, Thiele W. Tumor lymphatics. Semin Cancer Biol. 2009;19:285–97.
3. Halstead WS. The results of operations for the cure of cancer of the breast performed at the Johns Hopkins Hospital from June 1889 to 1894. Johns Hopkins Hop Bull. 1894;4:297–323.
4. Fisher B. Seminars of Bernard Fisher 1960—nature of cancer as systemic disease? Bull Soc Int Chir. 1972;31:604–9.
5. Nemoto T, Vana J, Bedwani RN, Baker HW, McGregor FH, Murphy GP. Management and survival of female breast cancer: results of a national survey by the American College of Surgeons. Cancer. 1980;45:2917–24.
6. Carter CL, Allen C, Henson DE. Relation of tumor size, lymph node status, and survival in 24,740 breast cancer cases. Cancer. 1989;63:181–7.
7. Fisher B, Montague E, Redmond C, Barton B, Borland D, Fisher ER, et al. Comparison of radical mastectomy with alternative treatments for primary breast cancer: a first report of results from a prospective randomized clinical trial. Cancer. 1977;39(6 Suppl):2827–39.
8. Fisher B, Jeong JH, Anderson S, Bryant J, Fisher ER, Wolmark N. Twenty-five-year follow-up of a randomized trial comparing radical mastectomy, total mastectomy, and total mastectomy followed by irradiation. N Engl J Med. 2002;347(8):567–75.
9. Cancer Research Campaign Working Party. Cancer Research Campaign (King's/Cambridge) trial for early breast cancer: a detailed update at the tenth year. Lancet. 1980;2:55–60.
10. Fisher B, Slack NH, Bross ID. Cancer of the breast: size of neoplasm and prognosis. Cancer. 1969;24(5):1071–80.
11. Patani NR, Dwek MV, Douek M. Predictors of axillary lymph node metastasis in breast cancer: a systematic review. Eur J Surg Oncol. 2007;33(4):409–19.
12. Yoshihara E, Smeets A, Laenen A, Reynders A, Soens J, Van Ongeval C, et al. Predictors of axillary lymph node metastases in early breast cancer and their applicability in clinical practice. Breast. 2013;22(3):357–61.

13. Jatoi I, Hilsenbeck SG, Clark GM, Osborne CK. Significance of axillary lymph node metastasis in primary breast cancer. J Clin Oncol. 1999;17(8):2334–40.
14. Smeets A, Ryckx A, Belmans A, Wildiers H, Neven P, Floris G, et al. Impact of tumor chronology and tumor biology on lymph node metastasis in breast cancer. Springerplus. 2013;2:480.
15. Early stage breast cancer: consensus statement. NIH consensus development conference, June 18–21, 1990. Cancer Treat Res. 1992;60:383–93.
16. Orr RK. The impact of prophylactic axillary node dissection on breast cancer survival—a Bayesian meta-analysis. Ann Surg Oncol. 1999;6:109–16.
17. Majid S, Tengrup I, Manjer J. Clinical assessment of axillary lymph nodes and tumor size in breast cancer compared with histopathological examination: a population-based analysis of 2,537 women. World J Surg. 2013;37(1):67–71.
18. Haron NH, Taib NA, Yip CH. Is clinical assessment of the axilla a reliable indicator for lymph node metastases in breast cancer? ANZ J Surg. 2008;78(11):943–4.
19. Cooper KL, Meng Y, Harnan S, Ward SE, Fitzgerald P, Papaioannou D, et al. Positron emission tomography (PET) and magnetic resonance imaging (MRI) for the assessment of axillary lymph node metastases in early breast cancer: systematic review and economic evaluation. Health Technol Assess. 2011;15:1–134.
20. Hwang SO, Lee SW, Kim HJ, Kim WW, Park HY, Jung JH. The comparative study of ultrasonography, contrast-enhanced MRI, and (18) F-FDG PET/CT for detecting axillary lymph node metastasis in T1 breast cancer. J Breast Cancer. 2013;16:315–21.
21. Caudle AS, Cupp JA, Kuerer HM. Management of axillary disease. Surg Oncol Clin N Am. 2014;23:473–86.
22. Schrenk P, Rieger R, Shamiyeh A, et al. Morbidity following sentinel lymph node biopsy versus axillary lymph node dissection for patients with breast carcinoma. Cancer. 2000;88:608–14.
23. Gilchrist RK. Fundamental factors governing lymphatic spread of carcinoma. Ann Surg. 1940;111:630–9.
24. Zeidman I, Buss JM. Experimental studies on the spread of cancer in the lymphatic system: I. effectiveness of the lymph node as a barrier to the passage of embolic tumor cells. Cancer Res. 1954;14:403–5.
25. Gould EA, Winship T, Philbin PH, Kerr HH. Observations on a 'sentinel node' in cancer of the parotid. Cancer. 1960;13:77–8.
26. Cabanas RM. An approach for the treatment of penile carcinoma. Cancer. 1977;39:456–66.
27. Morton DL, Wen DR, Wong JH, Economou JS, Cagle LA, Storm FK, Foshag LJ, Cochran AJ. Technical details of intraoperative lymphatic mapping for early stage melanoma. Arch Surg. 1992;127:392–9.
28. Kett K, Varga G, Lukács L. Direct lymphography of the breast. Lymphology. 1970;3:2–12.
29. Krag DN, Weaver DL, Alex JC, Fairbank JT. Surgical resection and radiolocalization of the sentinel lymph node in breast cancer using a gamma probe. Surg Oncol. 1993;2:335–9.
30. Guiliano AE, Kirgan DM, Guenther JM, Morton DL. Lymphatic mapping and sentinel lymphadenectomy for breast cancer. Ann Surg. 1994;220(3):391–8.
31. Mamounas ET. Optimal management of the axilla: a look at the evidence. Adv Surg. 2016;50:29–40.
32. Kim T, Giuliano AE, Lyman GH. Lymphatic mapping and sentinel lymph node biopsy in early-stage breast carcinoma: a metaanalysis. Cancer. 2006;106:4–16.
33. Hunt KK, Ballman KV, McCall LM, et al. Factors associated with local-regional recurrence after a negative sentinel node dissection: results of the ACOSOG Z0010 trial. Ann Surg. 2012;256:428–36.
34. Veronesi U, Paganelli G, Viale G, Luini A, Zurrida S, Galimberti V, et al. A randomized comparison of sentinel-node biopsy with routine axillary dissection in breast cancer. N Engl J Med. 2003;349:546–53.
35. Mansel RE, Fallowfield L, Kissin M, Goyal A, Newcombe RG, Dixon JM, et al. Randomized multicenter trial of sentinel node biopsy versus standard axillary treatment in operable breast cancer: the ALMANAC Trial. J Natl Cancer Inst. 2006;98:599–609.

36. Zavagno G, De Salvo GL, Scalco G, Bozza F, Barutta L, Del Bianco P, et al. A randomized clinical trial on sentinel lymph node biopsy versus axillary lymph node dissection in breast cancer: results of the Sentinella/GIVOM trial. Ann Surg. 2008;247:207–13.
37. Gill G, SNAC Trial Group of the Royal Australasian College of Surgeons (RACS) and NHMRC Clinical Trials Centre. Sentinel-lymph-node-based management or routine axillary clearance? One-year outcomes of sentinel node biopsy versus axillary clearance (SNAC): a randomized controlled surgical trial. Ann Surg Oncol. 2009;16:266–75.
38. Krag DN, Anderson SJ, Julian TB, Brown AM, Harlow SP, Ashikaga T, et al. Technical outcomes of sentinel-lymph-node resection and conventional axillary-lymph-node dissection in patients with clinically node-negative breast cancer: results from the NSABP B-32 randomised phase III trial. Lancet Oncol. 2007;8:881–8.
39. Canavese G, Catturich A, Vecchio C, Tomei D, Gipponi M, Villa G, et al. Sentinel node biopsy compared with complete axillary dissection for staging early breast cancer with clinically negative lymph nodes: results of randomized trial. Ann Oncol. 2009;20:1001–7.
40. Zahoor S, Haji A, Battoo A, Qurieshi M, Mir W, Shah M. Sentinel lymph node biopsy in breast cancer: a clinical review and update. J Breast Cancer. 2017;20(3):217–27.
41. Del Bianco P, Zavagno G, Burelli P, Scalco G, Barutta L, Carraro P, et al. Morbidity comparison of sentinel lymph node biopsy versus conventional axillary lymph node dissection for breast cancer patients: results of the sentinella-GIVOM Italian randomised clinical trial. Eur J Surg Oncol. 2008;34:508–13.
42. Purushotham AD, Upponi S, Klevesath MB, Bobrow L, Millar K, Myles JP, et al. Morbidity after sentinel lymph node biopsy in primary breast cancer: results from a randomized controlled trial. J Clin Oncol. 2005;23:4312–21.
43. Ashikaga T, Krag DN, Land SR, Julian TB, Anderson SJ, Brown AM, et al. Morbidity results from the NSABP B-32 trial comparing sentinel lymph node dissection versus axillary dissection. J Surg Oncol. 2010;102:111–8.
44. Veronesi U, Viale G, Paganelli G, Zurrida S, Luini A, Galimberti V, et al. Sentinel lymph node biopsy in breast cancer: ten-year results of a randomized controlled study. Ann Surg. 2010;251:595–600.
45. Krag DN, Anderson SJ, Julian TB, Brown AM, Harlow SP, Costantino JP, et al. Sentinel-lymph-node resection compared with conventional axillary-lymph-node dissection in clinically node-negative patients with breast cancer: overall survival findings from the NSABP B-32 randomised phase 3 trial. Lancet Oncol. 2010;11:927–33.
46. Wang Z, Wu LC, Chen JQ. Sentinel lymph node biopsy compared with axillary lymph node dissection in early breast cancer: a meta-analysis. Breast Cancer Res Treat. 2011;129:675–89.
47. Petrelli F, Lonati V, Barni S. Axillary dissection compared to sentinel node biopsy for the treatment of pathologically node-negative breast cancer: a meta-analysis of four randomized trials with long-term follow up. Oncol Rev. 2012;6:e20.
48. Lyman GH, Somerfield MR, Bosserman LD, Perkins CL, Weaver DL, Giuliano AE. Sentinel lymph node biopsy for patients with early-stage breast cancer: American society of clinical oncology clinical practice guideline update. J Clin Oncol. 2017;35(5):561–4.
49. Chagpar AB. Clinical significance of minimal sentinel node involvement and management options. Surg Oncol Clin N Am. 2010;19:493–505.
50. Cserni G, Gregori D, Merletti F, Sapino A, Mano MP, Ponti A, et al. Meta-analysis of non-sentinel node metastases associated with micrometastatic sentinel nodes in breast cancer. Br J Surg. 2004;91:1245–52.
51. van Deurzen CH, de Boer M, Monninkhof EM, Bult P, van der Wall E, Tjan-Heijnen VC, et al. Non-sentinel lymph node metastases associated with isolated breast cancer cells in the sentinel node. J Natl Cancer Inst. 2008;100:1574–80.
52. Shah-Khan M, Boughey JC. Evolution of axillary nodal staging in breast cancer: clinical implications of the ACOSOG Z0011 trial. Cancer Control. 2012;19(4):267–76.
53. Coutant C, Olivier C, Lambaudie E, Fondrinier E, Marchal F, Guillemin F, et al. Comparison of models to predict nonsentinel lymph node status in breast cancer patients with metastatic sentinel lymph nodes: a prospective multicenter study. J Clin Oncol. 2009;27(17):2800e8.

54. Fortunato L, Mascaro A, Amini M, Farina M, Vitelli CE. Sentinel lymph node biopsy in breast cancer. Surg Oncol Clin N Am. 2008;17:673–99.
55. Yi M, Giordano SH, Meric-Bernstam F, Mittendorf EA, Kuerer HM, Hwang RF, et al. Trends in and outcomes from sentinel lymph node biopsy (SLNB) alone vs. SLNB with axillary lymph node dissection for node-positive breast cancer patients: experience from the SEER database. Ann Surg Oncol. 2010;17 Suppl 3:343–51.
56. Bilimoria KY, Bentrem DJ, Hansen NM, Bethke KP, Rademaker AW, Ko CY, et al. Comparison of sentinel lymph node biopsy alone and completion axillary lymph node dissection for node-positive breast cancer. J Clin Oncol. 2009;27:2946–53.
57. Giuliano AE, Hunt KK, Ballman KV, Beitsch PD, Whitworth PW, Blumencranz PW, et al. Axillary dissection vs no axillary dissection in women with invasive breast cancer and sentinel node metastasis: a randomized clinical trial. JAMA. 2011;305:569–75.
58. Galimberti V, Cole BF, Zurrida S, Viale G, Luini A, Veronesi P, et al. Axillary dissection versus no axillary dissection in patients with sentinel-node micrometastases (IBCSG 23-01): a phase 3 randomised controlled trial. Lancet Oncol. 2013;14:297–305.
59. Solá M, Alberro JA, Fraile M, Santesteban P, Ramos M, Fabregas R, et al. Complete axillary lymph node dissection versus clinical follow-up in breast cancer patients with sentinel node micrometastasis: final results from the multicenter clinical trial AATRM 048/13/2000. Ann Surg Oncol. 2013;20(1):120–7.
60. Giuliano AE, Ballman KV, McCall L, Beitsch PD, Brennan MB, Kelemen PR, et al. Effect of axillary dissection vs no axillary dissection on 10-year overall survival among women with invasive breast cancer and sentinel node metastasis: the ACOSOG Z0011 (Alliance) randomized clinical trial. JAMA. 2017;318(10):918–26.
61. Galimberti V, Cole BF, Viale G, Veronesi P, Vicini E, Intra M, et al. Axillary dissection versus no axillary dissection in patients with breast cancer and sentinel-node micrometastases (IBCSG 23-01): 10-year follow-up of a randomised, controlled phase 3 trial. Lancet Oncol. 2018;19(10):1385–93.
62. Massimino KP, Hessman CJ, Ellis MC, Naik AM, Vetto JT. Impact of American College of Surgeons Oncology Group Z0011 and National Surgical Adjuvant Breast and Bowel Project B-32 trial results on surgeon practice in the Pacific Northwest. Am J Surg. 2012;203:618–22.
63. Caudle AS, Hunt KK, Tucker SL, Hoffman K, Gainer SM, Lucci A, et al. American College of Surgeons Oncology Group (ACOSOG) Z0011: impact on surgeon practice patterns. Ann Surg Oncol. 2012;19:3144–51.
64. Beek MA, Verheuvel NC, Luiten EJ, Klompenhouwer EG, Rutten HJ, Roumen RM, et al. Two decades of axillary management in breast cancer. Br J Surg. 2015;102:1658–64.
65. Wright GP, Mater ME, Sobel HL, Knoll GM, Oostendorp LD, Melnik MK, et al. Measuring the impact of the American College of Surgeons Oncology Group Z0011 trial on breast cancer surgery in a community health system. Am J Surg. 2015;209:240–5.
66. Yao K, Liederbach E, Pesce C, Wang CH, Winchester DJ. Impact of the American College of Surgeons Oncology Group Z0011 randomized trial on the number of axillary nodes removed for patients with early-stage breast cancer. J Am Coll Surg. 2015;221:71–81.
67. de Boniface J, Frisell J, Andersson Y, et al. Survival and axillary recurrence following sentinel node-positive breast cancer without completion axillary lymph node dissection: the randomized controlled SENOMAC trial. BMC Cancer. 2017;17(1):379.
68. Houvenaeghel G, Resbeut M, Boher J-M. Sentinel node invasion: is it necessary to perform axillary lymph node dissection? Randomized trial SERC. Bull Cancer. 2014;101(4):358–63.
69. Rubens RD, Sexton S, Tong D, Winter PJ, Knight RK, Hayward JL. Combined chemotherapy and radiotherapy for locally advanced breast cancer. Eur J Cancer. 1980;16:351–6.
70. Early Breast Cancer Trialists' Collaborative Group (EBCTCG). Long-term outcomes for neoadjuvant versus adjuvant chemotherapy in early breast cancer: meta-analysis of individual patient data from ten randomised trials. Lancet Oncol. 2018;19(1):27–39.
71. Qiu SQ, Zhang GJ, Jansen L, de Vries J, Schröder CP, de Vries EGE, et al. Evolution in sentinel lymph node biopsy in breast cancer. Crit Rev Oncol Hematol. 2018;123:83–94.

72. Mamounas EP, Brown A, Anderson S, Smith R, Julian T, Miller B, et al. Sentinel node biopsy after neoadjuvant chemotherapy in breast cancer: results from National Surgical Adjuvant Breast and Bowel Project Protocol B-27. J Clin Oncol. 2005;23:2694–702.
73. Classe JM, Bordes V, Campion L, Mignotte H, Dravet F, Leveque J, et al. Sentinel lymph node biopsy after neoadjuvant chemotherapy for advanced breast cancer: results of Ganglion SentinelleetChimiotherapieNeoadjuvante, a French prospective multicentric study. J Clin Oncol. 2009;27:726–32.
74. Mamounas EP. Impact of neoadjuvant chemotherapy on locoregional surgical treatment of breast cancer. Ann Surg Oncol. 2015;22:1425–33.
75. Fontein DB, van de Water W, Mieog JS, Liefers GJ, van de Velde CJ. Timing of the sentinel lymph node biopsy in breast cancer patients receiving neoadjuvant therapy - recommendations for clinical guidance. Eur J Surg Oncol. 2013;39(5):417–24.
76. Geng C, Chen X, Pan X, Li J. The feasibility and accuracy of sentinel lymph node biopsy in initially clinically node-negative breast cancer after neoadjuvant chemotherapy: a systematic review and meta-analysis. PLoS One. 2016;11(9):e0162605.
77. Tan VK, Goh BK, Fook-Chong S, Khin LW, Wong WK, Yong WS. The feasibility and accuracy of sentinel lymph node biopsy in clinically node-negative patients after neoadjuvant chemotherapy for breast cancer: a systematic review and meta-analysis. J Surg Oncol. 2011;104:97–103.
78. van der Heiden-van der Loo M, de Munck L, Sonke GS, van Dalen T, van Diest PJ, van den Bongard HJ, et al. Population based study on sentinel node biopsy before or after neoadjuvant chemotherapy in clinically node negative breast cancer patients: identification rate and influence on axillary treatment. Eur J Cancer. 2015;51:915–21.
79. Hunt KK, Yi M, Mittendorf EA, Guerrero C, Babiera GV, Bedrosian I, et al. Sentinel lymph node surgery after neoadjuvant chemotherapy is accurate and reduces the need for axillary dissection in breast cancer patients. Ann Surg. 2009;250(4):558–66.
80. Classe JM, Loaec C, Gimbergues P, Alran S, de Lara CT, Dupre PF, et al. Sentinel lymph node biopsy without axillary lymphadenectomy after neoadjuvant chemotherapy is accurate and safe for selected patients: the GANEA 2 study. Breast Cancer Res Treat. 2019;173(2):343–52.
81. Jatoi I, Benson JR, Toi M. De-escalation of axillary surgery in early breast cancer. Lancet Oncol. 2016;17(10):e430–41.
82. Shen J, Gilcrease MZ, Babiera GV, Ross MI, Meric-Bernstam F, Feig BW, et al. Feasibility and accuracy of sentinel lymph node biopsy after preoperative chemotherapy in breast cancer patients with documented axillary metastases. Cancer. 2007;109:1255–63.
83. Alvarado R, Yi M, Le-Petross H, Gilcrease M, Mittendorf EA, Bedrosian I, et al. The role for sentinel lymph node dissection after neoadjuvant chemotherapy in patients who present with node-positive breast cancer. Ann Surg Oncol. 2012;19:3177–84.
84. vanNijnatten TJ, Schipper RJ, Lobbes MB, Nelemans PJ, Beets-Tan RG, Smidt ML. The diagnostic performance of sentinel lymph node biopsy in pathologically confirmed node positive breast cancer patients after neoadjuvant systemic therapy: a systematic review and meta-analysis. Eur J Surg Oncol. 2015;41:1278–87.
85. Boughey JC, Suman VJ, Mittendorf EA, Ahrendt GM, Wilke LG, Taback B, et al. Sentinel lymph node surgery after neoadjuvant chemotherapy in patients with node-positive breast cancer: the ACOSOG Z1071 (Alliance) clinical trial. JAMA. 2013;310:1455–61.
86. Kuehn T, Bauerfeind I, Fehm T, Fleige B, Hausschild M, Helms G, et al. Sentinel-lymph-node biopsy in patients with breast cancer before and after neoadjuvant chemotherapy (SENTINA): a prospective, multicentre cohort study. Lancet Oncol. 2013;14:609–18.
87. Boileau JF, Poirier B, Basik M, Holloway CM, Gaboury L, Sideris L, et al. Sentinel node biopsy after neoadjuvant chemotherapy in biopsy-proven node-positive breast cancer: the SN FNAC study. J Clin Oncol. 2015;33:258–64.
88. El HageChehade H, Headon H, El Tokhy O, Heeney J, Kasem A, Mokbel K. Is sentinel lymph node biopsy a viable alternative to complete axillary dissection following neoadjuvant chemotherapy in women with node-positive breast cancer at diagnosis? An updated meta-analysis involving 3,398 patients. Am J Surg. 2016;212(5):969–81.

89. Boughey JC, Ballman KV, Hunt KK, McCall LM, Mittendorf EA, Ahrendt GM, et al. Axillary ultrasound afterneoadjuvant chemotherapy and its impact on sentinel lymph node surgery: results from the American College of Surgeons Oncology Group Z1071 Trial (Alliance). J Clin Oncol. 2015;33(30):3386–93.

90. Boughey JC, Ballman KV, Le-Petross HT, McCall LM, Mittendorf EA, Ahrendt GM, et al. Identification and resection of clipped node decreases the false-negative rate of sentinel lymph node surgery in patients presenting with node-positive breast cancer (T0-T4, N1-N2) who receive neoadjuvant chemotherapy: results from ACOSOG Z1071 (Alliance). Ann Surg. 2016;263(4):802–7.

91. Caudle AS, Yang WT, Krishnamurthy S, Mittendorf EA, Black DM, Gilcrease MZ, et al. Improved axillary evaluation following neoadjuvant therapy for patients with node-positive breast cancer using selective evaluation of clipped nodes: implementation of targeted axillary dissection. J Clin Oncol. 2016;34(10):1072–8.

92. Donker M, Straver ME, Wesseling J, Loo CE, Schot M, Drukker CA, et al. Marking axillary lymph nodes with radioactive iodine seeds for axillary staging after neoadjuvant systemic treatment in breast cancer patients: the MARI procedure. Ann Surg. 2015;261(2):378–82.

93. NCT01872975: Standard or comprehensive radiation therapy in treating patients with early-stage breast cancer previously treated with chemotherapy and surgery. https://clinicaltrials.gov/ct2/show/NCT01872975

94. NCT01901094: Comparison of axillary lymph node dissection with axillary radiation for patients with node-positive breast cancer treated with chemotherapy. https://clinicaltrials.gov/ct2/show/NCT01901094

95. Ernster VL, Ballard-Barbash R, Barlow WE, Zheng Y, Weaver DL, Cutter G, et al. Detection of ductal carcinoma in situ in women undergoing screening mammography. J Natl Cancer Inst. 2002;94:1546–54.

96. Ansari B, Ogston SA, Purdie CA, Adamson DJ, Brown DC, Thompson AM. Meta-analysis of sentinel node biopsy in ductal carcinoma in situ of the breast. Br J Surg. 2008;95(5):547–54.

97. Dupont EL, Kuhn MA, McCann C, Salud C, Spanton JL, Cox CE. The role of sentinel lymph node biopsy in women undergoing prophylactic mastectomy. Am J Surg. 2000;180:274–7.

98. Peralta EA, Ellenhorn JD, Wagman LD, Dagis A, Andersen JS, Chu DZ. Contralateral pro-phylactic mastectomy improves the outcome of selected patients undergoing mastectomy for breast cancer. Am J Surg. 2000;180:439–45.

99. Zhou WB, Liu XA, Dai JC, Wang S. Meta-analysis of sentinel lymph node biopsy at the time of prophylactic mastectomy of the breast. Can J Surg. 2011;54:300–6.

100. Nagaraja V, Edirimanne S, Eslick GD. Is sentinel lymph node biopsy necessary in patients undergoing prophylactic mastectomy? A systematic review and meta-analysis. Breast J. 2016;22:158–65.

101. Boughey JC, Cormier JN, Xing Y, Hunt KK, Meric-Bernstam F, Babiera GV, et al. Decision analysis to assess the efficacy of routine sentinel lymphadenectomy in patients undergoing prophylactic mastectomy. Cancer. 2007;110:2542–50.

102. Derkx F, Maaskant-Braat AJ, van der Sangen MJ, Nieuwenhuijzen GA, van de Poll-Franse LV, Roumen RM, et al. Staging and management of axillary lymph nodes in patients with local recurrence in the breast or chest wall after a previous negative sentinel node procedure. Eur J Surg Oncol. 2010;36:646–51.

103. Maaskant-Braat AJ, Voogd AC, Roumen RM, Nieuwenhuijzen GA. Repeat sentinel node biopsy in patients with locally recurrent breast cancer: a systematic review and meta-analysis of the literature. Breast Cancer Res Treat. 2013;138:13–20.

104. Port ER, Garcia-Etienne CA, Park J, Fey J, Borgen PI, Cody HS 3rd. Reoperative sentinel lymph node biopsy: a new frontier in the management of ipsilateral breast tumor recurrence. Ann Surg Oncol. 2007;14(8):2209–14.

105. Ahmed M, Baker R, Rubio IT. Meta-analysis of aberrant lymphatic drainage in recurrent breast cancer. Br J Surg. 2016;103:1579–88.

106. Gentilini O, Cremonesi M, Toesca A, Colombo N, Peccatori F, Sironi R, et al. Sentinel lymph node biopsy in pregnant patients with breast cancer. Eur J Nucl Med Mol Imaging. 2010;37(1):78–83.
107. Loibl S, Schmidt A, Gentilini O, Kaufman B, Kuhl C, Denkert C, et al. Breast cancer diagnosed during pregnancy: adapting recent advances in breast cancer care for pregnant patients. JAMA Oncol. 2015;1(8):1145–53.
108. Albertini JJ, Lyman GH, Cox C, Yeatman T, Balducci L, Ku N, et al. Lymphatic mapping and sentinel node biopsy in the patient with breast cancer. JAMA. 1996;276(22):1818–22.
109. Derossis AM, Fey J, Yeung H, Yeh SD, Heerdt AS, Petrek J, et al. A trend analysis of the relative value of blue dye and isotope localization in 2,000 consecutive cases of sentinel node biopsy for breast cancer. J Am Coll Surg. 2001;193(5):473–8.
110. Morrow M, Rademaker AW, Bethke KP, Talamonti MS, Dawes LG, Clauson J, et al. Learning sentinel node biopsy: results of a prospective randomized trial of two techniques. Surgery. 1999;126(4):714–20.
111. Pesek S, Ashikaga T, Krag LE, Krag D. The false-negative rate of sentinel node biopsy in patients with breast cancer: a meta-analysis. World J Surg. 2012;36(9):2239–51.
112. Rubio IT, Klimberg VS. Techniques of sentinel lymph node biopsy. Semin Surg Oncol. 2001;20(3):214–23.
113. Bleiweiss I. Sentinel lymph nodes in breast cancer after 10 years: rethinking basic principles. Lancet Oncol. 2006;7:686–92.
114. Ahmed M, Purushotham AD, Douek M. Novel techniques for sentinel lymph node biopsy in breast cancer: a systematic review. Lancet Oncol. 2014;15(8):e351–62.
115. Ferrucci M, Franceschini G, Douek M. New techniques for sentinel node biopsy in breast cancer. Transl Cancer Res. 2018;7(Suppl 3):S405–17.
116. Edge S, Byrd D, Compton C, Fritz AG, Greene F, Trotti A. AJCC cancer staging manual. 7th ed. New York: Springer; 2009.
117. de Boer M, van Deurzen CH, van Dijck JA, Borm GF, van Diest PJ, Adang EM, et al. Micrometastases or isolated tumor cells and the outcome of breast cancer. N Engl J Med. 2009;361:653–63.
118. International (Ludwig) Breast Cancer Study Group. Prognostic importance of occult axillary lymph node micrometastases from breast cancers. Lancet. 1990;335:1565–8.
119. Chen SL, Hoehne FM, Giuliano AE. The prognostic significance of micrometastases in breast cancer: a SEER population-based analysis. Ann Surg Oncol. 2007;14(12):3378–84.
120. Weaver DL, Ashikaga T, Krag DN, Skelly JM, Anderson SJ, Harlow SP, et al. Effect of occult metastases on survival in node negative breast cancer. N Engl J Med. 2011;364(5):412–21.
121. Giuliano AE, Hawes D, Ballman KV, Whitworth PW, Blumencranz PW, Reintgen DS, et al. Association of occult metastases in sentinel lymph nodes and bone marrow with survival among women with early-stage invasive breast cancer. JAMA. 2011;306(4):385–93.
122. Motomura K. Sentinel node biopsy for breast cancer: past, present, and future. Breast Cancer. 2015;22(3):212–20.

Oncoplastic Surgery in Early Breast Cancer

8

Arun Peter Mathew

8.1 Beyond Breast Conservation Surgery for Early Breast Cancer

The breast as an organ has been regarded in many cultures since antiquity as an anatomic structure embodying femininity and motherhood. Surgery for breast cancer results in bodily disfigurement negatively affecting the patient's sense of being whole and sexual well-being.

Advances in the understanding of the biology of breast cancer and progress in the fields of medical and radiation oncology have led to the development of a less mutilating approach of breast conservation surgery aimed to reduce the bodily disfigurement associated with surgery for breast cancer while maintaining the primary goal of disease eradication. Long-term results of the prospective, randomised trials in the 1970s and 1980s comparing the less extensive surgical approach of BCS with mastectomy for early breast cancer have reported no difference in overall survival and breast cancer mortality when BCS is performed with appropriate adjuvant therapy [1, 2].

BCS is based on the principle of en bloc removal of the tumour with adequate surgical margins with acceptable cosmetic outcome to be followed by external-beam radiotherapy to the remaining breast tissue, but the surgeon has to balance removing adequate breast volume to achieve clear margins and conserving as much breast tissue as possible to achieve cosmetically acceptable results. However, BCS results in poor cosmetic results in 20–30% of patients either immediately after surgery or over time, especially after radiotherapy [3].

A. P. Mathew (✉)
Division of Surgical Oncology, Department of Surgical Services, Regional Cancer Centre, Thiruvananthapuram, Kerala, India

© Springer Nature Singapore Pte Ltd. 2021
B. Kunheri, D. K. Vijaykumar (eds.), *Management of Early Stage Breast Cancer*, https://doi.org/10.1007/978-981-15-6171-9_8

In a standard BCS, the breast tumour is completely removed with a concentric margin of surrounding healthy breast, and the remaining defect is left open to be filled with seroma post-operatively to preserve normal breast contour, but seromas get reabsorbed over time, and especially in large-volume resections, the cavities collapse due to fibrosis pulling both parenchyma and skin towards the cavity resulting in deformity and nipple-areola complex (NAC) displacement. This alteration is magnified by post-operative radiotherapy resulting in breast deformity and asymmetry and poor long-term cosmetic outcome. For example, excision of tumours in the portions of the breast inferior to the nipple-areola complex (NAC) will pull down the NAC, producing nipple retraction inferiorly in the long term referred to as the bird's beak deformity.

8.1.1 What Is Oncoplastic Surgery and for Whom?

Oncoplastic surgery (OPS) or oncoplastic breast surgery refers to the optimal blending of surgical techniques from surgical oncology and reconstructive surgery with due consideration for control of cancer and breast aesthetics. It aims to reduce the negative impact of breast cancer surgery on the body image by improving the aesthetic outcomes and preserve the shape and appearance of the post-operative breast. The term 'oncoplastic' literally translated means 'moulding of tumour' [4]. Dr. Werner Audretsch, accepted by many as the father of oncoplastic surgery, referred to it as tumour-specific immediate reconstruction [5].

8.2 Indication

OPS is indicated for a patient with operable breast cancer who is keen on conserving her breast, but due to unfavourable tumour to breast size ratio or tumour location, the surgeon is unsure that wide excision with adequate margins will result in a major breast deformity.

8.3 Contraindications

OPS is contraindicated when [6].

- Clear margins cannot be assured without doing a mastectomy.
- T4 tumours.
- Inflammatory carcinoma.

- Extensive malignant mammary micro-calcification.
- Multicentric disease.

8.4   Factors to Be Evaluated Before Oncoplastic Surgery

In the patient who is a candidate for OPS, it is important in the preoperative period to establish expectations of both the patient and the surgeon. Often a patient is comfortable with small breast deformations and asymmetries in the post-operative period that a surgeon may not be 'proud of'. The primary aim should be to achieve a successful oncological outcome first and not necessarily a 'perfect' breast.

Ideally, a multidisciplinary evaluation with the breast surgeon and plastic surgeon in the preoperative period should be done, but this may not be possible all the time and hence any surgeon performing resections for breast cancer needs to have a minimum skill set, which includes knowledge and ability of basic techniques of surgical oncology and plastic surgery.

The following points should be evaluated before proceeding for any oncoplastic surgery: [7].

- Patient-related risk factors: Obesity, diabetes mellitus, smoking and previous breast surgeries can impair tissue viability and healing, resulting in an increased risk of post-operative complications.
- Volume of resection: It is the most important factor predicting surgical outcome and potential for breast deformity. For disease control, the largest possible specimen should be excised to achieve margins while the greater the amount of breast tissue resected, the higher the risk for a poor cosmetic result. Excisions of more than 20% of the breast result in a poor cosmetic score [8].
- Tumour location: BCS for lesions from the upper inner quadrants or lower pole of the breast are at high risk for post-operative deformity. The most favourable location for large-volume resections is the upper outer quadrant of the breast, where adequate adjacent tissue is available for mobilisation and correction of deformity.
- Glandular density: Breast density, as noted on a digital mammogram, predicts the fatty composition of the breast and restricts the ability to perform reshaping of the breast without complications by utilising extensive breast undermining. Breast tissue density is classified into four categories on the Breast Imaging Reporting and Data System (BIRADS) (Table 8.1) [9]. During reconstruction, undermining the breast from both the skin and pectoralis muscle may be required for which a low-density breast tissue with a major fatty composition (BIRADS a/b) has a higher risk of fat necrosis while a dense glandular breast (BIRADS c/d) can easily be mobilised without risk of necrosis.

Table 8.1 BIRADS breast composition categories	Breast composition categories
	a. Breasts are almost entirely fatty
	b. Scattered areas of fibroglandular density
	c. Breasts are heterogeneously dense
	d. Breasts are extremely dense

8.5   Oncoplastic Surgery Techniques

Various oncoplastic techniques have been described to reconstruct the defect following a wide local resection. Broadly, these are classified into two: volume displacement and volume replacement techniques.

8.5.1   Volume Displacement Techniques

These are used when excision of <50% of breast volume is done and utilise the remaining breast tissue to fill the resection cavity and reshape the breast. Different techniques have been proposed, and the Clough bi-level classification has been recommended for standard use in clinical practice for OPS [10].

Clough et al. have classified these surgeries into two levels (bi-level classification) depending on the volume of breast tissue excised: [7].

- *Level I OPS*: Resections where <20% of breast volume is excised. The general principle is to place skin incisions along Kraissl's lines of tension to limit scaring followed by undermining of the skin in the mastectomy plane. Full-thickness excision of the tumour with adequate margins is done from the subcutaneous fat underlying the skin down to the pectoralis fascia. The resulting cavity is closed by mobilising and approximating adjacent breast tissue. Nipple-areola complex (NAC) repositioning is done to avoid asymmetry.
- *Level II OPS*: Resections where 20–50% of breast volume is excised. These procedures are indicated in patients with large-sized breasts or ptotic breasts. The skin incision and breast parenchymal excisions are planned along reduction mammoplasty (breast reduction) or mastopexy (breast lift) techniques used in cosmetic breast surgery. After excision, reshaping of the breast is done by transposition of glandular or dermo-glandular flaps from adjacent breast and NAC repositioned to the centre of new breast mound (therapeutic mammoplasty) [11, 12]. There will be a net loss of breast volume resulting in a smaller breast after reconstruction, and a contralateral reduction mammoplasty procedure will be required to achieve symmetry. These procedures carry a higher rate of postoperative complications, mostly wound dehiscence and seromas (Table 8.2).

Depending on the location of the tumour, various OPS techniques have been proposed, as shown in Fig. 8.1 [7].

Table 8.2 Clough bi-level classification

	Level I	Level II
Maximum volume excision	20%	20–50%
Requirement of skin excision for reshaping	No	Yes
Mammaplasty/mastopexy	No	Yes
Glandular density preferred	Dense	Dense/fatty

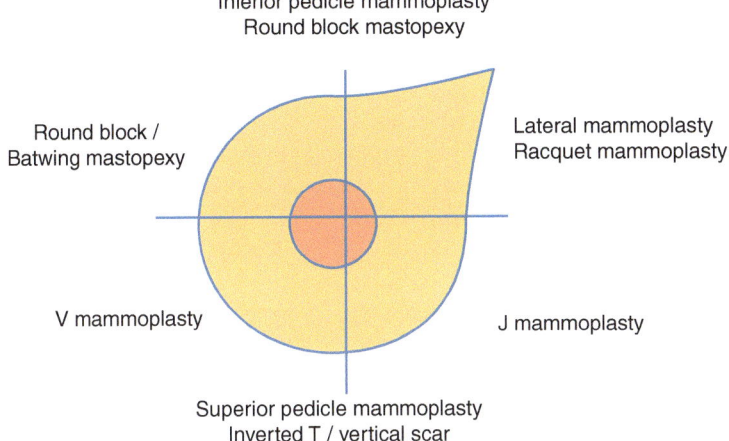

Fig. 8.1   Level II OPS procedures

8.5.2   Volume Replacement Techniques

Large-volume excisions, especially in patients with small- to medium-sized breasts, result in insufficient volumes for reconstruction and require the transfer of tissue from elsewhere via locoregional flaps or pedicled flaps to replace tissue volume and maintain breast shape. Commonly used locoregional flaps include intercostal artery perforator flaps and thoracodorsal flap [13, 14].

Latissimus dorsi (LD) flap is commonly used as a pedicled flap. If skin loss is present, it is harvested as a myocutaneous flap, and when adequate breast skin is available, it is harvested as a myocutaneous flap (mini LD) [15, 16]. Usually, higher volumes than required of muscle and subcutaneous fat are harvested to compensate for post-radiotherapy atrophy.

Options for volume replacement for medial tumours with local/pedicled flaps are limited in view of the reach and need for tunnelling the flap. Free flaps have been described like transverse upper gracilis (TUG) flap as it can avoid disruption of the remaining breast [17].

Table 8.3 Factors affecting OPS technique

	Volume displacement	Volume replacement
Breast size	Medium–large	Small–medium
Location	Central/lower pole	Any site
Scars	Bilateral breast	Breast and donor site
OT time	<2 h	>2 h
Complications	Glandular flap ischemia, fat necrosis	Donor site, flap loss

Though there is no need for contralateral breast surgery, volume replacement procedures have the disadvantage of requirement for a donor site and increased post-operative recovery time.

Various algorithms have been proposed to help determine the best oncoplastic technique [7, 18–20]. The choice of technique depends on multiple factors such as breast size, tumour location, breast-to-tumour ratio, surgical expertise available and the patients' expectations (Table 8.3).

8.5.3 Outcomes After Oncoplastic Surgery

The primary aim of OPS is to enable good cosmetic results without compromising oncologic outcomes in breast conservation surgery. Most of the reports on OPS are single-institution prospective or retrospective observational studies or prospective comparative studies limited by limited sample sizes and short follow-up period. In addition, lack of standardisation of techniques and variations in definitions of end points limit the generalisability of these reports.

8.5.4 Oncologic Outcomes

8.5.4.1 Margins

After standard BCS, involved surgical margins are noted in 20–40%, and approximately one-fourth of all patients undergo a second surgery (either re-excision or completion mastectomy) [21, 22]. OPS allows wider resections, and the reported margin positive rates after OPS in various reports vary from 0 to 36% depending on the definition of a positive margin [23]. Losken et al. in a meta-analysis comparing standard BCS with OPS reported that the positive margin rate was significantly lower in the oncoplastic group (12% vs 21%, $p < 0.0001$) [24]. There is no consensus regarding the definition of positive margins in the published reports on OPS, and future reports based on the Society of Surgical Oncology/American Society for Radiation Oncology (SSO/ASTRO) margin guidelines will provide clarification [25].

Intraoperative frozen section evaluation of the surgical margins is useful in reducing the rates of positive margins and reoperations. In the review by Piper et al., five studies in which intraoperative frozen section was utilised reported statistically significant lower re-excision rates and fewer completion mastectomies when compared to groups that did not use intraoperative frozen section [26].

Management of a positive margin after OPS can either be by a re-excision or a completion mastectomy. Due to the significant displacement of breast tissues in OPS, subsequent re excisions are difficult. In most reports, the reoperation rates vary between 0.7 and 18.9%, and positive margins were treated by completion mastectomy [27]. In the meta-analysis by Losken et al. comparing OPS with standard BCS, when positive margins are observed, a completion mastectomy was more common in the OPS group (6.5 vs. 3.8%) and re-excision is more common following standard BCS (4 vs 14.6%) [24].

8.5.4.2 Local Recurrence

In a review by Piper et al., the local recurrence rates after OPS was 3.1% in studies with a minimum of 2 years median follow-up [26]. In case series with a longer follow-up, it ranges from 2.2 to 6.8% at 5 years [28, 29]. The local recurrence rates after OPS are similar to standard BCS, and initial concerns regarding the risk of spreading cancer into unaffected breast by dissection into uninvolved breast tissue during OPS have not been confirmed.

8.5.5 Complications After OPS

The common complications noted after OPS are skin necrosis, delayed wound healing, NAC necrosis, fat necrosis, hematoma, wound infection and seroma formation [23]. Large-volume displacement surgeries carry a higher risk of fat necrosis with more complex reshaping, leading to more complications and potential delay in adjuvant therapy. In a large series by Fittousi of 540 patients, the complication rate was 16%, commonest being hematoma followed by seroma [28]. Surgical intervention was required in 3%, and complications delayed adjuvant therapy only in 1.9% [28]. Clough, in his report on 350 patients, reported a complication rate of 8.9%, commonest being fat necrosis with secondary infection and hematoma, and delay in adjuvant treatment in 4.6% [29]. In the meta-analysis by Losken, the complication rate in the oncoplastic reduction group was 16% and in the oncoplastic flap reconstruction group was 14%, and no delay in the initiation of adjuvant therapy was noted [24].

8.5.6 Cosmetic Outcomes

Most studies report good cosmetic outcome after OPS in nearly 90% of patients [30]. In a review of 25 studies that analysed cosmetic outcomes in OPS ($n = 1962$), OPS could achieve excellent, good, fair or poor outcomes in 55.2%, 31.0%, 9.4% and 4.4% of patients, respectively [31]. The main drawback of the reports on cosmetic outcomes is that most studies were retrospective and study population numbers low. In addition, there was variation in how cosmetic outcomes were evaluated with non-validated assessment tools. The timing of evaluation of the cosmetic outcome was also varied, and cosmetic failure rates were higher in studies with longer follow-up (Tables 8.4 and 8.5) [32].

8.6 Conclusion

Oncoplastic surgery aims to extend the indications for breast conservation surgery with improvement in the cosmetic outcomes without compromising the oncological outcomes. Proper patient selection and utilisation of the proper techniques can help in improving outcomes. The level of evidence supporting OPS is low, and prospective data collection with the use of validated assessment tools for assessment of cosmetic outcomes will contribute to the generation of stronger evidence and wider acceptance of oncoplastic surgeries for breast cancer patients.

Table 8.4 Outcomes after OPS: systematic reviews/meta-analysis

Systematic review/ meta-analysis	No. of patients	No. of studies	Follow-up – months	Positive margin	Re-excision/ mastectomy	Local recurrence	Complications	Cosmetic outcome
De La Cruz (2016) [31]	6011	55	50.5 mean (12–121 months)	9.8%	Re-excision 6% Mastectomy 6.2%	3.2%	14.3%	55.2% excellent 31% good 9.4% fair 4.4% poor
Piper (2016) [26]	1312	17	>36 months in >50% of studies	0–21%	Re-excision 0–16.4% Mastectomy 0–9.7%	3.1%	Wound dehiscence 4.6% Fat necrosis 4.3%	90% satisfactory (5 studies)
Yiannakopoulou (2016) [33]	2830	40	>60 months in 2 studies	0–36%	–	0–10.8%	–	–
Losken (2014) [24]	3165	41	37.1 mean (12–74)	12.3%	Re-excision 4% Mastectomy 6.5%	4.2%	15.5%	89.5% satisfactory
Haloua (2013) [30]	998	12	1–74	0–10%		0–7%		84–89% good cosmetic

Table 8.5 Outcomes after OPS case series with long follow-up

	No. of patients	Follow-up – months (median)	Median tumour size (mm)	Complications (%)	Positive margins (%)	Re-operation (%)	Local recurrence
Clough (2018) [29]	350	55 (0–138)	20 (0–180)	8.9	12.6	11.5	2.2% at 5 years
Losken (2017) [34]	353	24 (2–180)	20 (0–156)	16.4	6.2	9.9	5.2% at 2 years
Fitoussi (2010) [28]	540	49 (6–262)	29.1 (4–100)	16.3	18.9	9.4	6.8% at 5 years

References

1. Veronesi U, Cascinelli N, Mariani L, et al. Twenty-year follow-up of a randomized study comparing breast-conserving surgery with radical mastectomy for early breast cancer. N Engl J Med. 2002;347:1227–32.
2. Fisher B, Anderson S, Bryant J, et al. Twenty-year follow-up of a randomized trial comparing total mastectomy, lumpectomy, and lumpectomy plus irradiation for the treatment of invasive breast cancer. N Engl J Med. 2002;347:1233–41.
3. Clough KB, Cuminet J, Fitoussi A, et al. Cosmetic sequelae after conservative treatment for breast cancer: classification and results of surgical correction. Ann Plast Surg. 1998;41(5):471–81.
4. Mansfield L, Agrawal A, Cutress RI. Oncoplastic breast conserving surgery. Gland Surg. 2013;2(3):158–62.
5. Audretsch W. Tumor-specific immediate reconstruction in breast cancer patients. Perspect Plast Surg. 1998;11:71–100.
6. Association of Breast Surgery at BASO, BAPRAS and the Training Interface Group in Breast Surgery/EJSO. Oncoplastic breast surgery–a guide to good practice. Eur J Surg Oncol. 2007;33:S1–S23.
7. Clough KB, Kaufman GJ, Nos C, et al. Improving breast cancer surgery: a classification and quadrant per quadrant atlas for oncoplastic surgery. Ann Surg Oncol. 2010;17:1375–91.
8. Bulstrode NW, Shortri S. Prediction of cosmetic outcome following conservative breast surgery using breast volume measurements. Breast. 2001;10:124–6.
9. Sickles, EA, D'Orsi CJ, Bassett LW, et al. ACR BI-RADS® mammography. In: ACR BI-RADS® atlas, breast imaging reporting and data system. Reston, VA: American College of Radiology; 2013.
10. Weber WP, Soysal SD, El-Tamer M, et al. First international consensus conference on standardization of oncoplastic breast conserving surgery. Breast Cancer Res Treat. 2017;165:139–49.
11. Anderson BO, Masetti R, Silverstein MJ. Oncoplastic approaches to partial mastectomy: an overview of volume-displacement techniques. Lancet Oncol. 2005;6(3):145–57.
12. Iwuchukwu OC, Harvey JR, Dordea M, et al. The role of oncoplastic therapeutic mammoplasty in breast cancer surgery–a review. Surg Oncol. 2012;21(2):133–41.
13. Almasad JK, Salah B. Breast reconstruction by local flaps after conserving surgery for breast cancer: an added asset to oncoplastic techniques. Breast J. 2008;14:340–4.
14. Hamdi M, Rasheed MZ. Advances in autologous breast reconstruction with pedicled perforator flaps. Clin Plast Surg. 2012;39(4):477–90.
15. Noguchi M, Taniya T, Miyazaki I, et al. Immediate transposition of a latissimus dorsi muscle for correcting a postquadrantectomy breast deformity in Japanese patients. Int Surg. 1990;75:166–70.
16. Rainsbury RM. Breast-sparing reconstruction with latissimus dorsi miniflaps. Eur J Surg Oncol. 2002;28(8):891–5.
17. McCulley SJ, Macmillan RD, Rasheed T. Transverse Upper Gracilis (TUG) flap for volume replacement in breast conserving surgery for medial breast tumours in small to medium sized breasts. J Plast Reconstr Aesthet Surg. 2011;64(8):1056–60.
18. Losken A, Styblo TM, Carlson GW, et al. Management algorithm and outcome evaluation of partial mastectomy defects treated using reduction or mastopexy techniques. Ann Plast Surg. 2007;59:235–42.
19. Kronowitz SJ, Kuerer HM, Buchholz TA, et al. A management algorithm and practical oncoplastic surgical techniques for repairing partial mastectomy defects. Plast Reconstr Surg. 2008;122:1631–47.
20. Munhoz AM, Montag E, Arruda E, et al. Assessment of immediate conservative breast surgery reconstruction: a classification system of defects revisited and an algorithm for selecting the appropriate technique. Plast Reconstr Surg. 2008;121:716–27.

21. Jeevan R, Cromwell DA, Trivella M, et al. Reoperation rates after breast conserving surgery for breast cancer among women in England: retrospective study of hospital episode statistics. BMJ. 2012;345:e4505.
22. Wilke LG, Czechura T, Wang C, et al. Repeat surgery after breast conservation for the treatment of stage 0 to II breast carcinoma: a report from the National Cancer Data Base, 2004–2010. JAMA Surg. 2014;149:1296–305.
23. McIntosh JM, O'Donoghue JM. Therapeutic mammoplasty–a systematic review of the evidence. EJSO. 2012;38:196–202.
24. Losken A, Dugal CS, Styblo TM, et al. A meta-analysis comparing breast conservation therapy alone to the oncoplastic technique. Ann Plast Surg. 2014;72:145–9.
25. Moran MS, Schnitt SJ, Giuliano AE, et al. Society of Surgical Oncology-American Society for Radiation Oncology consensus guideline on margins for breast-conserving surgery with whole breast irradiation in stages I and II invasive breast cancer. J Clin Oncol. 2014;32(14):1507–15.
26. Piper ML, Esserman LJ, Sbitany H, et al. Outcomes following oncoplastic reduction mammoplasty: a systematic review. Ann Plast Surg. 2016;76 Suppl 3:S222–6.
27. Clough KB, Gouveia PF, Benyahi D, et al. Positive margins after oncoplastic surgery for breast cancer. Ann Surg Oncol. 2015;22(13):4247–53.
28. Fitoussi AD, Berry MG, Famà F, et al. Oncoplastic breast surgery for cancer: analysis of 540 consecutive cases [outcomes article]. Plast Reconstr Surg. 2010;125:454–62.
29. Clough KB, van la Parra RFD, Thygesen HH, et al. Longterm results after oncoplastic surgery for breast cancer: a 10-year follow-up. Ann Surg. 2018;268(1):165–71.
30. Haloua MH, Krekel NM, Winters HA, et al. A systematic review of oncoplastic breast-conserving surgery: current weaknesses and future prospects. Ann Surg. 2013;257(4):609–20.
31. De La Cruz L, Blankenship SA, Chatterjee A, et al. Outcomes after oncoplastic breast conserving surgery in breast cancer patients: a systematic literature review. Ann Surg Oncol. 2016;23:3247–58.
32. Rainsbury RM. Surgery insight: oncoplastic breast conserving reconstruction- indications, benefits, choices and outcomes. Nat Clin Pract Oncol. 2007;4(11):657–64.
33. Yiannakopoulou EC, Mathelin C. Oncoplastic breast conserving surgery and oncological outcome: systematic review. Eur J Surg Oncol. 2016;42(5):625–30.
34. Losken A, Hart AM, Broecker JS, et al. Oncoplastic breast reduction technique and outcomes: an evolution over 20 years. Plast Reconstr Surg. 2017;139:824–33.

Risk Stratification for Adjuvant Treatment in Early Breast Cancer

Wesley M. Jose

Molecular understanding of breast cancer pathology has brought about a sea change in clinical management schema of this disease. Availability of genomic assay tools has eased the implementation of tailored therapy for individual breast cancer patients. The latest adaptive changes in TNM staging manual (eighth edition) is a proof of the impact that has been created. This chapter discusses in brief the various genomic assays used and the pieces of evidence supporting them, in risk-stratifying patients with early breast cancer.

9.1   Introduction

The management of breast cancer is becoming increasingly complex over time. Over the years, with the advent of the information highway, increased mammographic screening, reflex biopsy of calcifications, and the landscape of breast cancers being seen in the clinics have drastically changed from presentation with advanced breast cancers to a current situation of majority patients reporting with early breast cancer. Given the amount of research data being generated year over year, it is understandable that oncologists need to be abreast of the evolving landscape, more so in early breast cancer scenarios.

Early breast cancer has conventionally been defined as tumors of not more than 5 cm diameter with either impalpable or palpable but not fixed lymph nodes and absence of distant metastases [1]. This includes ductal carcinoma in situ and stage

W. M. Jose (✉)
Department of Medical Oncology, Amrita Institute of Medical Sciences, Kochi, Kerala, India
e-mail: wesleymjose@aims.amrita.edu

© Springer Nature Singapore Pte Ltd. 2021
B. Kunheri, D. K. Vijaykumar (eds.), *Management of Early Stage Breast Cancer*,
https://doi.org/10.1007/978-981-15-6171-9_9

I, stage IIA, stage IIB, and stage IIIA breast cancers. The greatest concern in breast malignancy is the worry about recurrence. This varies over time according to the clinical and molecular features of the tumor. Hence, a method of risk stratification is a must to clinically triage patients for appropriate treatment.

9.2 Anatomical Considerations and Updated TNM Staging

The primary tumor, lymph node, and metastasis (TNM) staging system was introduced by Pierre Denoix in 1952 for all cancer types and has become the common language among cancer caregivers. The seventh edition of TNM staging by the American Joint Committee on Cancer (AJCC), which was in force until December 31, 2017, depended largely on the quantitative assessment of primary tumor, lymph node involvement, and metastasis to other sites. It has now been well understood that the increased probability of breast cancer metastasis or its recurrence is not primarily because of size progression of the primary or its capacity to acquire genetic changes to increase metastatic potential; instead, it is likely to be an inherent property of the tumor from its inception [2]. This has led to a biomarker-driven, AJCC eighth edition cancer staging manual, where there has been a seismic shift from purely anatomical staging to a more focused prognostic staging as an add-on to the anatomic staging, and this has impacted how breast cancer management is practiced now. It is now accepted that their combined use gives a better predictive synergy. The tumor grade and proliferation index, common tumor markers like estrogen and progesterone receptor expression, and human epidermal growth factor 2 (HER2) expressions allow for the assessment of intrinsic tumor biology. The immunohistochemical markers and molecular classification of breast cancer have already been discussed at length in the previous chapters of this book. These markers have already established themselves to be of practical importance in making treatment decisions; however, they were not being used objectively for prognostication. This anomaly has been addressed in the latest breast cancer staging. These markers are detected by simple immunohistochemical methods and help the staging system to refine prognosis. The current TNM staging has downstaged a few hormone expressing, node-negative tumors on the basis of genomic assays [3].

It is a fact that there are logistic concerns to incorporation of AJCC eighth edition of TNM staging since a large part of the developing nations still do not have access to reliable and consistent evaluations of these breast biomarkers.

The convention during the era of anatomical staging was to err towards administering chemotherapy for most breast cancers irrespective of their intrinsic biology due to a heightened fear of recurrence. The prognostic value of these intrinsic biological markers was only a matter of assumption in the absence of objective genomic marker studies and its implications. This always led to overtreatment of significant numbers of early breast cancer patients [4]. Among patients with early node-negative breast cancer, the potential side effects of systemic chemotherapy far outweigh the benefit [5]. Therefore, it is prudent on the part of the oncologist to individualize the management so as to avoid overtreatment wherever feasible. It is now not impossible to identify the subset of patients with invasive breast cancer who have a prognosis favorable enough to forgo systemic chemotherapy. Refining treatment to adequacy needs clear objective evidence for the same. To understand this, it is necessary to examine the salient changes that have taken shape in the AJCC TNM eighth edition. The significant changes in the AJCC eighth edition are summarized below [6].

1. Lobular carcinoma in situ (LCIS) is a benign entity and is no more considered to be in the pathologic tumor in situ (pTis) category. The pleomorphic LCIS, which has overlapping features with ductal carcinoma in situ (DCIS), is now classified as pTis (DCIS).
2. The definition of microinvasive carcinoma (pT1mi) has been explicitly fixed at less than and equal to 1 mm.
3. Microscopic satellites around the main tumor mass do not impact size, the volume, or the T classification.
4. T4b category is attributed to only those skin nodules which are macroscopically separate from the primary tumor. Microscopic identification of skin involvement without obvious ulceration or peau d'orange does not equate as T4b.
5. Lymph nodes with isolated tumor cells defined as malignant cell clusters no larger than 0.2 mm do not contribute to overall pN classification.
6. Biologically low-risk pT2N0 disease has been downstaged from prognostic clinical stage II to stage I based on low recurrence score obtained from the use of multigene assays such as oncotype DX and Mammaprint.
7. Multigene panel testing is not to be used to upstage the disease (Table 9.1).

Table 9.1 Example of stage changes from seventh to eighth edition

T	N	M	G	HER2	ER	PR	7th edition stage	8th edition stage
Biomarkers								
1	0	0	1	Neg	Neg	Neg	I A	II A
1	0	0	3	Neg	Pos	Neg	I A	II A
3	1–2	0	1	Pos	Pos	Pos	III A	I B
Oncotype DX recurrence score – <11 for ER-positive tumors								
2	0	0	Any	Neg	Pos	Any	II A	I B
1–2	1	0	Any	Neg	Pos	Any	II A / II B	I B
0–2	2	0	1–2	Pos	Pos	Pos	III A	I B

Abbreviations: *Neg* negative, *Pos* positive, *ER* estrogen receptor, *G* grade, *HER2* human epidermal growth factor receptor 2, *M* metastasis classification, *N* lymph node classification, *PR* progesterone receptor, *T* tumor classification

9.3   Molecular Classification of Breast Cancer

Breast cancer has been known to be a heterogeneous disease even in the histological era. This fact has been affirmed with the availability of immunohistochemical markers and molecular tests. The conventional method of prognosticating breast cancer was based on the histological subtypes (e.g., ductal, lobular, tubular, mucinous, and metaplastic), modified Bloom–Richardson grades (based on tumor tubule formation, number of mitotic figures in most active areas, and nuclear pleomorphism), lymphovascular and perineural invasion, and lymph node involvement. The advent of technology has allowed us to decipher the genetic, epigenetic, and transcriptome changes in breast cancer, which in turn has led to better understanding of varying clinical findings and treatment responses within tumors with the same TNM group and same histological subtype. In year 2000, based on the differences in gene expression, Perou and Sorlie proposed for the first time a "molecular classification" terminology for breast cancer [7]. They divided breast cancer into four subgroups based on the estrogen, progesterone, and ErbB2 expression.

1. *Luminal A*: Expression of luminal (low molecular weight) cytokeratins, high expression of hormone receptors and related genes.
2. *Luminal B*: Expression of luminal (low molecular weight) cytokeratins, moderate–low expression of hormone receptors and related genes.
3. *HER2/neu*: High expression of HER2/neu, low expression of ER and related genes.
4. *Basal-like*: High expression of basal epithelial genes and basal cytokeratins, low expression of ER and related genes, low expression of HER2/neu.

High-risk hormone receptor-negative, HER2/neu-enriched breast cancers have increased probability of recurrence and mortality within 1–3 years. Contrary to this, the hormone-positive, HER2/neu-negative breast cancers have lower mortality risk but has a persistent rate of recurrence even after the first 5 years [8]. HER2-enriched breast tumors are further subdivided into three subgroups based on clinical behavior and aggressiveness. Clinical determinants of these subgroups are under development [9].

Luminal, HER2/neu, and triple-negative tumors can be differentiated by basic IHC for ER, PR, HER2/neu, Ki67, epidermal growth factor receptor (EGFR), and basal cytokeratin (CK14, CK 5/6, etc.) [10]. There exist no prognostic signatures for hormone receptor-negative breast cancer. There are also no predictors of treatment response in this group. The HER2/neu-positive and triple-negative breast cancers are generally aggressive and mandate treatment with appropriate chemotherapy and targeted agents such as trastuzumab and poly (ADP-ribose) polymerase (PARP) inhibitors. This chapter focuses on objective risk stratification of luminal A and B subtypes of breast cancer where the decision of avoiding chemotherapy and its related toxicity has more relevance apart from prognosticating and deciding the appropriate duration of hormonal therapy.

The IHC4 score is a prognostic model that uses classical variables and the semi-quantitative information from four standard IHC markers (ER, PR, HER2/neu, and Ki67) to assess predictability of distant recurrence. These four IHC markers provide independent information about disease and treatment outcomes. The information in the IHC4 score was found to be similar to that in Oncotype DX [11]. The IHC4 is a simple, cost-effective test. However, there is a lack of standardization in the quantification of each of these four variables. Therefore, the local pathology results may not be as sensitive as described in the IHC assay used in the seminal paper [12].

9.4   Genomic Assays

Genomic assays are multigene prognostic tests that help improve prognostication. The AJCC eighth edition has incorporated Oncotype DX as the only multigene panel for prognostic stage grouping because that alone is supported by level 1 data. However, there are many other assays that have been developed and validated over the past two decades for the same purpose.

First-generation assays are more accurate in their recurrence prediction within the first 5 years but fall short in later years. This is a serious limitation in the era where extended adjuvant endocrine therapy has been found to be more effective than the historical 5-year hormonal treatments. The newer assays have solved this concern to a large extent by providing prognostic value for late recurrences as well as remaining accurate of early relapse (Table 9.2).

We briefly discuss these assays here.

Oncotype DX (Genomic Health Inc., Redwood City, CA): This genomic test became available in 2004 and has been primarily developed for estrogen receptor-positive, HER2/neu- and node-negative breast cancer. The test uses reverse transcription-polymerase chain reaction (RT PCR) to examine the activity of 21 genes (5 reference genes and 16 cancer-related genes including those associated with cell proliferation, invasion, and hormone response) in a patient's breast tumor tissue. This assay computes a quantitative recurrence score on a continuous scale of 0 to 100, which can be categorized into low-risk (<18), intermediate-risk (18–30), or high-risk (>31) groups. This test was validated on a cohort from the National Surgical Adjuvant Breast and Bowel Project (NSABP), trials B-14 and B-20 [13, 14]. A low recurrence score defined as 0–10 suggests a 2% chance of distant recurrence at 10 years. This group does not benefit from adjuvant chemotherapy [5, 15]. The *Trial Assigning*

Table 9.2 Generation of genomic assay

First-generation assays	Second-generation assays	Newer assays
Oncotype DX	Prosigna	OncoMasTR test
Mammaprint	EndoPredict	Curebest 95GC assay
Genomic Grade Index	Breast Cancer Index	95-gene assay

Individualized Options for Treatment (*Rx*) (TAILORx) study evaluated the benefit of chemotherapy in women who were hormone receptor-positive, HER2-negative, axillary node-negative breast cancer with an intermediate recurrence score of 11–25. It did not find any benefit of adjuvant chemoendocrine over endocrine therapy alone in this group except in some patients who were 50 years of age or younger [16]. This finding is corroborated by the SOFT [17] and TEXT [18] studies in which ovarian suppression after chemotherapy in premenopausal women with intermediate- or high-risk score had substantial improvement in outcome. The TransATAC study was conducted in samples from 1231 postmenopausal patients with ER+ node-negative and node-positive disease enrolled in the ATAC trial. It confirmed the NSABP B-14 results and also reported an increase in 9-year risk of distant recurrence proportionate to the number of positive nodes for all recurrence score values. The 9-year risk of distant recurrence among patients with low recurrence score and one to three positive nodes was similar to those with node-negative disease [19].

The shortcoming of this test is that it does not provide significant prognostic value for lymph node-positive breast cancer. It also suffers from the inability to predict late distant recurrences. The ongoing phase III RxPONDER trial is assessing standard adjuvant endocrine therapy with or without chemotherapy in patients with one to three positive nodes, hormone receptor-positive and HER2-negative breast cancer with recurrence score (RS) of 25 or less [20].

MammaPrint (Agendia, Amsterdam, The Netherlands): This genomic test became available in 2007 and has been primarily developed for estrogen receptor-positive, HER2/neu-negative, and node-negative or -positive breast cancer. This 70-gene signature classifies tumors into groups that are associated with a good prognosis or a poor prognosis on the basis of the risk of distant recurrence at 5 years and at 10 years. Unlike Oncotype DX, which classifies the risks into low, intermediate, and high risks, MammaPrint classifies them into low and high risks alone.

The MINDACT trial studied patients between 18 and 70 years of age with T1, T2, or operable T3 primary invasive breast cancer. Initially, the trial included only lymph node-negative patients, which was later amended to allow the enrolment of women with up to three positive axillary nodes [21]. Among the patients deemed to be high clinical risk and low genomic risk, the 5-year survival rate was 94.7% among those not receiving chemotherapy, which was only an absolute difference of 1.5 percentage points compared to those who received chemotherapy. This suggested that approximately 46% of women with breast cancer who are at high clinical risk might not require chemotherapy. The PROMIS trial (Patients with an Intermediate Recurrence Score) evaluated the impact of MammaPrint assay on treatment decisions in the subgroup of patients who were intermediate risk (39–67%) by Oncotype DX [22]. This multi-institutional study included 840 patients with early-stage breast cancer and a 21-gene assay recurrence score of 18–30. MammaPrint reclassified the intermediate score population into low risk in 44.5% and into high-risk in 55.5% of patients. Among the low-risk patients, 28.9% had chemotherapy removed from their treatment recommendation, and among the high-risk patients, 36.7% had chemotherapy added, making a change in treatment decision on 33.6% of the patients studied.

The STO-3 trial analyzed 652 patient samples with 20-year follow-up data from the prospective, randomized Stockholm tamoxifen trial [23]. These patients included postmenopausal women with clinically detected node-negative breast cancers treated with mastectomy or lumpectomy and radiation. This study identified a new MammaPrint threshold christened as ultralow risk comprising of patients with exceedingly low risk of cancer recurrence 20 years after diagnosis.

Prosigna (NanoString Technologies, Inc.): This genomic test became available in 2013. It is a second-generation multigene expression assay. This test is based on PAM50 gene signature, which measures the expression of 50 genes (50 discriminator genes +8 controls) to classify tumors into one of four intrinsic subtypes, namely luminal A, luminal B, HER2-enriched, and basal-like. It was primarily developed for postmenopausal women with estrogen receptor-positive, lymph node-negative, or node-positive disease who were treated with tamoxifen. This test generates a risk of recurrence (ROR) score, which is on a numerical scale of 0–100 and it gives an estimate of distant recurrence over 10 years. ROR is derived based on the PAM50 gene signature, intrinsic subtype, tumor size, nodal status, and proliferation score. The test classifies patients into three risk groups: low, intermediate, and high. The test has been validated for providing prognostic information regarding both early and late recurrences [24, 25]. The clinical utility of this assay was studied in the hormone receptor-positive, postmenopausal patient population treated with adjuvant systemic endocrine therapy alone in the large ABCSG-8 trial [26]. The study showed that ROR score significantly adds prognostic information to the clinical predictor. PAM50 assigned an intrinsic subtype to all cases, and the luminal A cohort had a significantly lower ROR at 10 years compared with luminal B. Significant and clinically relevant discrimination could be made between low- and high-risk groups. In a population-based study, the Prosigna assay was able to identify 37% of patients with a one positive lymph node and 15% of patients with two positive nodes as low risk, with very favorable outcomes when treated with adjuvant endocrine therapy alone [25]. In comparison to Oncotype DX, the PAM50 ROR score provides more prognostic information with fewer patients being categorized as intermediate risk and more as high risk [27]. The predictive ability of the Prosigna assay is currently being investigated in the OPTIMA trial [28].

EndoPredict (Myriad Genetics, Inc.): This is a second-generation breast cancer recurrence test and was made available in 2017. The EndoPredict (EP) is an RNA-based multigene test and is designed to predict the likelihood of distant recurrence in ER-positive, HER2-negative breast cancer patients on adjuvant endocrine therapy. This test was validated in ABCSG-6 and ABCSG-8 trials, which demonstrated that EndoPredict provides significant prognostic information [29, 30]. This test predicts both early and late recurrences. It also reliably identifies a subgroup of patients who have an excellent long-term prognosis after 5 years of endocrine therapy. This test has the ability for identification of women with an extremely low risk who can be spared a full decade of endocrine treatment as is the practice today and therefore provides significant clinical benefit. The low-risk group of women identified by the EndoPredict have an absolute risk of distant metastasis of 1.8% between 5 and 10 years of follow-up and might be sufficiently treated with 5 years of adjuvant endocrine therapy [31].

Breast Cancer Index (Biotheranostics, Inc.): This test is not cleared by the United States Food and Drug Administration (US FDA). This test is developed to predict late distant recurrence risk in patients with estrogen receptor-positive (ER+), lymph node-negative (LN−), or lymph node-positive (LN+; with one to three positive nodes) early-stage, invasive breast cancer, who are distant recurrence-free. It also provides prediction of likelihood of benefit from extended (>5 years) endocrine therapy. The BCI test is a quantitative molecular assessment of estrogen signaling pathways. It evaluates the expression ratio of two genes HOXB13/IL17BR (H/I) and produces a binary result as high or low. This test was validated on the MA.17 tumor samples. A high H/I identifies a subgroup of ER-positive patients disease-free after 5 years of tamoxifen, who are at risk for late recurrence. When extended endocrine therapy with letrozole is prescribed, high H/I predicts benefit from therapy and a decreased probability of late disease recurrence [32, 33].

Genomic Grade Index (MapQuant Dx, Ipsogen, France): Histologic grade in breast cancer provides clinically important prognostic information. However, 30–60% of tumors are classified as histologic grade 2. This grade is associated with an intermediate risk of recurrence and is thus not informative for clinical decision making. Genomic Grade Index (GGI) is a multigene index (97-gene measure), representing a genomic correlate of histologic tumor grade. GGI assigns breast cancers of intermediate grade into two groups as low or high genomic grade (GG-1 and GG-3, respectively), whose prognoses resemble those of either high or low histologic grade and predictive of higher risk of recurrence than a low index in both untreated and tamoxifen-treated patients [34]. A prospective study revealed that changes in treatment recommendations occurred mainly in the subset of histologic grade 2 tumors that were reclassified into GG-3, with the increased use of chemotherapy in this subset. They reported that the use of GGI is feasible in routine clinical practice, and it impacts treatment decisions in early-stage breast cancer [35].

OncoMasTR Test (OncoMark Ltd., Ireland): It is an RT-qPCR test. This is a continuous risk prediction model that provides a quantitative assessment of the likelihood of distant recurrence in patients with ER-positive HER2-negative early-stage breast cancer patients with up to three involved lymph nodes. It measures the expression of three prognostic genes plus three reference genes. The OncoMasTR Risk Score considers tumor size and lymph node status in addition to the three-gene expression [36]. It was validated in the TransATAC cohort, and it provided significant prognostic information for late distant recurrence and differential risk stratification (low versus high risk), in particular for node-negative disease and to a lesser extent in those with lymph node-positive disease [37].

Curebest 95GC Breast Assay: It is a multigene assay useful to predict prognosis of node-negative and estrogen receptor (ER)-positive breast cancer patients, developed using 95 gene-set without overlap with that used in Oncotype DX. The merit of 95GC is to divide the intermediate-risk patients of 21GC (Oncotype DX) further into the two risk groups (high/low-risk) [38]. This 95-gene classifier seems to perform better than the GGI, with approximately 58% of the patients classified into the low-risk group with this classifier and safely spared adjuvant chemotherapy. It is validated for the prognostic performance for the prediction of early recurrence only (<5 years).

95-Gene Assay: An mRNA abundance analysis using the Tamoxifen and Exemestane Adjuvant Multinational (TEAM) trial pathology cohort identified this signature of 95 genes, which in conjunction with nodal status was able to stratify patients into low- and high-risk groups, with significantly different 10-year distant recurrence risk. This assay needs to be further validated in an independent patient cohort. This assay further identifies several genes and pathways suitable for targeted therapies, suggesting that the test may predict response to drug-specific chemotherapy [39].

9.5 Comparative Performance of Multigene Signatures: Which Is the Most Appropriate Test?

A retrospective preplanned comparative biomarker study of data from the Anastrozole or Tamoxifen Alone or Combined (ATAC) randomized clinical trial in 774 postmenopausal women with ER-positive, HER2-negative breast cancer was done to assess the accuracy of prediction for distant recurrence for 0–10 years and 5–10 years after diagnosis. The biomarker signatures included the Oncotype DX recurrence score, PAM50-based Prosigna risk of recurrence (ROR), Breast Cancer Index (BCI), EndoPredict (EPclin), Clinical Treatment Score, and 4-marker immunohistochemical score. The signatures providing the most prognostic information were the ROR (hazard ratio [HR], 2.56; 95% CI, 1.96–3.35), followed by the BCI (HR, 2.46; 95% CI, 1.88–3.23) and EPclin (HR, 2.14; 95% CI, 1.71–2.68). Each of these provided substantially more information than Clinical Treatment Score (HR, 1.99; 95% CI, 1.58–2.50), the recurrence score (HR, 1.69; 95% CI, 1.40–2.03), and the 4-marker immunohistochemical score (HR, 1.95; 95% CI, 1.55–2.45). Substantially, less information was provided by all six molecular tests for the 183 patients with one to three positive nodes, but the BCI and EPclin provided more additional prognostic information than the other signatures [40].

9.6 Conclusions

Almost all guidelines recommend genomic assays. The majority of studies have been done on OncotypeDx Recurrence Score, Prosigna, and EndoPredict, and all three have been found equally useful in identifying a low risk population with a favorable outcome at five and ten years in whom chemotherapy can be deferred. On the contrary, the high-risk patients identified by these tests mandate systemic chemotherapy. Compared to Oncotype DX, which has been extensively studied and validated, the second-generation assays such as Prosigna and EndoPredict provide better information regarding the risk of recurrence, especially in node-positive patients.

The following should be considered before risk stratifying a patient with genomic assays:

1. Clinical parameters are still very important to determine prognosis, and genomic assays should be used in conjunction with these features.
2. Prognostic and predictive markers should not be used as part of the staging system without knowledge of basic tumor markers (ER, PR, and HER2) as a necessary prerequisite.
3. Multigene panels should be incorporated into the staging system only for selected subsets of breast cancer (e.g., hormone receptor-positive, HER2-negative, lymph node-negative).
4. Use of more than one multigene assay at a time is not recommended.

References

1. National Breast Cancer Centre. Clinical practice guidelines for the management of early breast cancer. 2nd ed. Commonwealth of Australia: Canberra; 2001.
2. Oakman C, Bessi S, Zafarana E. Recent advances in systemic therapy: new diagnostics and biological predictors of outcome in early breast cancer. Breast Cancer Res. 2009;11(2):205.
3. Giuliano AE, Connolly JL, Edge SB, Mittendorf EA, Rugo HS, Solin LJ, et al. Breast cancer—major changes in the American Joint Committee on Cancer Eighth Edition, Cancer Staging Manual. CA Cancer J Clin. 2017;67:290–303.
4. Alvarado M, Ozanne E, Esserman L. Overdiagnosis and overtreatment of breast cancer. Am Soc Clin Oncol Educ Book. 2012:e40–5. https://doi.org/10.14694/EdBook_AM.2012.32.e40.
5. Paik S, Tang G, Shak S. Gene expression and benefit of chemotherapy in women with node-negative, estrogen receptor-positive breast cancer. J Clin Oncol. 2006;24(23):3726–34.
6. Sestak I. Risk stratification in early breast cancer inpremenopausal and postmenopausal women: integrating genomic assays with clinicopathological features. Curr Opin Oncol. 2019;31:29–34.
7. Perou CM, Sorlie T, Eisen MB, van de Rijn M, Jeffrey SS, Rees CA, Pollack JR, Ross DT, Johnsen H, Akslen LA, Fluge O, Pergamenschikov A, Williams C, Zhu SX, Lonning PE, Borresen-Dale AL, Brown PO, Botstein D. Molecular portraits of human breast tumours. Nature. 2000;406:747–52.
8. Jatoi I, Anderson WF, Jeong JH, Redmond CK. Breast cancer adjuvant therapy: time to consider its time-dependent effects. J Clin Oncol. 2011;29(17):2301–4.
9. Staaf J, Ringnér M, Vallon-Christersson J, Jönsson G, Bendahl PO, Holm K, Arason A, Gunnarsson H, Hegardt C, Agnarsson BA, Luts L, Grabau D, Fernö M, Malmström PO, Johannsson OT, Loman N, Barkardottir RB, Borg A. Identification of subtypes in human epidermal growth factor receptor 2-positive breast cancer reveals a gene signature prognostic of outcome. J Clin Oncol. 2010;28:1813–20.
10. Eliyatkın N, Yalçın E, Zengel B, Aktaş S, Vardar E. Molecular classification of breast carcinoma: from traditional, old-fashioned way to a new age, and a new way. J Breast Health. 2015;11(2):59–66. https://doi.org/10.5152/tjbh.2015.1669.
11. Cuzick J, Dowsett M, Pineda S, Wale C, Salter J, Quinn E, et al. Prognostic value of a combined estrogen receptor, progesterone receptor, Ki-67, and human epidermal growth factor receptor 2 immunohistochemical score and comparison with the Genomic Health recurrence score in early breast cancer. J Clin Oncol. 2011;29(32):4273–8.

12. Győrffy B, Hatzis C, Sanft T, Hofstatter E, Aktas B, Pusztai L. Multigene prognostic tests in breast cancer: past, present, future. Breast Cancer Res. 2015;17(1):11. https://doi.org/10.1186/s13058-015-0514-2.
13. Cronin M, Pho M, Dutta D. Measurement of gene expression in archival paraffin-embedded tissues: development and performance of a 92-gene reverse transcriptase-polymerase chain reaction assay. Am J Pathol. 2004;164(1):35–42.
14. Paik S, Shak S, Tang G. A multigene assay to predict recurrence of tamoxifen-treated, node-negative breast cancer. N Engl J Med. 2004;351(27):2817–26.
15. Sparano JA, Paik S. Development of the 21-gene assay and its application in clinical practice and clinical trials. J Clin Oncol. 2008;26:721–8.
16. Sparano JA, Gray RJ, Makower DF, et al. Adjuvant chemotherapy guided by a21-gene expression assay in breast cancer. N Engl J Med. 2018;379:111–21.
17. Francis PA, Regan MM, Fleming GF, et al. Adjuvant ovarian suppression inpremenopausal breast cancer. N Engl J Med. 2015;372:436–46.
18. Pagani O, Regan MM, Walley BA, et al. Adjuvant exemestane with ovariansuppression in premenopausal breast cancer. N Engl J Med. 2014;371:107–18.
19. Dowsett M, Cuzick J, Wale CJ, et al. Prediction of risk of distant recurrence using the 21-gene recurrence score in node-negative and node-positive postmenopausal breast cancer patients treated with anastrozole or tamoxifen: a TransATAC study. J Clin Oncol. 2010;28:1829–34.
20. Kalinsky K. Tamoxifen citrate, letrozole, anastrozole, or exemestane with or without chemotherapy in treating patients with invasive RxPONDER breast cancer—full text view. https://clinicaltrials.gov/ct2/show/NCT01272037
21. Cardoso F, van't Veer LJ, Bogaerts J, et al. 70-gene signature as an aid to treatment decisions in early-stage breast cancer. N Engl J Med. 2016;375(8):717–29.
22. Tsai M, Lo S, Audeh W, et al. Association of 70-gene signature assay findings with physicians' treatment guidance for patients with early breast cancer classified as intermediate risk by the 21-gene assay. JAMA Oncol. 2018;4(1):e173470.
23. Esserman LJ, Yau C, Thompson CK, et al. Use of molecular tools to identify patients with indolent breast cancers with ultralow risk over 2 decades. JAMA Oncol. 2017;3(11):1503–10.
24. Sestak I, Cuzick J, Dowsett M, et al. Prediction of late distant recurrence after 5 years of endocrine treatment: a combined analysis of patients from the Austrian breast and colorectal cancer study group 8 and arimidex, tamoxifen alone or in combination randomized trials using the PAM50 risk of recurrence score. J Clin Oncol. 2015;33:916–22.
25. Laenkholm AV, Jensen MB, Eriksen JO, et al. PAM50 risk of recurrence score predicts 10-year distant recurrence in a comprehensive Danish cohort of postmenopausal women allocated to 5 years of endocrine therapy for hormone receptor-positive early breast cancer. J Clin Oncol. 2018;36:735–40.
26. Gnant M, Filipits M, Greil R, et al.; Austrian Breast and Colorectal Cancer Study Group. Predicting distant recurrence in receptor-positive breast cancer patients with limited clinicopathological risk: using the PAM50 Risk of Recurrence score in 1478 postmenopausal patients of the ABCSG-8 trial treated with adjuvant endocrine therapy alone. Ann Oncol. 2014;25(2):339–345.
27. Dowsett M, Sestak I, Lopez-Knowles E, et al. Comparison of PAM50 risk of recurrence score with Oncotype DX and IHC4 for predicting risk of distant recurrence after endocrine therapy. J Clin Oncol. 2013;31(22):2783–90.
28. Bartlett J, Canney P, Campbell A, et al. Selecting breast cancer patients for chemotherapy: the opening of the UKOPTIMA trial. Clin Oncol (R Coll Radiol). 2013;25:109–16.

29. Filipits M, Rudas M, Jakesz R, et al. EP Investigators: a new molecular predictor of distant recurrence in ER-positive, HER2–negative breast cancer adds independent information to conventional clinical risk factors. Clin Cancer Res. 2011;17:6012–20.
30. Dubsky P, Filipits M, Jakesz R, et al. Austrian Breast and Colorectal Cancer Study Group (ABCSG): EndoPredict improves the prognostic classification derived from common clinical guidelines in ER-positive, HER2–negative early breast cancer. Ann Oncol. 2013;24:640–7.
31. Dubsky P, Brase JC, Jakesz R, et al. The EndoPredict score provides prognostic information on late distant metastases in ER+/HER2- breast cancer patients. Br J Cancer. 2013;109(12):2959–64.
32. Sgroi DC, Carney E, Zarrella E, et al. Prediction of late disease recurrence and extended adjuvant letrozole benefit by the HOXB13/IL17BR biomarker. J Natl Cancer Inst. 2013;105(14):1036–42.
33. Sgroi DC, Sestak I, Cuzick J, et al. Prediction of late distant recurrence in patients with oestrogen-receptor-positive breast cancer: a prospective comparison of the breast-cancer index (BCI) assay, 21-gene recurrence score, and IHC4 in the TransATAC study population. Lancet Oncol. 2013;14:1067–76.
34. Liedtke C, Hatzis C, Symmans WF, et al. Genomic grade index is associated with response to chemotherapy in patients with breast cancer. J Clin Oncol. 2009;27(19):3185–91.
35. Metzger-Filho O, Catteau A, Michiels S, et al. Genomic Grade Index (GGI): feasibility in routine practice and impact on treatment decisions in early breast cancer. PLoS One. 2013;8(8):e66848. https://doi.org/10.1371/journal.pone.0066848.
36. Lanigan F, et al. Delineating transcriptional networks of prognostic gene signatures refines treatment recommendations for lymph node-negative breast cancer patients. FEBS. 2015;282(18):3455–73.
37. Sestak I, Buus R, Cuzick JM, et al. Evaluation of the OncoMasTR prognostic signature in postmenopausal women with primary ER-positive breast cancer. J Clin Oncol. 2018;36:553; suppl; abstr 553.
38. Naoi Y, Kishi K, Tanei T, Tsunashima R, Tominaga N, Baba Y, et al. Development of 95-gene classifier as a powerful predictor of recurrences in node-negative and ER-positive breast cancer patients. Breast Cancer Res Treat. 2011;128:632–41.
39. Bayani J, Yao CQ, Quintayo MA, et al. Molecular stratification of early breast cancer identifies drug targets to drive stratified medicine. NPJ Breast Cancer. 2017;3:3. https://doi.org/10.1038/s41523-016-0003-5.
40. Sestak I, Buus R, Cuzick J, et al. Comparison of the performance of 6 prognostic signatures for estrogen receptor–positive breast cancer: a secondary analysis of a randomized clinical trial. JAMA Oncol. 2018;4(4):545–53.

Adjuvant Chemotherapy in Early Breast Cancer

Arun Philip

10.1 Introduction

The basic idea of adjuvant cytotoxic therapy in breast cancer, as in any other malignancy, is to eradicate the residual microscopic disease, if any, and thus prevent recurrence. The role of adjuvant chemotherapy for an early breast cancer (EBC) patient often generates more discussion than other scenarios in most breast oncology tumour boards. The data in this regard have been evolving quite rapidly in the past decade, especially with more information coming from trials on tumour gene expression profiling. Many large trials have looked at the benefit of adjuvant chemotherapy in EBC, and data have been incorporated into guidelines. More recently, the focus has been on de-escalation of therapy, minimising long-term adverse events. Online tools such as Adjuvant online & Predict, which have been clinically validated, also help clinicians and patients take informed decisions on adjuvant therapy. This chapter looks at all the currently available evidence on adjuvant chemotherapy in EBC and hopes to arrive at a consensus on adjuvant therapy in different subsets of EBC.

10.2 Risk Stratification and Decision on Chemotherapy

The decision on adjuvant chemotherapy in EBC is primarily based on the presence or absence of certain high-risk clinico-pathological features. The tumour characteristics looked into while making decisions on adjuvant therapy include the tumour size, estrogen and progesterone receptor status (ER/PR), HER2-neu status along with the grade or the proliferation index (Ki67) and lymphovascular invasion (LVI).

A. Philip (✉)
Department of Medical Oncology, Amrita Institute of Medical Sciences, Kochi, Kerala, India

Regional Cancer Center, Thiruvananthapuram, Kerala, India
e-mail: arunp19955@aims.amrita.edu

The nodal stage is also a very significant factor in this regard, as proven by innumerable studies. Other important clinical parameters include the patient's age and comorbidities and very importantly the patient's preferences. It is now well known that ER/PR negativity and HER2-neu positivity confer a higher risk, as do a high proliferation index and LVI. Younger age is considered to be a high-risk factor. Many clinicians would prefer avoiding chemotherapy in elderly patients with multiple comorbidities even if otherwise indicated. In general, adjuvant chemotherapy is administered to medically fit patients with one or more of the above-mentioned high-risk features. In recent times, gene expression profiling has become more widely available, and more and more clinicians are utilising this tool to decide on adjuvant therapy.

10.3 Early Evidence on the Benefit of Adjuvant Chemotherapy

Strong evidence on the benefit of adjuvant chemotherapy in EBC first came from the meta-analysis of the Early Breast Cancer Trialists' Collaborative Group (EBCTCG). The preliminary results were reported for over 28,000 women from over 60 randomised trials who received adjuvant poly-chemotherapy vs no chemotherapy [1]. Women younger than 50 years who received adjuvant chemotherapy had a 10% absolute survival benefit over those who received no adjuvant chemotherapy. Although the benefit with adjuvant therapy was seen across the study population, it was more pronounced in the younger women, particularly those under 50 years and those who were ER negative [1]. A similar result was seen in more recent data from the retrospective analysis of multiple randomised controlled trials (RCTs) by the Cancer and Leukemia Group B [2]. Although even later trials did show benefit with chemotherapy for subsets of ER-positive patients, we still do not clearly know who. A caveat to the EBCTCG analysis in the present era is that the studies were conducted when taxane-based regimens were yet to be widely used and anti-HER2 therapy was evolving. As a result, the added benefit of newer generation of chemotherapeutic drugs and anti-HER2 therapy in the relevant EBC population was not factored in during the analysis.

10.4 Quality of Life Issues

Another very important consideration to be made while offering adjuvant therapy is the quality of life (QOL) concerns it brings along. Post EBCTCG, clinicians looked at the QOL. It was seen that, although the QOL was affected adversely to some extent due to the chemotherapy, the relative gain in survival it conferred was significant. To quote a figure, the net gain in survival from adjuvant chemotherapy after adjusting for QOL was 10 months of relapse-free survival (RFS) and 5 months of overall survival (OS) [3]. Hence, it became quite clear that adjuvant chemotherapy definitely improved survival in early breast cancer. The focus then slowly started shifting to identifying those patients in whom chemotherapy can be avoided without adversely affecting survival. Also, an effort was on to minimise the intensity and toxicity of the chemotherapy in the adjuvant setting.

10.5   Who Should Receive Adjuvant Chemotherapy in EBC

As discussed before, not every patient who undergoes a definitive surgery for EBC is a candidate for chemotherapy. In fact, a good number of these patients can safely forgo chemotherapy. It would be worthwhile to look at the benefit of therapy separately in the clinically relevant subgroups. The St Gallen consensus guidelines identify certain clinical subgroups which guide therapy [4].

The broad clinical groups are the following:

1. Triple negative (ER/PR negative and HER2 negative).
2. HER2 positive (ER/PR positive or negative).
3. Luminal-like tumours (ER/PR positive and HER2 negative).

The luminal-like group is further subdivided into the following:

(a) *Luminal A type* where the ER and PR are strongly expressed, the proliferation marker is low (Ki67 < 20%), and the multiparameter molecular marker shows low risk.
(b) *Intermediate type*, which consists of the multiparameter molecular marker showing intermediate risk.
(c) *Luminal B type* where the ER/PR receptors are weakly expressed and the proliferation index is high (Ki67 > 20%) or the multiparameter molecular marker shows a high-risk status [4].

It would be worthwhile to look at the different groups separately as far as their adjuvant therapy recommendations are concerned.

10.6   Triple-Negative Early Breast Cancer

Being hormone receptor negative, patients belonging to this group are not candidates for endocrine therapy. They are also not candidates for anti-HER2 therapy and hence chemotherapy is pretty much their only treatment option in the adjuvant setting. Consequently, the threshold among clinicians for suggesting chemo in this setting is also very low. Most guidelines including the National Comprehensive Cancer Network (NCCN) and the St Gallen guidelines recommend adjuvant chemotherapy for all TNBCs, which are more than 5 mm in size (≥T1b).

10.6.1 Cytotoxic Regimens Commonly Given for TNBC

Most authorities now feel that adjuvant treatment should consist of an anthracy-cline and taxane-based chemotherapy if indicated [4, 5]. Four cycles of adriamycin + cyclophosphamide (AC) followed by four cycles of taxane, either docetaxel or paclitaxel (T) given in a dose-dense fashion every 2 weeks (dd AC-T), is considered the standard. Recently published EBCTCG data showed that taxane, when added to an anthracycline-containing regimen, significantly improved recurrence-free sur-vival and survival [6]. The subgroup analysis from these data showed that added taxanes reduced the recurrence rate from 35% to 30% (RR-0.84) and improved the survival from 24% to 21% (RR-0.86) [6]. Further ahead, the dose-dense regimen of AC-T became the preferred regimen, especially in poorer biologies such as TNBC- and HER2-positive tumours. The data in this regard came from seven published trials, which compared dose-dense versus standard-dose chemotherapy. Published data from two independent meta-analysis, one of them with over 10,000 patients, showed significant improvements in disease-free survival and overall survival [7, 8]. Paclitaxel in the adjuvant setting should ideally be used either 175 mg/m^2 every 2 weeks × 4 doses or 80 mg/m^2 weekly × 12 doses. The extended schedule of dose-dense taxane beyond 4 cycles showed no benefit over the weekly taxane × 12 schedule [9]. Hence, dd AC-T became the standard adjuvant chemotherapy regimen advocated in TNBC.

10.6.2 Can Anthracyclines Be Avoided in TNBC

Anthracycline cardiotoxicity being a major worry in the long term, avoiding adri-amycin without compromising survival in triple-negative EBC, became the next research question. The most commonly used non-anthracycline-containing regimen is docetaxel plus cyclophosphamide (TC), which is given every 3 weeks. One of the early evidence in favour of TC over AC came from the United States Oncology Trial 9735, in which over 1000 women with HER2-negative EBC were randomised to receive 4 cycles of either of the two regimens [10]. However, only a third of these patients were TNBCs. The 7-year follow-up data revealed a significantly higher DFS (81% vs 75%) and OS (87% vs 82%) with TC when compared to AC [11]. Although this was good evidence to avoid anthracyclines in ER-positive node-negative and low-risk TNBC (T1 and node negative), it did not really answer the question as to whether adjuvant anthracyclines could be avoided in all triple-negative EBCs. A more recent analysis of Anthracyclines in Early Breast Cancer (ABC) tri-als compared TC versus an AC along with a taxane-based regimen in over 4000 HER2-negative EBC. The four-year invasive DFS was better in the anthracycline-containing cohort vs TC (88.2% vs 90.7%; HR 1.23) [12]. The results of the ABC trials seemed to suggest that adjuvant AC followed by taxanes still remains standard in TNBC, but one recently reported trial came up with a different finding. The West German study group in the Plan B trial, which was a phase III randomised con-trolled trial which randomised 2449 high-risk pN0 (T2–4, G2–3, <35 years) or pN+

HER2- EBC, to receive either 6 cycles of TC or 4EC (epirubicin plus cyclophos-phamide) followed by 4 cycles of docetaxel as an adjuvant [13]. Among these, 41% were node positive, 42% were grade 3 and 18% were triple negative. The 5-year DFS (89.9% vs 90.2%) and OS (94.7% vs 94.6%) were similar in both the groups. The conclusion of this potentially practice-changing study was that 6 cycles of TC was enough in high-risk EBC, even in TNBCs [13]. Therefore, we probably may avoid adjuvant anthracyclines in triple-negative EBC, but more studies in this regard are needed for further confirmation and change in guidelines.

10.7 HER2-Positive Early Breast Cancer (ER/PR Positive or Negative)

As with TNBC, a vast majority of HER2-positive EBC patients are candidates for adjuvant chemotherapy plus anti-HER2 therapy. Approximately 15–20% of newly diagnosed breast cases are HER2 positive [14]. The introduction of anti-HER2 agents was a milestone in the history of breast cancer therapy. The huge survival advantage it brought about in the metastatic setting was also found in the adjuvant setting through multiple trials (Table 10.1). A majority of these trials

Table 10.1 Trials on adjuvant trastuzumab therapy

Study	Number patients/median follow-up	Comparison treatment	DFS (compared to chemotherapy alone)	OS (compared to chemotherapy alone)
BCIRG 006 trial	3222/5 years	• AC → docetaxel	• HR 0.64, $p < 0.001$; 0.75, $p = 0.04$	• HR 0.63, $p < 0.001$; HR 0.77, $p = 0.04$
		• AC → docetaxel + trastuzumab → trastuzumab	• 75% versus 84% versus 81%	• 87% versus 92% versus 91%
		• Docetaxel + carboplatin + trastuzumab → trastuzumab	• 257 versus 185 versus 214 events	• 489 versus 290 events
NCCTG N9831 trial	2184/6 years (DFS analysis at 5 years follow-up)	• AC → paclitaxel	*Sequential arm*	*Sequential arm*
		• AC → paclitaxel → trastuzumab	• HR 0.69, $p < 0.001$	• HR 0.88, $p < 0.343$
			• 71.8% versus 80.1%	• 88.4% versus 89.3%
			• 225 versus 165 events	• 108 versus 96 events

(continued)

Table 10.1 (continued)

Study	Number patients/median follow-up	Comparison treatment	DFS (compared to chemotherapy alone)	OS (compared to chemotherapy alone)
NCCTG N9831 and NSABP B—31 trials	4046/8.4 years	• AC → paclitaxel	• HR 0.60, $p < 0.001$	• HR 0.63, $p < 0.001$
		• AC → paclitaxel + trastuzumab → trastuzumab	• 62.3% versus 73.7%	• 75.2% versus 84.0%
			• 680 versus 473 events	• 418 versus 286
HERA trial	3401/4 years	• Four cycles standard chemotherapy	• HR 0.76, $p < 0.001$	• HR 0.85, $p < 0.11$
		• Four cycles standard chemotherapy → trastuzumab	• 72.2% versus 78.6%	• 87.7% versus 89.3%
			• 458 versus 369 events	• 213 versus 182 events
FNCLCC— PACS04 trial	3010/3 years	• FEC or epirubicin plus docetaxel	• HR 0.86, $p = 0.41$	• HR 1.27, $p = NR$
		• FEC or epirubicin plus docetaxel → trastuzumab	• 77.9% versus 80.9%	• 96% versus 95%
			• 70 versus 59 events	• 18 versus 22 events
FinHer trial	232/5.1 years	• Docetaxel or vinorelbine → FEC	• HR 0.65, $p = 0.12$	• HR 0.55, $p = 0.09$
		• Docetaxel or vinorelbine with trastuzumab → FEC	• 73.3% versus 80.9%	• 82.3% versus 91.3%
			• 31 versus 22 events	• 21 versus 12 events

[Source: ecancer 9523/https://doi.org/10.3332/ecancer.2015.523]

proved survival advantage with adjuvant trastuzumab in tumours more than 1 cm; among them, the landmark trials were the NSABP-B31, HERA and BCIRG-006, which changed the paradigm of adjuvant therapy in HER2-positive breast cancer [15–17]. The dose of trastuzumab used was 8 mg/kg as a loading dose followed by 6 mg/kg 3 weekly for 1 year. These studies proved that adjuvant trastuzumab given for 1 year significantly improved survival. The adjuvant FINHER study was done in patients with a tumour size of >2 cm and who were given an abridged schedule of 9 weekly doses of trastuzumab [18]. This trial proved that even a shorter schedule conferred a disease-free survival benefit and a trend towards overall survival benefit.

The Cochrane database in their meta-analysis, including more than 12,000 HER2-positive breast cancer patients, reported a significant DFS and OS benefit with the use of adjuvant trastuzumab for a period of 1 year [19]. Future studies explored the use of shorter schedules of trastuzumab but were found to be inferior, and an extended schedule of up to 2 years of adjuvant therapy also failed to confer any benefit. Hence, adjuvant trastuzumab for 1 year became the standard of care and still continues to be. At the recently concluded ASCO, data from the PERSEPHONE trial were presented [20]. The trial looked at the efficacy of 6 months of trastuzumab vs 12 months of trastuzumab in the adjuvant setting. Over 4000 women with HER2-positive breast cancer were randomised to receive either 6 months or 12 months of adjuvant trastuzumab. Eighty-five percentage of the study population received chemotherapy. The trial demonstrated that 6 months of trastuzumab was non-inferior to 12 months in terms of the 4-year DFS (89.4% vs 89.8%; HR 1.07). The subgroup analysis showed that women who received a non-anthracycline chemotherapy did not fare as well with the 6-month regimen as with the 12-month regimen. Hence, it is probably too early to recommend the 6-month adjuvant trastuzumab as standard for all HER2-positive breast cancer patients.

10.7.1 Adjuvant Recommendations in Small HER2-Positive Tumours

The benefit of trastuzumab in small HER2-positive tumours has been a matter of debate. Several studies done in small tumours have shown that the HER2-positive subset has fared worse in terms of survival compared to the HER2-negative subset [21, 22]. While there are no randomised data with regard to the benefit of trastuzumab in small tumours, a single-arm phase 2 trial evaluating adjuvant trastuzumab and paclitaxel was reported recently [23]. The trial which enrolled over 400 women with T1 tumours showed that the 3-year invasive DFS and RFS were to the tune of nearly 99%. Tumours with a size of less than 1 cm seemed to benefit as much as bigger tumours. This trial has prompted many authorities to recommend paclitaxel and trastuzumab in small tumours [23]. T1a tumours consisted of just about 17% of the study group; hence, a definite recommendation cannot be made in this subset. However, T1a tumours with other risk factors, such as ER negativity, LVI, young age, and high-grade tumours, may be given the benefit of anti-HER2 agents based on this evidence.

10.7.2 Dual HER2 Blockade

The benefit of anti-HER2 agents prompted researchers to look into the benefit of intensifying anti-HER2 therapy. Trials looked at the oral dual HER2 kinase inhibitor lapatinib in addition to trastuzumab in the adjuvant setting. Lapatinib, as a single agent or in combination with trastuzumab, showed no improvements in DFS or OS, as shown by the adjuvant lapatinib and/or trastuzumab treatment optimisation (ALLTO) trial [24]. Hence, the agent lapatinib is not to be used in any form of adjuvant breast cancer. Another novel anti-HER2 agent is pertuzumab, which has made huge practice changes in HER2-positive metastatic breast cancers. The Adjuvant Pertuzumab and Trastuzumab in Early HER2-Positive Breast Cancer (APHINITY trial) looked at the use of concurrent trastuzumab and pertuzumab in the adjuvant setting for 1 year. Results from the trial showed that the addition of pertuzumab to trastuzumab improves invasive disease survival in the high-risk, node-positive and ER-negative subset [25]. The trial showed no significant difference in OS in the two groups. Based on the results of this trial, dual anti-HER2 therapy with trastuzumab and pertuzumab may be offered to high-risk individuals like node-positive, ER-negative tumours. Neratinib is another dual HER2 kinase inhibitor, which was approved by the FDA for use as an extended adjuvant therapeutic agent after 1 year of trastuzumab in EBC. The approval was based on the ExteNet study, in which this agent improved the invasive DFS in comparison to the placebo, although no OS benefit was observed [26]. Most authorities do not yet advocate the use of this drug as data are still evolving.

10.7.3 Choice of Cytotoxic Agents in HER2-Positive EBC
(Table 10.2)

As discussed, all tumours above T1b are candidates for adjuvant chemotherapy and trastuzumab. Smaller tumours, with a size of <2 cm, if node negative, may be treated with 12 weekly doses of single-agent paclitaxel given at a dose of 80 mg/m^2 along with weekly trastuzumab. All tumours > T2 or node positive are considered candidates for anthracycline-containing chemotherapy, based on the existing data. Another regimen which is popular in the adjuvant setting is TCH (docetaxel 75 mg/m^2 + carboplatin AUC 6 + trastuzumab). The main advantage of this schedule is that it is non-anthracycline based. The evidence for its efficacy came from the BCIRG-006 trial, which was one among the landmark trials which proved the benefit of adjuvant trastuzumab [17]. It randomised over 3200 women with HER2-positive/node-positive or high-risk node-negative disease to receive either AC-T or AC-TH or TCH to a total of 6 cycles followed by trastuzumab for a year in the latter two regimens. At 5 years, both TCH and AC-TH demonstrated better DFS (84% and 81% vs 75%) and OS (92% and 91% vs 87%) compared to AC-T [17]. Although the DFS and OS were numerically better in the AC-TH regimen compared to TCH, it was not statistically significant. It was not meant to be a non-inferiority

Table 10.2 Commonly used chemotherapy regimens in HER2 positive breast cancer

AC- TH	Doxorubicin 60 mg/m^2 IV D1 + Cyclophosphamide 600 mg/m^2 D1 every 21 days × 4 cycles → Paclitaxel 175 mg/m^2 every 21 days × 4 cycles + Trastuzumab 4 mg/kg loading with first dose of Paclitaxel followed by 2 mg/kg weekly for 1 year OR Trastuzumab 8 mg/kg loading with first dose of Paclitaxel followed by 6 mg/kg 3 weekly for 1 year
Dose dense AC- Weekly TH	Doxorubicin 60 mg/m^2 IV D1 + Cyclophosphamide 600 mg/m^2 D1 every 14 days × 4 cycles → Paclitaxel 80 mg/m^2 weekly × 12 doses + Trastuzumab 4 mg/kg loading with first dose of Paclitaxel followed by 2 mg/kg weekly for 1 year
TCH	Docetaxel 75 mg/m^2 D1 + Carboplatin AUC 6 D1 every 21 days × 4 cycles + Trastuzumab 8 mg/kg D1 followed by 6 mg/kg 3 weekly for 1 year OR Trastuzumab 4 mg/kg loading D1 followed by 2 mg/kg weekly for 1 year
Paclitaxel Trastuzumab	Paclitaxel 80 mg/m^2 weekly × 12 doses + Trastuzumab 4 mg/kg loading with first dose of Paclitaxel followed by 2 mg/kg weekly for 1 year OR 6 mg/kg 3 weekly for 1 year after completion of paclitaxel
AC- THP	Doxorubicin 60 mg/m^2 IV D1 + Cyclophosphamide 600 mg/m^2 D1 every 21 days × 4 cycles → Paclitaxel 175 mg/m^2 every 21 days × 4 cycles + Trastuzumab 8 mg/kg + Pertuzumab 840 mg loading with first dose of Paclitaxel followed by Trastuzumab 6 mg/kg + Pertuzumab 420 mg every 3 weeks for 1 year
TCHP	Docetaxel 75 mg/m^2 D1 + Carboplatin AUC 6 D1 every 21 days × 4 cycles + Trastuzumab 8 mg/kg + Pertuzumab 840 mg loading D1 followed by Trastuzumab 6 mg/kg + Pertuzumab 420mg every 3 weeks for 1 year

[Source: NCCN clinical practice guidelines Breast Cancer: 2018 ver 2.2018]

trial to answer the question of whether TCH is comparable to AC-TH; the results seemed to suggest that TCH may be used in this setting without significantly affecting survival.

10.8 Luminal-Like Tumours (ER/PR Positive and HER2 Negative)

This is the third clinical group and probably the most difficult one as far as decision on adjuvant chemotherapy is concerned. This subset of breast cancer is probably the most prevalent in clinical practice. The luminal tumours may be either luminal A (ER/PR strong positive and Ki67 < 20%) or luminal B (ER/PR weak positive and Ki67 > 20%). The factors considered while deciding on adjuvant therapy in these women mainly include the age (younger the age higher the risk), performance status, lymph node status (higher nodal stage confers higher risk), LVI, grade of the tumour or a genomic test recurrence risk score, if available [27].

It is fairly well accepted that T1 tumours which are luminal A and node negative with no additional high-risk features are not candidates for adjuvant chemotherapy and are for hormone therapy alone. A good majority of T2N0 patients will also be given hormones alone, but in the present era, a genomic risk score has to be obtained for the said population before they are offered only hormones. The majority of luminal B patients, T3 tumours or node-positive EBC patients are considered for chemotherapy. Data are now emerging on the role of genomic analysis for recurrence risk score like Oncotype DX in the node-positive (N1) EBC. Howevr, in a scenario where these advanced tests are out of the reach of most of our patients, a clinical decision is taken on adjuvant therapy.

10.8.1 Gene Expression Signatures: Changing Paradigms

The gene-based assays for the recurrence risk estimation is revolutionising decisions on adjuvant therapy at least in the west where its use is routine. The internationally accepted genomic expression signatures include the Oncotype DX (21-gene assay), the Mammaprint (70-gene assay) and the Prosigna – PAM50 (50-gene assay) and these have been endorsed by most of the guidelines for use in the adjuvant setting [28–30].

- *The Oncotype DX*: This is a 21-gene signature assay and is done on paraffin-embedded breast cancer tissue. It is probably the best validated of the existing assays. It gives a recurrence score ranging from 0 to 100. The test has been found to strongly predict the risk of relapse and survival and the benefit of chemotherapy. Patients with a low recurrence risk score (<11) can safely avoid chemotherapy. Prospective studies, findings of which were reported recently, show that even in node-positive disease (N1), patients with a low-risk score can safely avoid adjuvant chemotherapy [31]. Patients with a risk score of >25 derived significant benefit from the addition of chemotherapy [32]. The recently reported data from the TailorX trial showed that women with an intermediate score (12–25) did not benefit from the addition of chemotherapy to hormone therapy, except in the <50-year subgroup who seemed to have a marginal benefit from adjuvant chemo [33].
- *The Mammaprint*: It is a 70-gene signature assay that has been validated in clinics. In the prospective MINDACT trial (ER-positive, node-negative and 0–3 node-positive group), it was seen that the low-risk group had no benefit with the addition of chemotherapy and we could safely avoid chemotherapy in them [29].

10.8.2 Risk Calculators

These are another set of supportive tools which the clinician has at his disposal to decide on who benefits from adjuvant chemotherapy. The most popular one is the Adjuvant online, which is available online. It uses an algorithm to estimate the DFS and OS and subsequently the benefit of local therapy alone vs addition of chemotherapy to hormone therapy. A disadvantage of the tool is that it does not factor

Table 10.3 Commonly used chemotherapy regimens in HER2 negative breast cancer

Dose dense AC- Paclitaxel	Doxorubicin 60 mg/m^2 IV D1 + Cyclophosphamide 600 mg/m^2 D1 every 14 days × 4 cycles → Paclitaxel 175 mg/m^2 every 14 days × 4 cycles
Dose dense AC-Weekly Paclitaxel	Doxorubicin 60 mg/m^2 IV D1 + Cyclophosphamide 600 mg/m^2 D1 every 14 days × 4 cycles → Paclitaxel 80 mg/m^2 weekly × 12 doses
TC	Docetaxel 75 mg/m^2 + cyclophosphamide 600 mg/m^2 every 21 days × 4 cycles
AC	Doxorubicin 60 mg/m^2 IV D1 + Cyclophosphamide 600 mg/m^2 D1 either 2 weekly(dose dense) OR 3 weekly × 4 cycles
CMF	Cyclophosphamide 100 mg/m^2 D1–D14 oral + Methotrexate 40 mg/m^2 D1,D8 + Fluorourcil 600 mg/m^2 D1, D8 every 4 weeks × 6 cycles
AC - Docetaxel	Doxorubicin 60 mg/m^2 IV D1 + Cyclophosphamide 600 mg/m^2 D1 every 3 weeks × 4 cycles → Docetaxel 100 mg/m^2 every 3 weeks × 4 cycles
TAC	Doxorubicin 50 mg/m^2 IV D1 + Cyclophosphamide 500 mg/m^2 D1 + Docetaxel 75 mg/m^2 D1 every 3 weeks × 6 cycles

[Source: NCCN clinical practice guidelines Breast Cancer: 2018 ver 2.2018]

in HER2 in its algorithm, but many clinicians make use of this tool to discuss the benefits of adjuvant chemotherapy with their patients and take an informed joint decision.

10.8.3 Choice of Cytotoxics (Table 10.3)

The choice of chemotherapy, if required, is one of the standard regimens, as discussed previously. The AC-T is the classical one, especially if node positive. We have data in luminal-like EBCs, even ones with limited nodes to give 4 cycles of TC (preferred) or 4 cycles of AC. The US intergroup trial 9735 showed evidence in this regard. Therefore, in a good majority of EBC patients who are luminal-like, the chemotherapy schedule would be TC × 4. This regimen is becoming increasingly popular in HER2-negative EBC, considering the distressing long-term cardiac morbidity with anthracycline-containing regimens.

10.9   Conclusion

In conclusion, EBC is a very heterogeneous subset of breast cancers whose behaviour varies considerably based on the clinical characteristics and tumour biology. Adjuvant chemotherapy is a difficult decision in luminal-like tumours. In HER2-positive tumours as in TNBCs, all women with a tumour size of >1 cm are candidates for adjuvant chemotherapy. The dose-dense AC-T is the preferred schedule. In smaller tumours, single-agent paclitaxel may be adequate with standard-schedule trastuzumab. In high-risk HER2-positive EBCs, like young patients with node-positive disease and LVI, dual HER2 blockade with pertuzumab and trastuzumab may be considered. The duration of trastuzumab therapy is 12 months. We also have recent information which suggests that 6 months of adjuvant trastuzumab may be an equivalent option, but we still do not know who are the right patients eligible for the abridged schedule. Adjuvant chemotherapy in TNBC is indicated in all women with a tumour size of >5 mm. Data are emerging that smaller node-negative TNBC patients may be offered non-anthracycline-based chemotherapy (TC × 6), although not incorporated into any guidelines. In luminal-like tumours, the genomic expression signatures are increasingly being utilised to aid in deciding on adjuvant therapy. In a resource-starved setting like ours, we would continue to rely on the age-old clinico-pathological factors to base our decisions on adjuvant therapy.

References

1. Early Breast Cancer Trialists' Collaborative Group (EBCTCG). Effects of chemotherapy and hormonal therapy for early breast cancer on recurrence and 15-year survival: an overview of the randomised trials. Lancet. 2005;365:1687.
2. Berry DA, Cirrincione C, Henderson IC, et al. Estrogen-receptor status and outcomes of modern chemotherapy for patients with node-positive breast cancer. JAMA. 2006;295:1658.
3. Cole BF, Gelber RD, Gelber S, et al. Polychemotherapy for early breast cancer: an overview of the randomised clinical trials with quality-adjusted survival analysis. Lancet. 2001;358:277.
4. Curigliano G, Burstein HJ, Winer EP, et al. De-escalating and escalating treatments for early-stage breast cancer: the St. Gallen international expert consensus conference on the primary therapy of early breast cancer 2017. Ann Oncol. 2017;28:1700–12.
5. National comprehensive cancer network guidelines. Breast Cancer: ver 2.2018.
6. Early Breast Cancer Trialists' Collaborative Group (EBCTCG), Peto R, Davies C, et al. Comparisons between different polychemotherapy regimens for early breast cancer: meta-analyses of long-term outcome among 100,000 women in 123 randomised trials. Lancet. 2012;379:432.
7. Gray R, Bradley R, Braybrooke J, et al. Increasing the dose density of adjuvant chemotherapy by shortening intervals between courses or by sequential drug. SABCS. 2017:GS1-01.
8. Bonilla L, Ben-Aharon I, Vidal L, et al. Dose-dense chemotherapy in nonmetastatic breast cancer: a systematic review and meta-analysis of randomized controlled trials. J Natl Cancer Inst. 2010;102:1845.
9. Budd GT, Barlow WE, Moore HC, et al. SWOG S0221: a phase III trial comparing chemotherapy schedules in high-risk early-stage breast cancer. J Clin Oncol. 2015;33:58.
10. Jones SE, Savin MA, Holmes FA, et al. Phase III trial comparing doxorubicin plus cyclophosphamide with docetaxel plus cyclophosphamide as adjuvant therapy for operable breast cancer. J Clin Oncol. 2006;24:5381.
11. Jones S, Holmes FA, O'Shaughnessy J, et al. Docetaxel with cyclophosphamide is associated with an overall survival benefit compared with doxorubicin and cyclophosphamide: 7-year follow-up of US oncology research trial 9735. J Clin Oncol. 2009;27:1177.
12. Blum JL, Flynn PJ, Yothers G, et al. Anthracyclines in early breast cancer: the abc trials-USOR 06-090, NSABP B-46-I/USOR 07132, and NSABP B-49 (NRG Oncology). J Clin Oncol. 2017;35:2647.
13. Harbeck N, Gluz O, Michael R, et al. Prospective WSG phase III planB trial: final analysis of adjuvant 4xEC→4x doc vs. 6x docetaxel/cyclophosphamide in patients with high clinical risk and intermediate-to-high genomic risk HER2-negative, early breast cancer. J Clin Oncol. 35(15_suppl):504. https://doi.org/10.1200/JCO.2017.35.15_suppl.504.

14. Noone AM, Cronin KA, Altekruse SF, et al. Cancer incidence and survival trends by subtype using data from the surveillance epidemiology and end results program, 1992-2013. Cancer Epidemiol Biomark Prev. 2017;26:632.
15. Romond EH, Perez EA, Bryant J, et al. Trastuzumab plus adjuvant chemotherapy for operable HER2-positive breast cancer. N Engl J Med. 2005;353:1673.
16. Piccart-Gebhart MJ, Procter M, Leyland-Jones B, et al. Trastuzumab after adjuvant chemotherapy in HER2-positive breast cancer. N Engl J Med. 2005;353:1659.
17. Slamon D, Eiermann W, Robert N, et al. Adjuvant trastuzumab in HER2-positive breast cancer. N Engl J Med. 2011;365:1273.
18. Joensuu H, Kellokumpu-Lehtinen PL, Bono P, et al. Adjuvant docetaxel or vinorelbine with or without trastuzumab for breast cancer. N Engl J Med. 2006;354:809.
19. Moja L, Tagliabue L, Balduzzi S, et al. Trastuzumab containing regimens for early breast cancer. Cochrane Database Syst Rev. 2012:CD006243.
20. Earl HM, Hiller L, Vallier AL. Persephone: 6 versus 12 months (m) of adjuvant trastuzumab in patients (pts) with HER2 positive (+) early breast cancer (EBC): randomised phase 3 non-inferiority trial with definitive 4-year (yr) disease-free survival (DFS) results. J Clin Oncol. 2018;36(suppl; 506 abstr).
21. Curigliano G, Viale G, Bagnardi V, et al. Clinical relevance of HER2 overexpression/amplification in patients with small tumor size and node-negative breast cancer. J Clin Oncol. 2009;27:5693.
22. Gonzalez-Angulo AM, Litton JK, Broglio KR, et al. High risk of recurrence for patients with breast cancer who have human epidermal growth factor receptor 2-positive, node-negative tumors 1 cm or smaller. J Clin Oncol. 2009;27:5700.
23. Tolaney SM, Barry WT, Dang CT, et al. Adjuvant paclitaxel and trastuzumab for node-negative, HER2-positive breast cancer. N Engl J Med. 2015;372:134.
24. Piccart-Gebhart M, Holmes E, Baselga J, et al. Adjuvant lapatinib and trastuzumab for early human epidermal growth factor receptor 2-positive breast cancer: results from the randomized phase III adjuvant lapatinib and/or trastuzumab treatment optimization trial. J Clin Oncol. 2016;34:1034.
25. Von Minckwitz G, Procter M, de Azambuja E, et al. Adjuvant pertuzumab and trastuzumab in early HER2-positive breast cancer. N Engl J Med. 2017;377(2):122–31.
26. https://www.accessdata.fda.gov/drugsatfda_docs/label/2017/208051s000lbl.pdf. Accessed 19 July 2017.
27. Henry NL, Somerfield MR, Abramson VG, et al. Role of patient and disease factors in adjuvant systemic therapy decision making for early-stage, operable breast cancer: American society of clinical oncology endorsement of cancer care ontario guideline recommendations. J Clin Oncol. 2016;34:2303.
28. Sparano JA, Gray RJ, Makower DF, et al. Prospective validation of a 21-gene expression assay in breast cancer. N Engl J Med. 2015;373:2005–14.
29. Cardoso F, van't Veer LJ, Bogaerts J, et al., MINDACT Investigators. 70-Gene signature as an aid to treatment decisions in early-stage breast cancer. N Engl J Med 2016;375:717–729.
30. Gnant M, Filipits M, Greil R, et al., Austrian Breast and Colorectal Cancer Study Group. Predicting distant recurrence in receptor-positive breast cancer patients with limited clinicopathological risk: using the PAM50 risk of recurrence score in 1478 postmenopausal patients of the ABCSG-8 trial treated with adjuvant endocrine therapy alone. Ann Oncol 2014; 25: 339–345.
31. Gluz O, Nitz UA, Christgen M, et al. West German Study Group phase III planB trial: first prospective outcome data for the 21-gene recurrence score assay and concordance of prognostic markers by central and local pathology assessment. J Clin Oncol. 2016;34:2341.
32. Paik S, Tang G, Shak S, et al. Gene expression and benefit of chemotherapy in women with node-negative, estrogen receptor-positive breast cancer. J Clin Oncol. 2006;24:3726.
33. Sparano JA, Gray RJ, Makower DF, et al. Adjuvant chemotherapy guided by a 21-gene expression assay in breast cancer. N Engl J Med. 2018;379:111.

Role of Anti-HER2/Neu Molecules in the Management of HER2-Positive Early Breast Cancer

11

K. Pavithran

Human epidermal growth factor receptor 2 (HER2) is overexpressed in approximately 20% of breast cancers and is usually linked to a more aggressive natural history with poor response rates and decreased survival [1]. HER2-targeted therapies have changed this landscape as has been proven by an improvement in progression-free survival (PFS) and overall survival (OS) with the addition of trastuzumab as compared to chemotherapy in patients with early as well as advanced disease [2]. Although survival rates have improved after the use of trastuzumab, still we are unable to predict the response to treatment. Further understanding of the biology of HER2-positive breast cancer would help in choosing the most suitable treatment regimen for our patients and in developing new ways to combat HER2 resistance.

11.1 HER2 Biology

HER2 was first described as a proto-oncogene for breast cancer in 1989. The HER2 receptor family consists of four members: HER1 (ErbB1), HER2 (ErbB2), HER3 (ErbB3) and HER4 (ErbB4). They are involved in the control of cell proliferation, differentiation and survival. No known ligand directly activates HER2. HER2 gets activated either constitutively or after homo- or heterodimerisation of two ErbB receptors, followed by stimulation of downstream signalling pathways resulting in cell proliferation [3].

Anti-HER 2 therapy is very important in the treatment for HER2-positive breast cancer, and many agents were brought to clinical practice after the first approval of trastuzumab in 1998 for metastatic cancers. Table 11.1 indicates how rapidly newer agents are changing the way we now treat a patient with HER2-positive breast cancer.

K. Pavithran (✉)
Department of Medical Oncology, Amrita Institute of Medical Sciences and Research Centre, Kochi, Kerala, India
e-mail: pavithrank@aims.amrita.edu

© Springer Nature Singapore Pte Ltd. 2021
B. Kunheri, D. K. Vijaykumar (eds.), *Management of Early Stage Breast Cancer*,
https://doi.org/10.1007/978-981-15-6171-9_11

Table 11.1 Approved anti-Her2 agents in breast cancer

Drug	Year of FDA approval	Indication in breast cancer
Trastuzumab	1998	Metastatic
Trastuzumab	2005	Adjuvant
Lapatinib	2005	Metastatic
Pertuzumab	2012	Metastatic
T-DM1	2013	Metastatic
Pertuzumab	2013	Neoadjuvant
Pertuzumab	2017	Adjuvant
Neratinib	2017	Adjuvant
T-DM1	2019	Adjuvant
Tucatinib	2020	Metastatic

11.2   Drugs Used for HER2-Targeted Therapy [4]

Trastuzumab: Trastuzumab is a recombinant monoclonal antibody. It binds to the extracellular subdomain IV of HER2 and acts through various mechanisms to inhibit cell proliferation. Reversible cardiotoxicity is the only major side effect.

Pertuzumab: Pertuzumab is a humanised monoclonal antibody. It gets attached to the subdomain II of HER2 and blocks the extracellular dimerisation of HER2 with other HER family members. Known adverse effects include fatigue, nausea, increased lacrimation, flu-like symptoms, alopecia, skin rash, diarrhoea, neutropenia and rarely cardiotoxicity.

Ado-Trastuzumab Emtansine (T-DM1): T-DM1 is an antibody–drug conjugate. It is formed by linking trastuzumab to the microtubule-inhibiting chemotherapeutic agent DM1 (emtansine—a microtubule inhibitor that is 400-fold more potent than paclitaxel). T-DM1 undergoes receptor-mediated internalisation into cells followed by degradation by lysosomes where DM1-containing catabolites are released. DM1 binds to tubulin, causing disruption of microtubule networks leading to arrest of mitosis and cell death [6]. Adverse events reported with T-DM1 are fatigue, nausea, altered liver enzymes, musculoskeletal pain, constipation, headache, anaemia, thrombocytopenia and peripheral neuropathy

Lapatinib: Lapatinib is a reversible dual tyrosine kinase inhibitor that blocks EGFR and HER2 pathways. Main adverse effects are diarrhoea, skin rashes, interstitial lung disease and hepatotoxicity.

Neratinib: Neratinib is an irreversible inhibitor of EGFR, HER2, and HER4. It is more potent than lapatinib in blocking HER2 activation. Diarrhoea is the major side effect.

Tucatinib: Tucatinib is an orally active and highly potent tyrosine kinase inhibitor, which selectively inhibits HER2 phosphorylation. The common side effects are diarrhoea, hand-foot syndrome, nausea, fatigue and altered liver function.

11.3   Neoadjuvant Setting

Neoadjuvant chemotherapy (NACT) is a well-established approach used in the treatment of early as well as locally advanced or inflammatory breast cancer. Following NACT, chances of breast conservation are better and objective evaluation of the response to treatment is possible. Survival benefit with NACT is the same as with postoperative adjuvant therapy [5]. Several studies have shown that the addition of anti-HER2 treatment in HER2-positive tumours demonstrated a higher pathological complete response rate (pCR) after neoadjuvant therapy. pCR is defined as no evidence of residual invasive as well as in situ cancer in the breast and all sampled regional lymph nodes on pathological examination after NACT. Progression-free survival (PFS) and overall survival (OS) are higher in HER2-positive patients, whose tumours achieve a pCR following NACT, and the effect is more pronounced in hormone receptor-negative tumors [5]. pCR rates can be up to 45–66% if dual anti-HER2 treatment using trastuzumab plus lapatinib or trastuzumab plus pertuzumab combined with chemotherapy is used. The NeoALTTO (Neo-Adjuvant Lapatinib and/or trastuzumab treatment optimisation) and the GeparQuinto trials studied the combination of trastuzumab with lapatinib. The NeoALTTO study was a three-arm study, and the pCR rate was much higher in the combination (paclitaxel plus lapatinib plus trastuzumab) (51.3%) group when compared to the trastuzumab group (29.5%) or the lapatinib group (24.7%). This suggests that dual HER2 blockade is better than single anti-HER2 therapy [6]. Neoadjuvant Study of Pertuzumab and Herceptin in an Early Regimen Evaluation (NeoSphere) study was a randomised phase II trial that studied neoadjuvant docetaxel with either pertuzumab, trastuzumab or both in women with early, locally advanced or inflammatory HER2+ breast cancer. There was a significant improvement in the pCR rate (45.8% *versus* 29.0%) with the pertuzumab, trastuzumab and docetaxel combination arm [7]. In the TRYPHAENA study, pCR rates were 66.2% for docetaxel/carboplatin/trastuzumab/pertuzumab versus 57.3% for 5-fluorouracil/epirubicin/cyclophosphamide followed by docetaxel/trastuzumab/pertuzumab [8]. This pCR rate was confirmed in the GeparSepto study (pCR rate 57.8%) [9], KRISTINE (pCR rate was 55.7% in the chemotherapy-containing arm) [10] and Symphony (pCR 53%) [11] studies. TRAIN-2 study showed high pathological complete responses (67 vs 68% in the non-anthracycline group) and more frequent febrile neutropenia in the anthracycline group (10% vs 1%). Therefore, this study showed that when dual HER2 blockade is used, omitting anthracyclines from neoadjuvant treatment regimens might be a preferred approach [12].

Following the neoadjuvant use of dual HER2 blockade concurrently or sequentially with anthracycline-based chemotherapy, the incidence of left ventricular systolic dysfunction is low [13]. Established neoadjuvant protocols in HER2+ EBC are either an anthracycline and taxane sequentially with trastuzumab/pertuzumab or docetaxel–carboplatin plus dual Her2 blockade.

11.4 Adjuvant Therapy

It was observed from the data from the adjuvant trials and the meta-analysis that combining trastuzumab with standard chemotherapy reduces the risk of recurrence by approximately 40% and the risk for death up to 34%.

These benefits are independent of the patient's age and pathological characteristics such as tumour size, the status of the lymph node or hormone receptor (HR) status [14, 15].

Both anthracycline and non-anthracycline-based chemo (Breast Cancer International Research Group 006 study) with trastuzumab is an option in the adjuvant setting. Results from the North Central Cancer Treatment Group N9831 study and meta-analysis showed that there was a trend towards better outcomes when patients receive doxorubicin and cyclophosphamide followed by trastuzumab concurrently with taxanes.

For HER2+ EBC patients who are having low-risk disease, data from the adjuvant paclitaxel and trastuzumab (APT) trial demonstrated very good outcome (7-year recurrence-free survival of 97.5%) with 12 weeks of adjuvant paclitaxel with trastuzumab followed by trastuzumab for nine months. It is also a well-tolerated regimen [16].

In the KATHERINRE trial, patients having residual invasive disease in the breast or axillary nodes following taxane-based neoadjuvant chemotherapy along with trastuzumab were randomly allotted to continue trastuzumab or be changed to T-DM1. Adjuvant treatment with T-DM1 lowered the risk of developing recurrence of invasive breast cancer or death by 50%. The benefit was seen in all prespecified subgroups (patients with operable or inoperable cancers at initial presentation, hormone receptor-negative or -positive tumours as well as post-neoadjuvant node-positive and node-negative disease). This study established a new standard of care for adjuvant therapy for patients not achieving a pCR after NACT [17].

ALTTO (Adjuvant Lapatinib and/or Trastuzumab Treatment Optimisation trial) evaluated lapatinib with and without trastuzumab. The results of this trial were negative, and there was severe toxicity with lapatinib [18]. The ExteNET study evaluated the role of neratinib in patients who already had completed one year of adjuvant trastuzumab. Neratinib reduced the risk of relapse by 27%. Neratinib is approved for patients with early-stage HER2-positive breast cancer who have finished 1 year of adjuvant trastuzumab. The benefit was more for patients with hormone receptor-positive cancer. More than one-third of the patients on neratinib had grade 3 diarrhoea [19]. The APHINITY study tested pertuzumab and trastuzumab combination with chemotherapy. Pertuzumab reduced the risk of recurrence by 19% with a good safety profile [20]. The pertuzumab and trastuzumab combination is preferred in EBC patients who are node-positive (in whom the absolute invasive disease-free survival benefit was 3.2%) or estrogen receptor-negative.

11.5   Optimal Duration of Anti-HER2 Treatment

In the adjuvant setting, 12-months of treatment remains the standard of care [21, 22]. The HERA trial demonstrated that 24 months of treatment was not superior to 12 months [23]. Heavy treatment costs and trastuzumab-related cardiac toxicity were major concerns regarding the duration of treatment. This led to seven de-escalation trials—addressing whether a shorter duration regimen would be non-inferior to the standard regimen. In four of these trials, trastuzumab was given concurrently with chemotherapy in the experimental arm (FinHer [24], E2198 [25], SOLD [26] and Short-HER [27] trials). Results of the FinHER trial showed that 9-week course of trastuzumab was associated with an improvement in recurrence-free survival benefit [24]. Short-HER and SOLD studies used nine weeks versus one year of adjuvant trastuzumab and three trials compared 6-month versus 12-month duration of trastuzumab (PHARE [28], HORG [29] and PERSEPHONE [30]). Of these, all except the PERSEPHONE study failed to prove non-inferiority. The PERSEPHONE trial demonstrated that a trastuzumab regimen shorter than one year could provide non-inferior disease-free survival (DFS) and OS. Four-year DFS was 89.8% in the 1-year arm vs 89.4% in the 6-months arm; 4-year OS was 94.8% vs 93.8%. Cardiac adverse events were significantly less in the 6-month arm. Patients with ER+ and node-negative disease who received full anthracycline and taxane-based chemotherapy are probably the ideal candidates for such an approach [30].

11.6   Conclusion

Since the identification of HER2 and development of trastuzumab, many other drugs (antibodies, antibody–drug conjugates and tyrosine kinase inhibitors) have become an important part of the treatment of HER2-over-expressing breast cancer. This has improved the survival of these patients in the adjuvant as well as the metastatic setting considerably. Availability of biosimilar trastuzumab has considerably increased the access to trastuzumab in low- and middle-income counties. Combination of chemotherapy and dual anti-HER2 blockade resulted in the highest rate of pCR in the NACT setting. The current standard adjuvant treatment for patients with early HER2-positive breast cancer is chemotherapy plus trastuzumab administered for 1 year. Financial and cardiac toxicity associated with trastuzumab was a major concern regarding the duration of treatment, leading to many de-escalation trials. Still, the majority failed to show non-inferiority to the standard regimen.

References

1. Moasser MM, Krop IE. The evolving landscape of HER2 targeting in breast cancer. JAMA Oncol. 2015;1:1154–61.
2. Slamon DJ, Leyland-Jones B, Shak S, Fuchs H, Paton V, Bajamonde A, et al. Use of chemotherapy plus a monoclonal antibody against HER2 for metastatic breast cancer that overexpresses HER2. N Engl J Med. 2001;344:783–92.
3. Yarden Y. Biology of HER2 and its importance in breast cancer. Oncology. 2001;61(Suppl 2):1–13.
4. Rimawi MF, Schiff R, Osborne CK. Targeting HER2 for the treatment of breast cancer. Annu Rev Med. 2015;66:111–28.
5. Wuerstlein R, Harbeck N. Neoadjuvant therapy for HER2-positive breast cancer. Rev Recent Clin Trials. 2017;12:81–92.
6. Baselga J, Bradbury I, Eidtmann H, Di Cosimo S, de Azambuja E, Aura C, et al.; NeoALTTO Study Team. Lapatinib with trastuzumab for HER2-positive early breast cancer(neoALTTO): a randomised, open-label, multicentre, phase 3 trial. Lancet. 2012;379:633–640.
7. Gianni L, Pienkowski T, Im YH, Roman L, Tseng LM, Liu MC, et al. Efficacy and safety of neoadjuvant pertuzumab and trastuzumab in women with locally advanced, inflammatory, or early HER2-positive breast cancer(NeoSphere): a randomised multicentre, open-label, phase 2 trial. Lancet Oncol. 2012;13:25–32.
8. Schneeweiss A, Chia S, Hickish T, Harvey V, Eniu A, Hegg R. Pertuzumab plus trastuzumab in combination with standard neoadjuvant anthracycline-containing and anthracycline-free chemotherapy regimens in patients with HER2-positive early breast cancer: a randomized phase II cardiac safety study (TRYPHAENA). Ann Oncol. 2013;24:2278–84.
9. Loibl S, Jackisch C, Schneeweiss A, Schmatloch S, Aktas B, Denkert C, et al.; Investigators of the German Breast Group (GBG) and the Arbeitsgemeinschaft Gynäkologische Onkologie—Breast (AGO-B) studygroups. Dual HER2-blockade with pertuzumab and trastuzumab in HER2-positive early breast cancer: a subanalysis of data from the randomized phase III GeparSepto trial. Ann Oncol. 2017;28:497–504.
10. Hurvitz SA, Martin M, Symmans WF, Jung KH, Huang CS, Thompson AM, et al. Neoadjuvant trastuzumab, pertuzumab, and chemotherapy versus trastuzumab emtansine plus pertuzumab in patients with HER2-positive breast cancer (KRISTINE): a randomised, open-label, multicentre, phase 3 trial. Lancet Oncol. 2018;19(1):115–26.
11. Whitworth P, Stork-Sloots L, de Snoo FA, Richards P, Rotkis M, Beatty J, et al. Chemosensitivity predicted by BluePrint 80-gene functional subtype and MammaPrint in the Prospective Neoadjuvant Breast Registry Symphony Trial (NBRST). Ann Surg Oncol. 2014;21:3261–7.
12. van Ramshorst MS, van der Voort A, van Werkhoven ED, Mandjes IA, Kemper I, Dezentjé VO, et al. Neoadjuvant chemotherapy with or without anthracyclines in the presence of dual HER2 blockade for HER2-positive breast cancer (TRAIN-2): a multicentre, open-label, randomised, phase 3 trial. Dutch Breast Cancer Research Group (BOOG). Lancet Oncol. 2018;19:1630–40.
13. Yu AF, Singh JC, Wang R, Liu JE, Eaton A, Oeffinger KC, et al. Cardiac safety of dual anti-HER2 therapy in the neoadjuvant setting for treatment of HER2-positive breast cancer. Oncologist. 2017;22:642–7.
14. Dahabreh IJ, Linardou H, Siannis F, et al. Trastuzumab in the adjuvant treatment of early-stage breast cancer: a systematic review and meta-analysis of randomized controlled trials. Oncologist. 2008;13:620–30.
15. Shen Y, Fujii T, Ueno NT, Tripathy D, Fu N, Zhou H, et al. Comparative efficacy of adjuvant trastuzumab-containing chemotherapies for patients with early HER2-positive primary breast cancer: a network meta-analysis. Breast Cancer Res Treat. 2019;173:1–9.
16. Tolaney SM, Guo H, Pernas S, Barry WT, Dillon DA, Ritterhouse L, et al. Seven-year follow-up analysis of adjuvant paclitaxel and trastuzumab trial for node-negative, human epidermal growth factor receptor 2-positive breast cancer. J Clin Oncol. 2019;37:1868–75.

17. von Minckwitz G, Huang CS, Mano MS, Loibl S, Mamounas EP, Untch M, et al.; KATHERINE Investigators. Trastuzumab emtansine for residual invasive HER2-positive breast cancer. N Engl J Med. 2019;380:617–28.
18. Piccart-Gebhart M, Holmes E, Baselga J, de Azambuja E, Dueck AC, Viale G, et al. Adjuvant lapatinib and trastuzumab for early human epidermal growth factor receptor 2 positive breast cancer: results from the randomized phase III adjuvant lapatinib and/or trastuzumab treatment optimization trial. J Clin Oncol. 2016;34:1034–42.
19. Martin M, Holmes FA, Ejlertsen B, Delaloge S, Moy B, Iwata H, et al.; ExteNET StudyGroup. Neratinib after trastuzumab-based adjuvant therapy in HER2-positive breast cancer (ExteNET): 5-year analysis of a randomised, double-blind, placebo-controlled, phase 3 trial. Lancet Oncol. 2017;18:1688-1700.
20. von Minckwitz G, Procter M, de Azambuja E, Zardavas D, Benyunes M, Viale G, et al. Adjuvant pertuzumab and trastuzumab in early HER2-positive breast cancer; APHINITY Steering Committee and Investigators. N Engl J Med. 2017;377:122–31.
21. Niraula S, Gyawali B. Optimal duration of adjuvant trastuzumab in treatment of early breast cancer: a meta-analysis of randomized controlled trials. Breast Cancer Res Treat. 2019;173:103–9.
22. Esposito A, Viale G, Criscitiello C, Curigliano G. Clinical perspective on escalating or de-escalating adjuvant therapy in HER2+ breast cancer. Expert Rev Clin Pharmacol. 2019;12:9–16.
23. Cameron D, Piccart-Gebhart MJ, Gelber RD, Procter M, Goldhirsch A, de Azambuja E, et al. 11 years' follow-up of trastuzumab after adjuvant chemotherapy in HER2-positive early breast cancer: final analysis of the HERceptin adjuvant (HERA) trial. Lancet. 2017;389:1195–2105.
24. Joensuu H, Bono P, Kataja V, Alanko T, Kokko R, Asola R, et al. Fluorouracil, epirubicin, and cyclophosphamide with either docetaxel or vinorelbine, with or without trastuzumab, as adjuvant treatments of breast cancer: final results of the FinHer trial. J Clin Oncol. 2009;27:5685–92.
25. Schneider BP, O'Neill A, Shen F, Sledge GW, Thor AD, Kahanic SP, et al. Pilot trial of paclitaxel-trastuzumab adjuvant therapy for early stage breast cancer: a trial of the ECOG-ACRIN cancer research group (E2198). Br J Cancer. 2015;113:1651–7.
26. Joensuu H, Fraser J, Wildiers H, Huovinen R, Auvinen P, Utriainen M, et al. Effect of adjuvant trastuzumab for a duration of 9 weeks vs 1 year with concomitant chemotherapy for early human epidermal growth factor receptor 2-positive breast cancer: the SOLD randomized clinical trial. JAMA Oncol. 2018;4:1199–206.
27. Conte P, Frassoldati A, Bisagni G, Brandes AA, Donadio M, Garrone O, et al.; Reader study level-I and level-II Groups. Nine weeks versus 1 year adjuvant trastuzumab in combination with chemotherapy: final results of the phase III randomized Short-HER study. Ann Oncol. 2018;29:2328–2333.
28. Pivot X, Romieu G, Debled M, Pierga JY, Kerbrat P, Bachelot T, et al. 6 months versus 12 months of adjuvant trastuzumab for patients with HER2-positive early breast cancer (PHARE): a randomised phase 3 trial. Lancet Oncol. 2013;14:741–8.
29. Mavroudis D, Saloustros E, Malamos N, Kakolyris S, Boukovinas I, Papakotoulas P, et al. Six versus 12 months of adjuvant trastuzumab in combination with dose-dense chemotherapy for women with HER2-positive breast cancer: a multicenter randomized study by the Hellenic Oncology Research Group (HORG). Ann Oncol. 2015;26:1333–40.
30. Earl HM, Hiller L, Vallier AL, Loi S, McAdam K, Hughes-Davies L, et al.; PERSEPHONE Steering Committee and Trial Investigators. 6 versus 12 months of adjuvant trastuzumab for HER2-positive early breast cancer (PERSEPHONE): 4-year disease-free survival results of a randomised phase 3 non-inferiority trial. Lancet. 2019;393:2599–2612.

Adjuvant Endocrine Therapy in Early Breast Cancer

Ashok S. Komaranchath

12.1 Introduction

It is thought that 20–30% of early breast cancers (EBCs) will ultimately develop distant metastases, and many of these patients will then succumb to their disease. These clinically inapparent metastases comprising of small numbers of individual or clumps of malignant cells can sometimes be found circulating in the blood and are referred to as micrometastases. There was a change in the concept of the natural history of breast cancer in the 1970s from the early Halstedian theory, which said that breast cancer was a local disease that turned systemic, to an alternative theory, which hypothesized that breast cancer was a systemic disease from its very beginning. This lead to a large number of clinical trials with various adjuvant therapies with hormonal agents, chemotherapeutic agents, or both. These trials indirectly supported the idea that micrometastases are indeed present in many patients at its onset and that adjuvant therapy to eradicate them improves disease-free survival and overall survival of patients to a remarkable extent. Even so, late recurrences do occur and in cases of hormone-positive breast cancer, may occur even decades after treatment of the primary tumor. It is postulated that these micrometastases may lie dormant and then get reactivated later on by unknown factors, or they grow so slowly that it may take years to decades for them to become clinically apparent. Breast cancer mortality rates have been falling steadily by approximately 2% per year since the 1990s with the widespread use of systemic adjuvant chemotherapy, endocrine therapy, and recently, with biological therapy. This chapter will be dealing with the clinical utility of hormonal manipulation in EBC.

A. S. Komaranchath (✉)
Aster Medcity, Kochi, Kerala, India

© Springer Nature Singapore Pte Ltd. 2021
B. Kunheri, D. K. Vijaykumar (eds.), *Management of Early Stage Breast Cancer*,
https://doi.org/10.1007/978-981-15-6171-9_12

12.2   History of Hormonal Manipulation

The potential role of hormone manipulation was first explored by George Thomas Bateson, who noticed that there was a loss of lactation in rabbits when bilateral oophorectomy was performed on them. Based on this, Beatson performed a bilateral oophorectomy on a premenopausal lady with unresectable breast cancer on October 3, 1895, after which she went into complete clinical remission and went on to live for another 40 years [1]. Stanley Boyd of Charing Cross Hospital compiled a series of 46 cases who underwent oophorectomy for breast cancer and found that only one-third of women had an objective response to the procedure and that the response lasted around a year [2]. Years later, in 1923, Edgar Allen and Edward Doisy discovered estrogen, an ovarian hormone that was found to play a pivotal role in regulating mammary tissue [3]. It took several decades of research into ablative hormonal methods before tamoxifen, a selective estrogen uptake modulator (SERM), was discovered by Harper and Walpole in 1967 [4]. The early concept of ovarian ablation explored by Beatson and Boyd was implemented into a randomized trial in the adjuvant setting by Cole in 1975 using ovarian irradiation. He found that there was a statistically significant reduction in the rates of distant metastases in patients whose ovaries were ablated and a slight increase in crude survival rates as well [5].

Definitive evidence for the benefit of adjuvant hormonal manipulation in early breast cancer was brought forth by the meta-analyses conducted by the Early Breast Cancer Trialists' Collaborative Group (EBCTCG), which established 5 years of tamoxifen as the standard of care. Later on, the aTTom and ATLAS trials confirmed the benefit of 10 years of tamoxifen over 5 years even in light of slightly increased adverse events. For postmenopausal breast cancer patients, the advent of aromatase inhibitors provided an even more effective method of hormonal manipulation. Three aromatase inhibitors were discovered in quick succession: anastrozole in 1995, letrozole in 1997, and exemestane in 1999. A first-in-class selective estrogen receptor degrader (SERD) called Fulvestrant, was approved for use in 2002 in metastatic breast cancer, but it has limited benefit in the adjuvant setting and has not been approved for the same. Everolimus, a derivative of sirolimus, which works as an mTOR (mammalian target of rapamycin) inhibitor, was found to have benefit in reversing hormonal resistance in metastatic breast cancer and was approved for use in July 2012 in conjunction with exemestane. Finally, after over a decade since the approval of fulvestrant, a new class of drugs called CDK4/6 inhibitors were discovered with the first of its kind, palbociclib, being approved for use in 2015. However, all CDK4/6 inhibitors are approved for use only in the metastatic setting and hence is outside the scope of this chapter.

12.3   Biology of Endocrine Therapy

The estrogen receptor (ER) protein is present in three-fourths of all postmenopausal breast cancers and 60% of all premenopausal patients. The estrogen receptor itself is a nuclear transcription factor, which is phosphorylated on binding with estrogen.

ER then homodimerizes and recruits CoA protein, and this receptor complex binds to target genes at specific estrogen response elements at their respective promoter sites [6]. Phosphorylation and activation of ER can also be achieved in the absence of estrogen via other signaling pathways. This is called ligand-independent ER activation [6]. Most of the ERs are present on the nucleus of the cell. However, studies have shown that in some breast cancer cells, a small subset of ERs lies outside the nucleus tethered to the cell membrane. This nonnuclear ER is thought to mediate what has been termed as nongenomic effects of estrogen and participates in activation of various growth factor pathways such as HER2, EGFR, and IGF1.

All forms of hormonal manipulation target the main ER pathways at one or more levels. Aromatase inhibitors and ovarian function suppression lower estrogen levels and block both genomic and nongenomic ligand-dependant activation of ER. SERMs such as tamoxifen alter the conformal state of estrogen receptor and hence produce either agonistic or antagonistic effects depending on the tissue in question. Hence, tamoxifen acts as an estrogen agonist at the liver, endometrium, bone, and even some genes in the breast. It acts as an antagonist in the breast tissue, blood vessels, and peripheral sites. Pure antagonists, such as fulvestrant, which acts as an ER downregulator, have no agonistic activity. This class of drugs have limited clinical data in the adjuvant setting, and a recent phase III trial, the GEICAM/2006-10, which was published in September 2017, showed no benefit of adding fulvestrant to anastrozole in the adjuvant setting in HR+/HER2− early breast cancers [7].

12.4 Selective Estrogen Receptor Modulators

The advantage of adjuvant tamoxifen, specifically in the node-negative setting, was established by the NSABP B-14 trial, which had over 2600 patients with histologically negative axillary nodes [8]. There were patients both above and below 50 years of age, and they were randomly assigned to receive placebo or tamoxifen for 5 years. There was a significant reduction in local and distant recurrences (78% vs. 65%, $p < 0.0001$) as well as overall survival (71% vs. 65%, $p = 0.0008$) with tamoxifen. Tamoxifen-treated patients also had an impressive 50% reduction in contralateral breast cancer. Long-term results showed that these benefits persist beyond 15 years of follow-up.

The landmark meta-analysis for adjuvant tamoxifen was put forward by the Early Breast Cancer Trialists' Collaborative Group (EBCTCG). In their publication in 2011, which covered over 70 trials including 20 trials of 5 years of tamoxifen spanning a total number of 21,457 patients, it was found that there was a significant increase in both DFS and OS in ER-positive patients who received at least 5 years of tamoxifen [9]. There was a significant reduction in disease recurrence from 0 to 4 years (while on tamoxifen) and to a lesser extent from 5 to 9 years (for 5 years after completion of tamoxifen). There was no further reduction in recurrence from 10 to 14 years after starting tamoxifen. In contrast to this, there was a significant reduction in mortality in these patients from 0 to 4 years, 5 to 9 years, and 10 to

Table 12.1 Results of 5 years of tamoxifen in patients with ER-positive tumors by years of follow-up

Years	Recurrence (*p*-value)	Mortality (*p*-value)
0–4	0.53 (<0.00001)	0.71 (<0.0001)
5–9	0.68 (<0.00001)	0.66 (<0.0001)
10–14	0.97 (NS)	0.68 (<0.0001)

Adapted from: Early Breast Cancer Trialists' Collaborative Group. Relevance of breast cancer hormone receptors and other factors to the efficacy of adjuvant tamoxifen: patient-level meta-analysis of randomized trials. Lancet. 2011;378:771–784. (Ref. no. [9])

14 years as well (Table 12.1). Another interesting conclusion was that there was a significant benefit with 5 years of tamoxifen in both pre- and postmenopausal women. In this meta-analysis, tamoxifen was also shown to be effective in node-positive breast cancers. The reduction in the odds of recurrence was 40%, 36%, and 44% for patients with negative nodes, one to three positive nodes, or four or more positive nodes, respectively. The 10-year recurrence rate for node-negative patients was 19% with tamoxifen versus 35% without tamoxifen, while the recurrence rate for node-positive patients was 42% with tamoxifen and 57% without tamoxifen. With these data, 5 years of adjuvant tamoxifen became the standard of care at that time for premenopausal women.

Over a decade after the NSABP B-14 trial was published, two trials assessing even longer use of tamoxifen (10 years vs. 5 years) were presented. The aTTom (adjuvant Tamoxifen—To offer more?) trial from the United Kingdom randomized nearly 7000 patients to 5 years of tamoxifen compared to extended tamoxifen for 10 years. It concluded that in ER-positive disease, continuing tamoxifen to year 10 rather than just to year 5 produced further reductions in recurrence from year 7 onward, and in breast cancer mortality after the tenth year [10]. A similar trial in the United States called ATLAS (Adjuvant Tamoxifen: Longer Against Shorter), which had recruited nearly 13,000 women, was published in the *Lancet* in 2012 [11]. By continuing tamoxifen for 10 years, there was significant reduction in recurrence ($p = 0.002$), overall mortality ($p = 0.01$), and breast cancer-specific deaths ($p = 0.01$). A reduction in breast cancer mortality for extended tamoxifen was only seen after 10 years (RR = 0.97 vs. 0.71), perhaps due to the known carryover effect of just 5 years of tamoxifen during years 5–9. The cumulative risk for recurrence during years 5–14 for extended tamoxifen was 21% compared to 25% for patients stopping at 5 years. The risk of breast cancer death during years 5–14 was 12% for continued tamoxifen compared to 15% for the control group. Well-known tamoxifen side effects were higher in women assigned to 10 years of tamoxifen as expected. However, these were counterbalanced by the favorable effects. Relative risks for pulmonary embolus (1.87) and endometrial cancer (1.74) were higher, but mortality was not significantly affected. There was a significant reduction in ischemic heart disease (0.76, $p = 0.02$) for continuing tamoxifen for 10 years. An interesting fact was that for both these trials, a large proportion of trial patients were not ER positive or ER status was unknown.

Due to these reasons, currently, both NCCN and ESMO guidelines [12] recommend 5 years of tamoxifen as adjuvant therapy, and if the patient remains premenopausal during the first 5 years of therapy, then one may "consider" giving another 5 years of tamoxifen for the patient.

12.5   Tamoxifen in the Elderly

An early study by the Eastern Cooperative Oncology Group (ECOG) in 1993 randomized 180 patients more than or equal to 65 years of age to tamoxifen or placebo for 2 years [13]. There were significant reductions in recurrence and borderline significant reductions in mortality, and it was well tolerated. Tamoxifen also reduced the incidence of contralateral breast cancers. However, nonadherence was found to be quite high, and there was also found to be an increase in other-cause mortality. There have been many small trials that have assessed the role of tamoxifen as the sole therapy without surgery in elderly operable primary breast cancer patients [14, 15], which have found that there was no difference in overall survival or time to distant metastases when tamoxifen alone was compared to mastectomy alone. This was confirmed in a large Cochrane review of seven trials [16]. Hence, hormonal therapy alone in the elderly should only be used for temporary disease control, and even then, in view of a relatively higher risk of thromboembolic phenomena, an AI may be preferred.

12.6   Ancillary Benefits and Adverse Events of Tamoxifen

Benefits: Tamoxifen has been found to have a beneficial effect on serum lipids and cardiovascular health. Long-term follow-up of the Cancer Research UK "Over 50s" trial showed a significant reduction in cardiovascular disease in women aged 50–59 years of age when they took 5 years of tamoxifen as compared to 2 years as adjuvant [17]. The Breast Cancer Prevention Trial (BCPT) run by the NSABP gave further evidence that tamoxifen reduced cardiovascular mortality [18]. Tamoxifen has estrogen receptor agonistic properties in the bone. In postmenopausal women, long-term tamoxifen treatment stabilizes the bone density of the peripheral skeleton and increases the bone density of the axial skeleton [19]. In premenopausal women, however, tamoxifen may decrease bone mineral density by antagonizing the more potent activity of endogenous estrogen [20]. Incidence of fractures was found to be markedly reduced with tamoxifen as compared to an aromatase inhibitor [21]. The 2005 EBCTCG meta-analysis has shown that 5 years of tamoxifen can also reduce contralateral breast cancer incidence by as much as 50% in ER-positive patients [22].

Toxicity: In general, tamoxifen is well tolerated, and only <5% of patients usually stop the drug due to its toxicity. The most frequent adverse events of tamoxifen are menopausal symptoms, including hot flashes, insomnia, arthralgia, depression, and fatigue. Vaginal dryness and dyspareunia, along with reduced libido, are also common complaints. There is a definite increase in thromboembolic events with tamoxifen, and this occurs even more frequently when used in combination with chemotherapy and when patients on tamoxifen undergo surgery. This was documented in the BIG 1–98 trial when compared to letrozole [23]. However, severe thromboembolic events occur in <1% of all patients. Leucopenia and thrombocytopenia have also been reported with tamoxifen but with very little clinical significance. Long-term follow-up of the NSABP B-14 trial showed that tamoxifen was associated with a relative risk of 2.2 compared with population-based rates of endometrial cancer from SEER data [24].

The risk of endometrial cancer with tamoxifen is related to the duration of therapy and is higher in obese women and women who have received prior hormone replacement therapy [25]. This was confirmed in the ATLAS trial where the cumulative risk of endometrial cancer was 3.1% with 10 years of tamoxifen and only 1.6% for patients treated with 5 years [11]. Mortality, however, was very low in both arms, 0.4% versus 0.2%, respectively. After several studies, it was determined that neither transvaginal ultrasound (TVUS) nor regular screening endometrial biopsies were effective in diagnosing endometrial cancer at an early stage. Routine TVUS had a significant number of false positives and thereby increased iatrogenic morbidity. Hence, these procedures are reserved for only for patients with symptoms such as abnormal uterine bleeding. The role of systemic or intrauterine progestins has not been determined so far.

Tamoxifen was found to be a hepatocarcinogen in rats, but no such effects except for mild steatohepatitis and transaminitis have been observed in humans. Potential for increased cerebrovascular accidents was also explored, and the ATLAS as well as the ATAC and BIG 1–98 showed no increase in CVAs as compared to an aromatase inhibitor.

12.7   Aromatase Inhibitors

Aromatase inhibitors (AIs) block aromatase and thereby the synthesis of estrogen in various tissues. This enzyme is normally present in fat, muscle, and brain, as well as tumor tissue, and it converts adrenal androgens to estrogen. There are two different types of AIs: the nonsteroidal aromatase inhibitors (anastrozole and letrozole), which bind to aromatase in a reversible fashion, and the steroidal aromatase inhibitors (exemestane), which form an irreversible complex with aromatase. As there is a small difference in the mechanism of action, there is incomplete cross-resistance and hence breast cancer patients who progress on a reversible inhibitor may frequently respond to an irreversible aromatase inhibitor.

Aromatase inhibitors have little or no action on the estrogen production in the ovary and hence are generally ineffective in premenopausal ladies. In fact, the reduced feedback of estrogen to the hypothalamus and pituitary increases gonadotropin secretion, which in turn may stimulate the premenopausal ovary and lead to an increase in aromatase and subsequently estrogen production in the ovary [26].

The current guidelines mandate that patients should be confirmed to be postmenopausal by estimating the FSH/LH levels as well as serum estradiol levels before starting on aromatase inhibitors.

There have been several phase III RCTs on the use of adjuvant aromatase inhibitors. The ATAC (Arimidex, Tamoxifen, Alone or in Combination) trial was the first of them. There were over 9000 patients randomized after surgery to receive anastrozole, tamoxifen, or their combination. However, the combination arm was discontinued at 33 months of follow-up after this group was found to be inferior to anastrozole monotherapy [27]. This trial reported a DFS benefit for the anastrozole arm over the tamoxifen arm in 2002 as well as in multiple updates of the trial (HR = 0.85; p = 0.003). There was also a significantly lower rate of ipsilateral and contralateral breast cancer recurrences in the anastrozole arm. However, long-term follow-up of the trial has not shown any clear OS benefit (HR = 0.97; p = 0.7). The next large trial recruited over 8000 postmenopausal women and compared letrozole with tamoxifen in a four-arm study called BIG (Breast International Group) 1–98 trial. The study arms were tamoxifen for 5 years, letrozole for 5 years, tamoxifen for 2 years followed by letrozole for 3 years, and finally, letrozole for 2 years followed by tamoxifen for 3 years [23]. There was a significant DFS (HR = 0.86) and OS (HR = 0.87) benefit for letrozole monotherapy as compared to tamoxifen in these patients. Moreover, they found that the addition of letrozole at any stage of the 5 years of adjuvant hormonal therapy was superior to 5 years of tamoxifen alone. This cemented the place of AIs as the drugs of choice in postmenopausal women with HR-positive invasive breast cancer. However, a large RCT comparing tamoxifen versus exemestane (Tamoxifen Exemestane Adjuvant Multinational—TEAM trial) failed to show a clear-cut DFS advantage for exemestane over tamoxifen (p = 0.12) [28]. There have been a few studies that assessed the sequential administration of an AI following a few years of tamoxifen. The first of these called the Intergroup Exemestane Study (IES) enrolled nearly 5000 patients and randomized them to taking 5 years of tamoxifen vs taking 2–3 years of tamoxifen followed by 2–3 years of exemestane. There was a clear DFS benefit when exemestane was used (HR = 0.76; p = 0.0001) and an absolute benefit of 3.3% [29]. Both ARNO95/ABCSG8 and ITA (Italian Tamoxifen Anastrozole) trials used anastrozole in sequence with tamoxifen and were reported in a combined analysis with over 4000 patients and showed a significant benefit in both DFS (HR 0.59; p < 0.0001) and OS (HR 0.71; p = 0.04) [30].

Several trials evaluated extending adjuvant therapy with AIs in postmenopausal women to a total of 10 years. The largest was the NCIC-MA17 trial, where over 5000 women who had completed 5 years of tamoxifen were randomly assigned to placebo versus letrozole. The study showed a significant improvement in DFS in the letrozole group in the first interim analysis and was terminated early. This benefit was confirmed on longer follow-up (HR = 0.58; p < 0.0001) [31]. An even longer extension of hormonal treatment was studied in the MA17R trial published in July 2016 in which 1900 women who received 5 years of letrozole following 5 years of tamoxifen were randomized to 5 more years of letrozole versus placebo. The results showed a significant reduction in DFS (HR = 0.66; p = 0.01) but no benefit in OS (HR = 0.97; p = 0.83) [32]. In an ASCO practice update published in the *Journal of Clinical Oncology* in 2014, it was recommended that all women who are pre- or perimenopausal and have received 5 years of adjuvant tamoxifen must be offered 10 years (total duration) of tamoxifen. If women happen to be postmenopausal and have received 5 years of adjuvant tamoxifen, they should be offered the choice of continuing tamoxifen or switching to an aromatase inhibitor for 10 years of total adjuvant endocrine therapy [33].

In an oral presentation at the San Antonio Breast Cancer Symposium 2017 of the ABCSG-16 trial by Gnant et al., he concluded that after 5 years of adjuvant endocrine therapy (tamoxifen or AI or sequence), 2 additional years of anastrozole are sufficient for extended adjuvant therapy and that a further extension to 5 additional years did not yield additional outcome benefit but added toxicity [34]. Hence, a total of 7 years of hormonal therapy may become the new standard for postmenopausal patients with hormone-positive cancers in the adjuvant setting once more matured data is released.

Toxicity: AIs significantly suppress plasma estrogen levels but do not bind to ER. Hence, the partial agonistic activity seen with tamoxifen and the consequent adverse events are not seen with AIs. However, they also lack the desirable effects of tamoxifen on lipid levels and the skeletal system. It is important to note that even with a detrimental effect on serum lipids, AIs seem to have a lower incidence of ischemic cerebrovascular events. AIs also have lower rates of venous thromboembolic events, hot flashes, and vaginal bleeding. However, fractures, disorders of lipid metabolism, and musculoskeletal pain are more frequent with aromatase inhibitors. Table 12.2 outlines the various adverse events noted in the ATAC trial and the *p*-value denoting its significance in comparison to the same events with tamoxifen. The ATAC trial did not study the difference in cardiovascular disease, but a meta-analysis of seven trials showed that there was a 26% increase in risk of CVS disease

Table 12.2 Adverse events of tamoxifen vs anastrozole observed in the ATAC trial

Adverse event	Anastrozole (%)	Tamoxifen (%)	Comparative *p*-value
Hot flushes	35.7	40.9	<0.0001
Fatigue/tiredness	15.6	15.1	0.5
Mood disturbances	15.5	15.2	0.7
Nausea and vomiting	10.5	10.2	0.7
Musculoskeletal	35.6	29.4	<0.0001
Vaginal bleeding	5.4	10.2	<0.0001
Vaginal discharge	3.5	13.2	<0.0001
Endometrial cancer	0.2	0.8	0.02
Fractures	11.0	7.7	<0.0001
Ischemic heart disease	4.1	3.4	NS
Cerebrovascular events	2.0	2.8	0.03
Any venous thromboembolic events	2.8	4.5	<0.0004

Adapted from: Baum M, Budzar AU, Cuzick J, et al. Anastrozole alone or in combination with tamoxifen versus tamoxifen alone for adjuvant treatment of postmenopausal women with early breast cancer: first results of the ATAC randomised trial. Lancet 2002;359(9324): 2131–2139

with AIs [35]. The incidence of arthralgias, joint stiffness, and musculoskeletal disorders are also increased in patients taking AIs and are collectively termed as AI-associated musculoskeletal syndrome (AIMSS). There have also been reports of higher incidence of cognitive dysfunction in patients taking AIs as compared with those not on any hormonal treatment.

Which AI to use in postmenopausal women? All three AIs are thought to have comparable efficacy and side-effect profiles in the adjuvant setting. This has been proven by multiple trials such as the NCIC-MA.27 trial, which compared exemestane to anastrozole [36], and the Femara Versus Anastrozole Clinical Evaluation (FACE) trial, which compared letrozole and anastrozole [37]. However, as a large adjuvant trial with exemestane versus tamoxifen (TEAM) has failed to show a DFS difference, it may be prudent to start with a nonsteroidal AI, i.e., either letrozole or anastrozole.

12.8   Ovarian Ablation in the Adjuvant Setting

In premenopausal women, the utility of ovarian ablation in the adjuvant setting was also studied. Ovarian ablation could be achieved in one of three ways: temporary ovarian function suppression using GnRH agonists or permanent ablation with either bilateral oophorectomy or ovarian irradiation. The earliest data concerning ovarian function suppression (OFS) came from the 2005 EBCTCG meta-analysis where nearly 8000 women younger than 50 years of age with ER-positive or ER-unknown disease were randomized into trials of ovarian ablation by surgery or irradiation, or of ovarian suppression by treatment with a GnRH agonist [38]. There was found to be a definite benefit of ovarian ablation or suppression on both recurrence and breast cancer mortality.

The most recent evidence in favor of OFS came from two large phase III RCTs involving premenopausal women with operable, hormone-positive early breast cancer: the TEXT (Tamoxifen and EXemestane Trial) and the SOFT (Suppression of Ovarian Function Trial) trials [39]. There were over 2500 patients in each trial, and the use of chemotherapy was optional. In the SOFT trial, 3000 premenopausal women were randomized into one of three arms: tamoxifen alone, tamoxifen plus OFS, or exemestane plus OFS. OFS was achieved by a choice of bilateral oophorectomy, ovarian irradiation, or triptorelin at a dose of 3.75 mg intramuscular once in 28 days. In the TEXT trial, around 2600 premenopausal women were randomized to one of two arms: tamoxifen plus OFS or exemestane plus OFS after surgery. In both trials, women did not receive any bone-modifying agents. After a median follow-up of 8 years, the SOFT trial reported improved 8-year DFS rate in tamoxifen plus OFS as compared to tamoxifen alone (83% vs 79%; HR = 0.76), as well as for exemestane plus OFS compared to tamoxifen alone (86% vs 79%; HR 0.65). There was also a modest improvement in overall survival for both tamoxifen plus OFS and exemestane plus OFS as compared to tamoxifen alone (93.3% vs 92.1% vs 91.5%). However, the 8-year freedom from distant recurrence was similar in patients receiving tamoxifen plus OFS as compared to tamoxifen alone and only a modest improvement for exemestane plus OFS compared to tamoxifen alone [40].

It was seen that toxicities were more among those receiving OFS across both the TEXT and SOFT trials. Of these, osteoporosis and musculoskeletal adverse events were more common in those patients receiving exemestane plus OFS. Grade III and IV toxicities were also more common in patients who received OFS with 32% in the exemestane plus OFS group, 31% in tamoxifen plus OFS group, and about 25% in the tamoxifen-only group.

Several exploratory and subgroup analyses within TEXT and SOFT have indicated that patients with a higher risk of relapse may have an enhanced benefit with ovarian function suppression when added to either tamoxifen or AIs [39–41]. In these trials, a composite risk score was calculated using a method similar to that used in the BIG 1–98 trial to determine the patients at a higher risk of recurrence. In general, younger age (≤35 years), large tumor size, high grade, presence of lymphovascular invasion, and/or a high-risk score in a genomic assay (Oncotype DX, Mammaprint, etc.) can be considered to have a higher risk of recurrence.

12.9   Conclusions and Future Directions

Hormonal therapy is perhaps the oldest form of targeted therapy and has been around in the form of tamoxifen for over 50 years now. In western countries, there has been a nearly 25% reduction in population-based mortality over the past 20 years, and it has largely been attributed to the widespread use of adjuvant therapy, especially hormonal agents such as tamoxifen, and to a lesser extent, chemotherapy [42]. Current management standards in adjuvant hormonal therapy may be summarized as follows:
Premenopausal women:

- Adjuvant therapy with at least 5 years of tamoxifen is mandatory, and with patients likely to have a higher risk of recurrence, a total of 10 years of tamoxifen must be offered.
- Ovarian function suppression may be offered to patients with high recurrence risk and may be combined with either tamoxifen or an AI. However, as there is a lack of robust data to support AIs over tamoxifen, a combination of OFS with tamoxifen may be preferred.
- Aromatase inhibitors and pure ER degraders such as fulvestrant have no role in premenopausal women at present.
- Patients need not undergo TVS or endometrial biopsy unless they present with symptoms of abnormal uterine bleeding while on tamoxifen.

Postmenopausal women:

- Aromatase inhibitors have been proven to have a modest but clear advantage over tamoxifen in postmenopausal women. If a patient has been started on tamoxifen initially, AIs should be added in sequence after 2–3 years of tamoxifen.
- Total duration of therapy is controversial at present, but the 2014 ASCO practice update recommends continuing hormonal therapy for 10 years in postmeno-

pausal women. There are emerging data to suggest that 5 years of AIs following 2 years of tamoxifen (total of 7 years of therapy) may have equal efficacy and reduced adverse events.

- It is better to start tamoxifen for those patients who are perimenopausal and those who develop amenorrhea after chemotherapy. If they remain amenorrheic with hormonal assays in the postmenopausal range after 2 years, they may be switched to aromatase inhibitors.
- Patients on aromatase inhibitors should monitor their serum lipids and bone mineral density periodically.

There are still many unanswered questions regarding adjuvant hormonal therapy such as the exact role of ovarian ablation and in which subset of patients, the optimal duration of adjuvant hormonal therapy, and the role of selective ER degraders in the adjuvant setting. In this era of targeted therapy and immuno-oncology, the respective roles of targeted agents such as mTOR or PI3K inhibitors as well as immunotherapeutic agents need to be defined in future clinical trials.

References

1. Beatson GT. On the treatment of inoperable cases of carcinoma of the mamma: suggestions for a new method of treatment, with illustrative cases. Lancet. 1896;148(3803):162–5.
2. Boyd S. On oophorectomy in the treatment of cancer. Br Med J. 1897;2(1918):890–6.
3. Allen E, Doisy EA. Landmark article Sept 8, 1923: an ovarian hormone: preliminary report on its localization, extraction and partial purification, and action in test animals. JAMA. 1983;250(19):2681–3.
4. Harper MJ, Walpole AL. A new derivative of triphenylethylene: effect on implantation and mode of action in rats. J Reprod Fertil. 1967;13(1):101–19.
5. Cole M. A clinical trial of an artificial menopause in carcinoma of the breast. INSERM. 1975:143–50.
6. Osborne CK, Schiff R. Mechanisms of endocrine resistance in breast cancer. Annu Rev Med. 2011;62:233–47.
7. Ruiz-Borrego M, Martin Jimenez M, Ruiz A, Lluch A, Ramos M, Cruz Jurado J, et al. Phase III evaluating the addition of fulvestrant (F) to anastrozol (A) as adjuvant therapy in postmenopausal women with hormone receptor positive HER2 negative (HR+/HER2-) early breast cancer (EBC): results from the GEICAM/2006–10 study. Ann Oncol. 2017;28(issue suppl_5).
8. Fisher B, Jeong JH, Dignam J, et al. Findings from recent National Surgical Adjuvant Breast and Bowel Project adjuvant studies in stage I breast cancer. J Natl Cancer Inst Monogr. 2001;30:62–6.
9. Early Breast Cancer Trialists' Collaborative Group (EBCTCG), Davies C, Goodwin J, et al. Relevance of breast cancer hormone receptors and other factors to the efficacy of adjuvant tamoxifen: patient-level meta-analysis of randomised trials. Lancet. 2011;378(9793):771–84.
10. Gray RG, Rea D, Handley K, et al. aTTom: long-term effects of continuing adjuvant tamoxifen to 10 years versus stopping at 5 years in 6,953 women with early breast cancer. American society of clinical oncology annual meeting 2013. Chicago, IL.
11. Davies C, Pan H, Godwin J, et al. Long-term effects of continuing adjuvant tamoxifen to 10 years versus stopping at 5 years after diagnosis of oestrogen receptor-positive breast cancer: ATLAS, a randomised trial. Lancet. 2012;381(9869):805–16.
12. Senkus E, Kyriakides S, Ohno S, Penault-Llorca F, Poortmans P, Rutgers E, Zackrisson S, Cardoso F. Primary breast cancer: ESMO clinical practice guidelines for diagnosis, treat-

ment and follow-up on behalf of the ESMO guidelines committee. Ann Oncol. 2015;26(issue suppl_5):v8–v30.

13. Cummings FJ, Gray R, Tormey DC, et al. Adjuvant tamoxifen versus placebo in elderly women with node-positive breast cancer: long-term followup and causes of death. J Clin Oncol. 1993;11(1):29–35.

14. Mustacchi G, Ceccherini R, Pluchinotta A, et al. Results of adjuvant treatment in breast cancer women aged more than 70: Italian cooperative group experience. Tumori. 2002;88(1 Suppl 1):S83–5.

15. Chakrabarti J, Kenny FS, Syed BM, et al. A randomised trial of mastectomy only versus tamoxifen for treating elderly patients with operable primary breast cancer—final results at 20-year follow-up. Crit Rev Oncol Hematol. 2011;78(3):260–4.

16. Hind D, Wyld L, Beverley CB, et al. Surgery versus primary endocrine therapy for operable primary breast cancer in elderly women (70 years plus). Cochrane Database Syst Rev. 2006;(1):CD004272.

17. Hackshaw A, Roughton M, Forsyth S, et al. Long-term benefits of 5 years of tamoxifen: 10-year follow-up of a large randomized trial in women at least 50 years of age with early breast cancer. J Clin Oncol. 2011;29(13):1657–63.

18. Reis SE, Costantino JP, Wickerham DL, et al. Cardiovascular effects of tamoxifen in women with and without heart disease: breast cancer prevention trial. National Surgical Adjuvant Breast and Bowel Project Breast Cancer Prevention Trial Investigators. J Natl Cancer Inst. 2001;93(1):16–21.

19. Love RR, Mazess RB, Barden HS, et al. Effects of tamoxifen on bone mineral density in post-menopausal women with breast cancer. N Engl J Med. 1992;326(13):852–6.

20. Powles TJ, Hickish T, Kanis JA, et al. Effect of tamoxifen on bone mineral density measured by dual-energy x-ray absorptiometry in healthy premenopausal and postmenopausal women. J Clin Oncol. 1996;14(1):78–84.

21. Amir E, Seruga B, Niraula S, et al. Toxicity of adjuvant endocrine therapy in postmenopausal breast cancer patients: a systematic review and meta-analysis. J Natl Cancer Inst. 2011;103(17):1299–309.

22. Group, E.B.C.T.C. Effects of chemotherapy and hormonal therapy for early breast cancer on recurrence and 15-year survival: an overview of the randomised trials. Lancet. 2005;365(9472):1687–717.

23. Regan MM, Neven P, Giobbie-Harder A, et al. Assessment of letrozole and tamoxifen alone and in sequence for postmenopausal women with steroid hormone receptor-positive breast cancer: the BIG 1-98 randomised clinical trial at 8.1 years median follow-up. Lancet Oncol. 2011;12(12):1101–8.

24. Fisher B, Costantino JP, Redmond CK, et al. Endometrial cancer in tamoxifen treated breast cancer patients: findings from the National Surgical Adjuvant Breast and Bowel Project (NSABP) B-14. J Natl Cancer Inst. 1994;86(7):527–37.

25. Bernstein L, Deapen D, Cerhan JR, et al. Tamoxifen therapy for breast cancer and endometrial cancer risk. J Natl Cancer Inst. 1999;91(19):1654–62.

26. Miller WR. Biological rationale for endocrine therapy in breast cancer. Best Pract Res Clin Endocrinol Metab. 2004;18(1):1–32.

27. Forbes JF, Cuzick J, Buzdar A, et al. Effect of anastrozole and tamoxifen as adjuvant treatment for early-stage breast cancer: 100-month analysis of the ATAC trial. Lancet Oncol. 2008;9(1):45–53.

28. van de Velde CJ, Rea D, Seynaeve C, et al. Adjuvant tamoxifen and exemestane in early breast cancer (TEAM): a randomised phase 3 trial. Lancet. 2011;377(9762):321–31.

29. Coombes RC, Kilburn LS, Snowdon CF, et al. Survival and safety of exemestane versus tamoxifen after 2–3 years' tamoxifen treatment (Intergroup Exemestane Study): a randomised controlled trial. Lancet. 2007;369(9561):559–70.

30. Jonat W, Gnant M, Boccardo F, et al. Effectiveness of switching from adjuvant tamoxifen to anastrozole in postmenopausal women with hormone-sensitive early-stage breast cancer: a meta-analysis. Lancet Oncol. 2006;7(12):991–6.

31. Goss PE, Ingle JN, Martino S, et al. Randomized trial of letrozole following tamoxifen as extended adjuvant therapy in receptor-positive breast cancer: updated findings from NCIC CTG MA.17. J Natl Cancer Inst. 2005;97(17):1262–71.
32. Goss PE, Ingle JN, Pritchard KI, et al. Extending aromatase-inhibitor adjuvant therapy to 10 years. N Engl J Med. 2016;375:209.
33. Burstein HJ, Temin S, Anderson H, et al. Adjuvant endocrine therapy for women with hormone receptor–positive breast cancer: American society of clinical oncology clinical practice guideline focused update. J Clin Oncol. 2014;32(21):2255–69.
34. Gnant M, Steger G, Greil R, Fitzal F, Mlineritsch B, Manfreda D, et al. A prospective randomized multi-center phase-III trial of additional 2 versus additional 5 years of Anastrozole after initial 5 years of adjuvant endocrine therapy—results from 3,484 postmenopausal women in the ABCSG-16 trial. SABCS. 2017:GS3-01.
35. Amir E, Seruga B, Niraula S, et al. Toxicity of adjuvant endocrine therapy in postmenopausal breast cancer patients: a systematic review and metaanalysis. J Natl Cancer Inst. 2011;103(17):1299–309.
36. Goss PE, Ingle JN, Pritchard KI, et al. Exemestane versus anastrozole in postmenopausal women with early breast cancer: NCIC CTG MA.27—a randomized controlled phase III trial. J Clin Oncol. 2013;31:1398.
37. Smith I, Yardley D, Burris H, et al. Comparative efficacy and safety of adjuvant letrozole versus anastrozole in postmenopausal patients with hormone receptor-positive, node- positive early breast cancer: final results of the randomized phase III femara versus anastrozole clinical evaluation (FACE) trial. J Clin Oncol. 2017;35:1041.
38. Early Breast Cancer Trialists' Collaborative Group. Effects of chemotherapy and hormonal therapy for early breast cancer on recurrence and 15-year survival: an overview of the randomised trials. Lancet. 2005;365(9472):1687–717.
39. Pagani O, Regan MM, Walley BA, et al. Adjuvant exemestane with ovarian suppression in premenopausal breast cancer. N Engl J Med. 2014;371:107.
40. Francis PA, Pagani O, Fleming GF, et al. Tailoring adjuvant endocrine therapy for premenopausal breast cancer. N Engl J Med. 2018;379:122.
41. Regan MM, Francis PA, Pagani O, et al. Absolute benefit of adjuvant endocrine therapies for premenopausal women with hormone receptor-positive, human epidermal growth factor receptor 2-negative early breast cancer: TEXT and SOFT trials. J Clin Oncol. 2016;34:2221.
42. Peto R, Boreham J, Clarke M, et al. UK and USA breast cancer deaths down 25% in year 2000 at ages 20–69 years. Lancet. 2000;355(9217):1822.

.

Ductal Carcinoma In Situ: Current Consensus in Management

13

Vineeta Goel and Deepti Sharma

13.1 Introduction

Ductal carcinoma in situ (DCIS) is characterized as the proliferation of abnormal cells of mammary ductal epithelial with neither evidence of invasion beyond the basement membrane nor involvement of the surrounding breast stroma. It is usually confined to the breast with involvement of axillary lymph node in 0–5% of cases and lacks the ability to metastasize [1].

Due to far-reaching utilization of screening mammography, the rate of DCIS has increased [2]. Earlier, <5% of mammary cancers were DCIS. At present, 15–30% of the cancers detected in mammography screening programs are DCIS. The incidence of DCIS in the United States has markedly increased from 5.8 per 100,000 females in the 1970s to 32.5 per 100,000 females in 2004 and afterward arrived at a plateau [2].

13.2 Epidemiology

Risk factors: Risk factors for the development of DCIS are similar to those for invasive carcinoma, including family history, early menarche, late menopause, delayed age of first live birth, nulliparity, history of breast biopsy for benign disease, obesity, increased breast density, and BRCA1/2 gene mutation [3, 4].

V. Goel
Radiation Oncology, Max Institute of Oncology, Delhi, India

D. Sharma (✉)
Max Institute of Oncology, Delhi, India

Radiation Oncology, Institute of Liver and Biliary Sciences, New Delhi, India

© Springer Nature Singapore Pte Ltd. 2021
B. Kunheri, D. K. Vijaykumar (eds.), *Management of Early Stage Breast Cancer*,
https://doi.org/10.1007/978-981-15-6171-9_13

13.3   Clinical Features

The majority of patients with DCIS are screen detected with no palpable breast lump.

13.4   Imaging Studies

1. Mammography

    Abnormal mammography findings are present in approximately 95% of new cases of DCIS, of which microcalcifications are most common (Fig. 13.1a, b), followed by noncalcified abnormalities, with asymmetric densities identified in 10%, dominant masses in 8%, and abnormal galactograms (performed for evaluation of nipple discharge) in 6% of cases [5]. The typical forms of calcifications related to DCIS are amorphous, coarse and fine pleomorphic, and fine linear. Linear and branching calcifications are often associated with high-grade DCIS and necrosis, whereas fine and granular calcifications are commonly associated with low-grade DCIS (Figs. 13.2 and 13.3).

2. Breast ultrasound

    Breast ultrasound findings are used to guide interventional procedures such as hookwire localization biopsy/excision. As per the JABTS (Japanese Association of Breast and Thyroid Sonology) classification system, the hypoechoic areas in the mammary gland (48.6%) was the most common finding followed by solid masses (28.0%) and duct abnormalities (10.2%) or mixed masses (8.1%). Distortion (1.3%), clustered microcysts (1.4%), and echogenic foci without a hypoechoic area (2.5%) were less frequent [6].

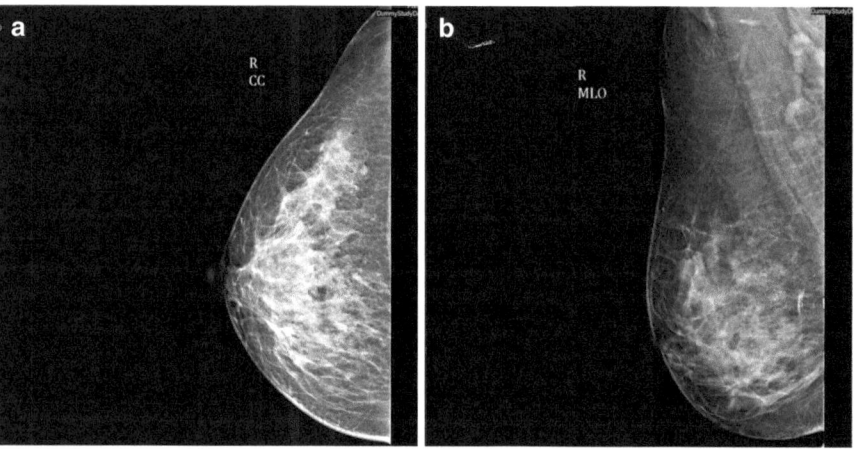

Fig. 13.1 (**a**, **b**) Mammography of right breast in craniocaudal view and right medial lateral oblique view showing microcalcification

Fig. 13.2 Linear and branching calcifications associated with high-grade DCIS

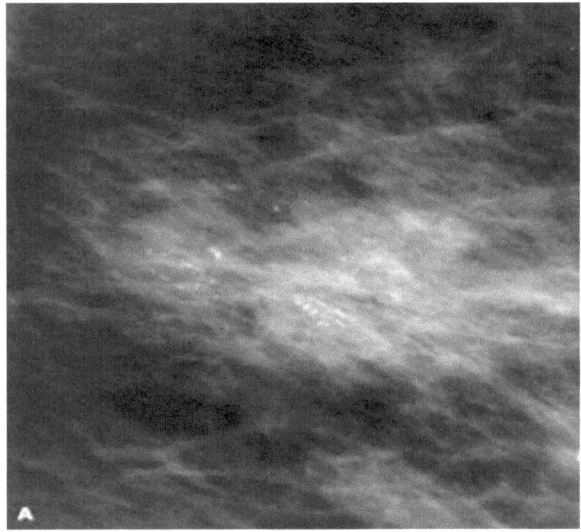

Fig. 13.3 Fine and granular calcifications associated with low-grade DCIS

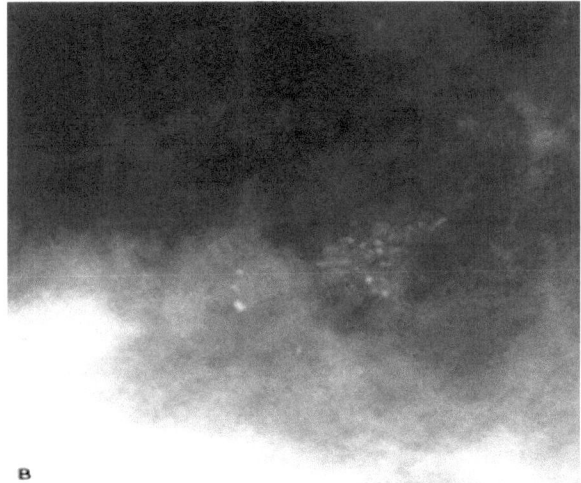

3. Breast MRI

Sometimes, contrast-enhanced dynamic MRI of the breast is used to complement mammography in the detection of DCIS because it is more sensitive to detect high-grade lesions. On MRI, DCIS frequently manifests as clumped non-masslike enhancement, in a ductal or segmental distribution, with rapid initial contrast uptake with plateau, persistent, or washout kinetics in the delayed phase. MRI is often used in patients with dense breasts and in high-risk groups such as patients with a family history of BRCA1/2 mutation.

13.5   Diagnosis

The diagnosis of DCIS is confirmed by a breast biopsy, such as a core or excisional biopsy, typically for an abnormal lesion detected by a screening mammogram. Stereotactic core biopsy is an option for individuals with microcalcification detected on mammogram or MRI [7]. Ultrasound-guided biopsies can be performed for evaluation of a palpable or nonpalpable mass with or without calcification.

- *Pathology*

  Historically, DCIS has been divided into five architectural subtypes: the majority of cases show a mixture of patterns [8].

1. Comedo DCIS (Fig. 13.4).
2. Noncomedo DCIS (Figs. 13.5 and 13.6).
   (a) Papillary DCIS.
   (b) Solid DCIS.
   (c) Cribriform DCIS.
   (d) Micropapillary DCIS.

   Diagnostic criteria for grade:

- Low grade (Fig. 13.7a).
   - Round, regular to mildly irregular nuclei up to 2–3 times the size of an RBC.
   - No comedo necrosis.
- Intermediate grade
   - Round, regular to mildly irregular nuclei up to 2–3 times the size of an RBC.
   - Substantial comedo necrosis.
- High grade (Fig. 13.7b).
   - Pleomorphic nuclei >3 times the size of an RBC.
   - Substantial comedo necrosis usually present.

Fig. 13.4 DCIS: Comedo pattern with necrosis and microcalcification (H&E ×100)

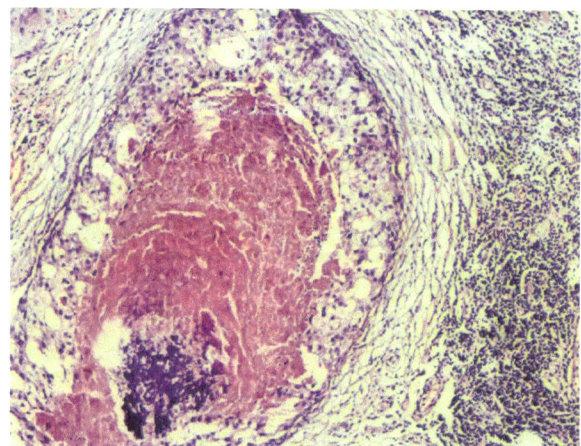

Fig. 13.5 DCIS:
Noncomedo papillary
pattern (H&E ×100)

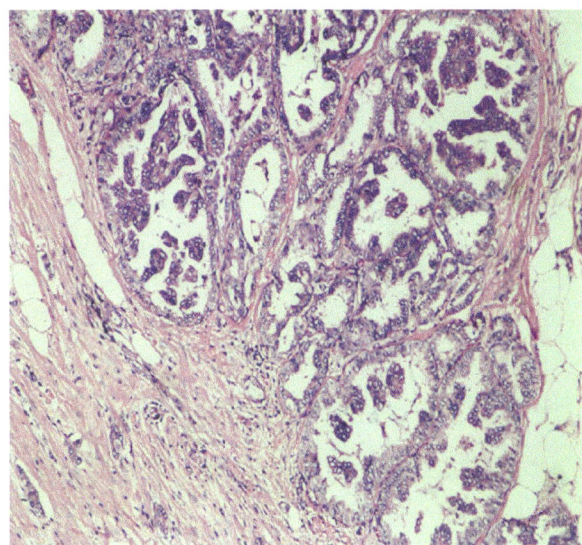

Fig. 13.6 DCIS:
Noncomedo cribriform
pattern (H&E ×100)

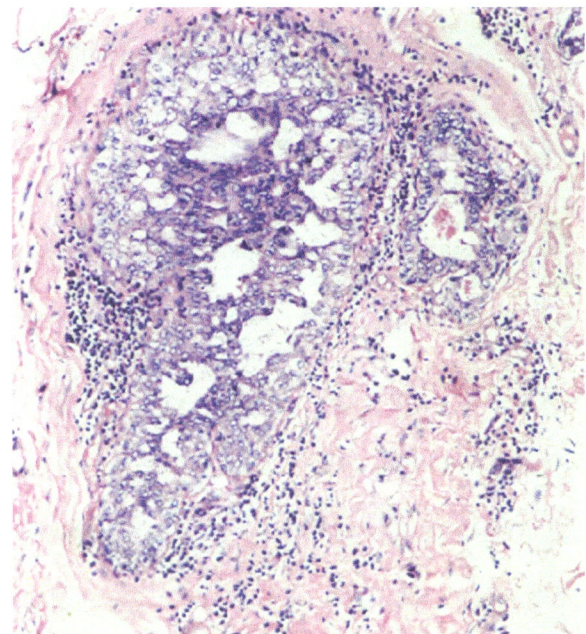

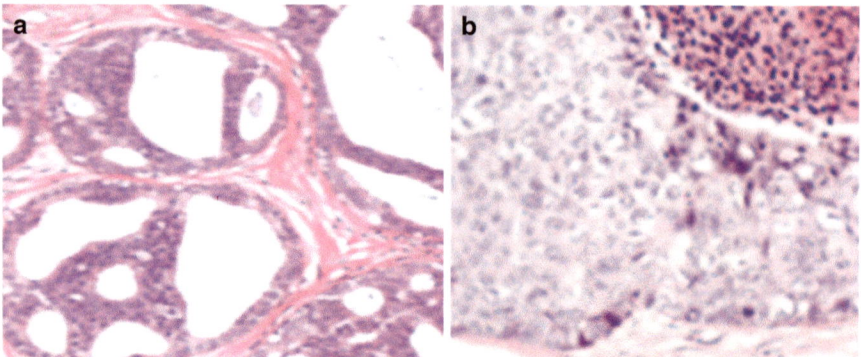

Fig. 13.7 (**a, b**) Low-grade vs high-grade DCIS

Common differential diagnosis for DCIS includes the following:

- Microinvasive carcinoma: It is defined as invasion of tumor cells beyond the basement membrane into adjacent stroma to a depth of 1 mm or less.
- Atypical ductal hyperplasia: It is defined as proliferation of uniform epithelial cells with monomorphic round nuclei that either partially fill an involved duct or completely fill a duct <2 mm in aggregate dimension.

13.6   Assessment of Margins

Adequate margin assessment is very difficult for surgeons as DCIS is often not palpable and is difficult for pathologists too as it grows three dimentionally along the ducts. Procedures such as frozen section and imprint cytology have reported encouraging results for intraoperative margin assessment. [9]

13.7   Molecular Markers

Commonly, DCIS is ER/PR positive and HER2/neu negative [10]. HER2/neu expression is inversely correlated with ER and PR status and positively associated with p53 expression. HER2/neu is often present in comedo subtypes of DCIS [10].

13.8   Natural History and Risk Assessment for DCIS

Studies of DCIS (biopsy proven) with long-term follow-up have shown an incidence of invasive carcinoma of >36% [11]. Usually, these malignancies occur within 10 years but may develop even after 15 years of diagnosis. Women with DCIS are at risk for a second malignancy (either invasive or in situ) in the contralateral breast too; the rate at which such tumors develop is approximately 0.5–1% per year [12].

Sometimes, DCIS occurs as part of the breast/ovarian cancer syndromes defined by BRCA1 and BRCA2 mutation [4].

13.8.1 Staging

As per TNM staging system by the American Joint Committee on Cancer (AJCC) and the International Union for Cancer Control (UICC) eighth edition, ductal carcinoma in situ (DCIS) is designated as Tis (DCIS) and stage 0, as it is confined within the ducts (TisN0M0) [13].

13.8.2 Prognostic Factors

The aim of the treatment of DCIS is prevention of local recurrence and progression to invasive breast cancer. A number of clinicopathological factors have been demonstrated to influence the rate of local recurrence (LR) following treatment [14]. Poor prognostic factors include the following:

- Diagnosis at young age.
- High tumor grade.
- Comedo-type necrosis.
- Large tumor size.
- Positive surgical margins.
- ER negativity.
- HER2 positivity.

The Van Nuys Prognostic Index (VNPI) has classified patients with DCIS in three risk groups to determine the aggressiveness of DCIS in terms of the likelihood of "local recurrence" following "breast-conserving" surgeries. The index uses factors such as patient age, tumor size, tumor growth patterns (histological grade) and resection margin width to predict the risk of cancer recurrence and accordingly plan their adjuvant treatment [14] (Table 13.1)

- Low risk: VNPI score of 4–6.
- Intermediate risk: VNPI score 7–9.
- High risk: VNPI score of 10–12.

Table 13.1 VNPI scoring system (California modification of DCIS)

Score	Age	DCIS size (mm)	Histological grade	Margin width (mm)
1	More than 60 years	Less than 16 mm	1–2, no necrosis	10 mm or more
2	40–60 years	16–40 mm	1–2, necrosis	1–9 mm
3	Less than 40 years	More than 40 mm	3	Less than 1 mm

Oncotype DX: The Oncotype DX is a genome-based test that analyzes the activity of 12 cancer-related genes so as to predict how DCIS is likely to behave and respond to treatment. Depending on the recurrence score number, DCIS has a low, intermediate, or high risk of recurrence. A low-risk score is <39, a high-risk score is ≥55, and a score of 39–54 is intermediate risk.

The recurrence score is considered in combination with other factors, including the size and grade of the DCIS, to make a decision regarding adjuvant therapy after surgery. So far, Oncotype DX has been used in invasive carcinomas, but recent studies show that it also helps in predicting the 10-year risk of developing an invasive cancer in patients with DCIS treated with BCS without adjuvant RT [14, 15].

13.9 Treatment

Local treatment of DCIS includes either mastectomy or breast-conserving therapy (BCT), followed in most cases by adjuvant radiation therapy (RT) and/or hormone therapy. In patients with clinically positive nodes, sentinel lymph node biopsy can also be done.

13.9.1 Surgery

Mastectomy is curative for DCIS. Silverstein et al. have shown a locoregional control rate of ≥96% and cancer-specific mortality rates of ≤4% in patients of DCIS post-mastectomy [16]. Local treatment failure after mastectomy is either due to incomplete removal of breast tissue or due to invasive carcinoma that has been missed during histopathology resulting in local or metastatic disease.

Breast-conserving surgery: Breast-conserving surgery (BCS) with R0 resection is another approach to treat invasive and in situ breast carcinomas with equivalent survival outcomes as compared to mastectomy [17]. To achieve clear margins along with an optimal cosmetic result is the challenge of BCS [18].

Criteria for BCS: Following criteria must be met for BCS:

- Cosmetically acceptable resection: The size of disease must be small as compared to the size of the breast.
- R0 resection should be the priority for BCS.
- Although multifocal disease is not considered as a contraindication, but multicentric disease is a relative contraindication for BCS.

Axillary surgery: Sentinel LN biopsy has become a standard of surgical care for patients with DCIS irrespective of BCS or mastectomy as there are chances of axillary lymph node metastasis with microinvasive carcinoma or high-grade DCIS. Some associations, such as the National Comprehensive Cancer Network (NCCN) and ASCO, have recommended its use in certain situations, such as palpable axillary lymph node and DCIS size >5 cm, and imaging is highly suggestive of invasive lesion [19].

13.9.1.1 Intraoperative Imaging

Although intraoperative margin status of the specimen can be assessed by intraoperative cytology, frozen section, etc., still approximately 20–30% of patients need to undergo revision surgery to obtain clear margins. Specimen radiography (SR) is widely used to ascertain the adequacy of surgical biopsy and removal of nonpalpable breast and in turn has reduced positive margin rates in several studies [20]. However, a recent meta-analysis and systemic review showed that cytology and frozen section are superior as compared to SR for intraoperative margin assessment [21].

As there is a lack of consensus on adequate margin criteria for patients with DCIS undergoing BCS, the Society of Surgical Oncology (SSO), American Society for Radiation Oncology (ASTRO), and American Society of Clinical Oncology (ASCO) convened a multidisciplinary panel to evaluate the effect of margin width and LR and also to define a minimum negative margin to maximize local control [22, 23]. The SSO, ASTRO, and ASCO multidisciplinary panel defined a positive margin as ink present on the resection surface. It has been seen that a minimum margin of 2 mm is associated with a reduced risk of LR, whereas margins wider than 2 mm are not associated with lower LR, thus the current practice supports the routine practice of obtaining margin width of 2 mm [24, 25].

13.9.2 Adjuvant Treatment

13.9.2.1 Radiation Therapy

Radiation therapy is used as adjuvant therapy after BCS. However, it may be omitted in a few selected patients under the conditions such as advanced age, extensive comorbidities, or small foci of low-grade disease resected with negative margins. Right now, we do not have clear scientific evidence to suggest who can do well without RT after BCS.

Several trials have demonstrated the benefit of adjuvant WBRT by decreasing the rate of local recurrence [26–31].

At a follow-up period of 7 years, the RTOG 9804 trial has demonstrated that the local recurrence rate was 0.9% in the radiation therapy arm as compared to 6.7% in the observation arm ($P < 0.001$) in patients with good risk disease features such as size measuring less than 2.5 cm with margins $\geq$3 mm [31]. At a median follow-up of 12.4 years, the 12-year cumulative incidence of LR was 2.8% with WBRT as compared to 11.4% in the observation group. The 12-year cumulative incidence of invasive LR was 1.5% with WBRT and 5.8% (3.2, 9.5) with observation. On multivariable analysis, only WBRT and the use of tamoxifen were associated with reduced LR [32]. Goodwin et al. also demonstrated that adjuvant radiation therapy after lumpectomy leads to statistically significant reduction in local recurrence ($P < 0.00001$) without overall survival benefit [33]. The long-term follow-up of the NSABP B-17 trial showed that at 15 years, adjuvant RT resulted in a 52% reduction of ipsilateral invasive recurrence as compared to excision alone ($P < 0.001$). However, overall survival (OS) and cumulative all-cause mortality rates were similar between the two arms [30].

Table 13.2 Studies depicting the impact of RT versus no radiotherapy on recurrence

	Ipsilateral breast tumor recurrence (IBTR)	NO XRT	XRT	
NSABP B-17 (12 years) [30] (n = 813)	Overall	31.4%	15.7%	P < 0.000005
	Invasive	16.8%	7.7%	P < 0.00001
	Non Invasive	14.6%	8%	P = < 0.001
EORTC 10853 [28] (10 years) (n = 1010)	Overall	26%	15%	P < 0.0001
	Invasive	13%	8%	P = 0.0065
	Noninvasive	14%	7%	P = 0.0011
UK/ANZ (n = 1030) [29]	Overall	23.2%	10.6%	P < 0.0001
	Invasive	10.1%	5.6%	P = 0.001
	NonInvasive	11.6%	4%	P < 0.0001
SweDCIS (n = 1016) [27]	Overall	0.22%	0.07%	P < 0.0001

A study by Narod et al., in which 60,000 women were treated with breast-conserving therapy, with or without radiation therapy, has also shown that radiation therapy was associated with a 50% reduction in the risk of ipsilateral recurrence (adjusted HR, 0.47 [95% CI, 0.42–0.53]; $P < 0.001$), with similar breast cancer-specific mortality in both groups ($P = 0.22$) [34] (Table 13.2).

Sagara et al. also demonstrated a statistically significant improvement in survival with adjuvant radiation therapy in patients with high-risk DCIS (e.g., higher nuclear grade, younger age, and larger tumor size) [35].

Researches have shown the benefit of a radiation boost in DCIS patients who have life expectancies of 10 or more years following breast-conserving surgery and WBRT. In an analysis from ten institutions, patients who received a WBRT followed by boost experienced lesser local recurrence. The ipsilateral breast tumor recurrence (IBTR) free survival for boost vs. no boost, respectively, was 97.1% vs. 96.3% at 5 years, 94.1% vs. 92.5% at 10 years, and 91.6% vs. 88.0% at 15 years following treatment, with these differences achieving statistical significance ($p = 0.013$) [36]. The benefit in reducing in-breast recurrence was demonstrated across all DCIS age subgroups. Furthermore, on multivariable analysis, boost treatment was an independent predictor for decreasing IBTR inspite of disease characteristics (i.e., grade, necrosis, margin status, patient age, tumor size, and use of tamoxifen).

BCT without WBRT: Several retrospective studies have demonstrated that there is no advantage of post-BCS radiation therapy in low-risk DCIS. In these studies, patients with a low VNPI score (scores 3–4) were considered as low-risk DCIS. [14, 37] Gilleard et al. have also demonstrated no benefit of radiation therapy in low-risk DCIS. In this study, the recurrence rate over 8 years was 0%, 21.5%, and 32.1% in patients with low-, intermediate-, or high-risk DCIS, respectively [38].

In a review by Di Saverio et al., 10-year disease-free survival (DFS) rates in DCIS treated with lumpectomy alone was 94% for patients with low-risk DCIS and 83% for patients with both intermediate- and high-risk DCIS [38]. VNPI scores of 4–6 were considered as low-risk DCIS as compared to VNPI scores of 7–9 and 10–12 as intermediate- and high-risk DCIS, respectively.

Contradictory to the above studies, Hughes et al. have demonstrated that the rate of developing an IBTR was 14.4% for low/intermediate grade as compared to 24.6% for high-grade DCIS ($P = 0.003$). This suggests that IBTR events may be delayed but not prevented in the seemingly low-risk population [39].

Doses of whole breast radiation therapy used in different studies range from 45 to 50 Gy in 25 fractions @ 1.8 to 2 Gy per fraction [27–30]. In some studies, a boost of 10 Gy in 5 fractions is given. A study by Chao et al. has suggested that earlier initiation of RT (i.e., ≤8 weeks) was associated with a lower incidence of ipsilateral breast tumor recurrence (i.e., >12 weeks) [40].

Alternative radiation therapy schedules such as hypofractionation or accelerated partial-breast RT have been studied. In hypofractionation technique, a dose of 42 Gy in 15 fractions is usually used as compared to 34 Gy in 10 fractions over 5 days for interstitial therapy and 38.5 Gy in 10 fractions twice daily for external-beam based treatment [41, 42]. NSABP B 39/ RTOG 0413 is an ongoing trial to assess the role of APBI in patients with DCIS as well as stage I and II breast cancer with tumors ≤3 cm and 3≤LNs.

As per the updated version of ASTRO guidelines for early breast cancer published in 2018, hypofractionated WBI may be used as an alternative to conventional field WBI in patients with DCIS to a dose of 40 Gy in 15 fractions or 42.5 Gy in 16 fractions [43].

It also stated that a tumor bed boost may be omitted in patients >50 years who meet the following criteria: (a) age ≤ 50 years, (b) high grade, and (c) close (≤ 2 mm) or positive margins to a dose of 10 Gy in 4–5 fractions.

A tumor bed boost may be omitted in patients with DCIS who, if age >50 years, meet the following criteria: screen detected, total size ≤2.5 cm, low-to-intermediate nuclear grade, and negative surgical margins (≥3 mm).

13.9.2.2 Systemic Therapy

The primary intent of the use of systemic treatment is to reduce the risk of ipsilateral and/or contralateral invasive breast cancer. Still, the use of chemotherapy and human epidermal growth factor receptor 2 (HER2)-directed therapy in DCIS is debatable. As DCIS patients are usually hormone receptor positive, endocrine therapy is usually offered to the majority of patients, if indicated.

Endocrine therapy: About 50–75% of DCIS lesions express estrogen receptors (ER) and/or progesterone receptors (PR) [12, 44]. Of the endocrine agents, tamoxifen is being approved to prevent invasive breast cancer. The role of aromatase inhibitors such as anastrozole is also being studied.

Current National Comprehensive Cancer Network guidelines also recommend tamoxifen for patients with ER+ disease or those who underwent BCS without radiation [45].

The use of postoperative tamoxifen is effective in reducing the risk of invasive breast cancer, with or without adjuvant radiotherapy, with no apparent benefit for survival. A meta-analysis of two randomized trials, National Surgical Adjuvant Breast and Bowel Project (NSABP) B-24 and United Kingdom, Australia, and New Zealand DCIS (UK/ANZ DCIS), has demonstrated that the addition of tamoxifen to BCT for DCIS not only reduces recurrence risk of ipsilateral DCIS and contralateral DCIS but also lowers the risk of ipsilateral and contralateral invasive carcinoma, although there was no benefit of tamoxifen in all-cause mortality [46].

The benefit of postoperative tamoxifen is primarily in patients with ER-positive DCIS. In a review of data from the NSABP B-24 trial at 10 years of follow-up, patients with ER expressing DCIS treated with tamoxifen had a significant decrease in subsequent (invasive and/or noninvasive; ipsilateral and/or contralateral) breast cancer events as compared to patients receiving placebo [47].

The aromatase inhibitor anastrozole is used as an alternative to tamoxifen in postmenopausal women with ER-expressing DCIS.

In the NRG Oncology/NSABP B-35 trial, hormone-receptor-positive, postmenopausal, post-BCT patients demonstrated that anastrozole resulted in a decreased rate of breast cancer events at 10 years compared with tamoxifen. At a median follow-up of 9 years, when compared with tamoxifen, anastrozole resulted in a lower incidence of subsequent breast cancer events (i.e., recurrent DCIS or subsequent invasive breast cancer) (90 versus 122 events, respectively; HR 0.73), including a lower rate of invasive breast cancer (43 versus 69 cases; HR 0.62) and an improved estimated breast cancer-free survival at 10 years (93.1 versus 89.1%) [48].

The results of the IBIS-II study have also indicated that anastrozole provides at least a comparable benefit as adjuvant treatment for postmenopausal women with hormone-receptor-positive DCIS, with a different toxicity profile [49].

13.10   Post-treatment Surveillance

The aims of follow-up after treatment for ductal carcinoma in situ (DCIS) are early recognition and treatment of potentially curable disease recurrences and second primary breast cancers, evaluation for therapy-related complications, and detection of symptoms consistent with metastatic disease. During follow-up, a detailed history with physical examination and routine mammography (if applicable) form the cornerstone.

References

1. Consensus conference on the classification of ductal carcinoma in situ. Cancer. 1997;80:1798–1802.
2. National Institutes of Health State-of-the-Science Conference Statement: diagnosis and management of ductal carcinoma in situ (DCIS). http://consensus.nih.gov/2009/dcis.htm. Accessed 05 Apr 2012.
3. Trentham-Dietz A, Newcomb PA, Storer BE, Remington PL. Risk factors for carcinoma in situ of the breast. Cancer Epidemiol Biomarkers Prev. 2000;9(7):697–703.
4. Hwang ES, McLennan JL, Moore DH, Crawford BB, Esserman LJ, Ziegler JL. Ductal carcinoma in situ in BRCA mutation carriers. J Clin Oncol. 2007;25(6):642–7.

5. Tabar L, Gad A, Parsons WC, et al. Mammographic appearances of in situ carcinomas. In: Silverstein MJ, editor. Ductal carcinoma in situ of the breast. Baltimore, MD: Williams & Wilkins; 1997. p. 413–20.

6. Watanabe T, Yamaguchi T, Tsunoda H, Kaoku S, Tohno E, Yasuda H, et al. Ultrasound image classification of ductal carcinoma in situ (DCIS) of the breast: analysis of 705 DCIS Lesions1. Ultrasound Med Biol. 2017;43(5):918–25.

7. Nori J, Meattini I, Giannotti E, Abdulcadir D, Mariscotti G, Calabrese M, et al. Role of preoperative breast MRI in ductal carcinoma in situ for prediction of the presence and assessment of the extent of occult invasive component. Breast J. 2014;20(3):243–8.

8. Gorringe KL, Fox SB. Ductal carcinoma in situ biology, biomarkers, and diagnosis. Front Oncol. 2017;7:248.

9. Creager AJ, Shaw JA, Young PR, Geisinger KR. Intraoperative evaluation of lumpectomy margins by imprint cytology with histologic correlation: a community hospital experience. Arch Pathol Lab Med. 2002;126(7):846–8.

10. Lari SA, Kuerer HM. Biological markers in DCIS and risk of breast recurrence: a systematic review. J Cancer. 2011;2:232–61.

11. Habel LA, Moe RE, Daling JR, Holte S, Rossing MA, Weiss NS. Risk of contralateral breast cancer among women with carcinoma in situ of the breast. Ann Surg. 1997;225(1):69.

12. Amin MB, Edge SB, Greene FL, et al., editors. AJCC (American Joint Committee on Cancer) Cancer staging manual; 8th edition, 3rd printing. Chicago: Springer; 2018.

13. Silverstein MJ, Lagios MD, Craig PH, Waisman JR, Lewinsky BS, Colburn WJ, Poller DN. A prognostic index for ductal carcinoma in situ of the breast. Cancer. 1996;77(11):2267–74.

14. Solin LJ, Gray R, Baehner FL, Butler SM, Hughes LL, Yoshizawa C, et al. A multigene expression assay to predict local recurrence risk for ductal carcinoma in situ of the breast. J Natl Cancer Inst. 2013;105(10):701–10.

15. Rakovitch E, Nofech-Mozes S, Hanna W, Baehner FL, Saskin R, Butler SM, et al. A population-based validation study of the DCIS score predicting recurrence risk in individuals treated by breast-conserving surgery alone. Breast Cancer Res Treat. 2015;152(2):389–98.

16. Silverstein MJ. Van Nuys experience by treatment. In: Silverstein MJ, Lagios MD, Poller DN, et al., editors. Ductal carcinoma in situ of the breast. Philadelphia, PA: Williams & Wilkins; 1997. p. 443–7.

17. Fisher B, Anderson S, Bryant J, Margolese RG, Deutsch M, Fisher ER, et al. Twenty-year follow-up of a randomized trial comparing total mastectomy, lumpectomy, and lumpectomy plus irradiation for the treatment of invasive breast cancer. N Engl J Med. 2002;347(16):1233–41.

18. Cutuli B, de Lafontan B, Mignotte H, Fichet V, Fay R, Servent V, et al. Breast-conserving therapy for ductal carcinoma in situ of the breast: the French Cancer Centers' experience. Int J Radiat Oncol Biol Phys. 2002;53(4):868–79.

19. Zahoor S, Haji A, Battoo A, Qurieshi M, Mir W, Shah M. Sentinel lymph node biopsy in breast Cancer: a clinical review and update. J Breast Cancer. 2017;20(3):217–27.

20. Bathla L, Harris A, Davey M, Sharma P, Silva E. High resolution intra-operative two-dimensional specimen mammography and its impact on second operation for re-excision of positive margins at final pathology after breast conservation surgery. Am J Surg. 2011;202(4):387–94.

21. Versteegden DP, Keizer LG, Schlooz-Vries MS, Duijm LE, Wauters CA, Strobbe LJ. Performance characteristics of specimen radiography for margin assessment for ductal carcinoma in situ: a systematic review. Breast Cancer Res Treat. 2017;166(3):669–79.

22. Morrow M, Van Zee KJ, Solin LJ, Houssami N, Chavez-MacGregor M, Harris JR, et al. Oncology-American Society of Clinical Oncology consensus guideline on margins for breast-conserving surgery with whole-breast irradiation in ductal carcinoma in situ. Ann Surg Oncol. 2016;23:3801–10.

23. Marinovich ML, Azizi L, Macaskill P, Irwig L, Morrow M, Solin LJ, et al. The Association of Surgical Margins and Local Recurrence in women with ductal carcinoma in situ treated with breast-conserving therapy: a meta-analysis. Ann Surg Oncol. 2016;23:3811–21.

24. National Institute of Health and Clinical Excellence. Early and locally advanced breast cancer: diagnosis and treatment. NICE clinical guideline. Surgery to the Breast chapter/1-Guidance#surgery-to-the-breast. 2009.
25. New Zealand Guidelines Group (NZGG). Ductal carcinoma in situ.Management of early breast cancer. Wellington: New Zealand Guidelines Group (NZGG); 2009. p. 133–41.
26. Bijker N, Meijnen P, Peterse JL, Bogaerts J, Van Hoorebeeck I, Julien JP, et al. Breast-conserving treatment with or without radiotherapy in ductal carcinoma-in-situ: ten-year results of European Organisation for Research and Treatment of Cancer randomized phase III trial 10853—a study by the EORTC breast Cancer cooperative group and EORTC radiotherapy group. J Clin Oncol. 2006;24(21):3381–7.
27. Emdin SO, Granstrand B, Ringberg A, Sandelin K, Arnesson LG, Nordgren H, et al. (Swedish breast Cancer group). SweDCIS: radiotherapy after sector resection for ductal carcinoma in situ of the breast. Results of a randomised trial in a population offered mammography screening. Acta Oncol. 2006;45(5):536–43.
28. Bijker N, Meijnen P, Peterse JL, Bogaerts J, Van Hoorebeeck I, Julien JP, Gennaro M, Rouanet P, Avril A, Fentiman IS, Bartelink H. Breast-conserving treatment with or without radiotherapy in ductal carcinoma-in-situ: ten-year results of European Organisation for Research and Treatment of Cancer randomized phase III trial 10853—a study by the EORTC Breast Cancer Cooperative Group and EORTC Radiotherapy Group. Journal of clinical oncology. 2006 Jul 20;24(21):3381–7.
29. Cuzick J, Sestak I, Pinder SE, Ellis IO, Forsyth S, Bundred NJ, et al. Effect of tamoxifen and radiotherapy in women with locally excised ductal carcinoma in situ: long-term results from the UK/ANZ DCIS trial. Lancet Oncol. 2011;12(1):21–9.
30. Wapnir IL, Dignam JJ, Fisher B, Mamounas EP, Anderson SJ, Julian TB, et al. Long-term outcomes of invasive ipsilateral breast tumor recurrences after lumpectomy in NSABP B-17 and B-24 randomized clinical trials for DCIS. J Natl Cancer Inst. 2011;103(6):478–88.
31. McCormick B, Winter K, Hudis C, Kuerer HM, Rakovitch E, Smith BL, et al. RTOG 9804: a prospective randomized trial for good-risk ductal carcinoma in situ comparing radiotherapy with observation. J Clin Oncol. 2015;33(7):709.
32. McCormick B. Randomized trial evaluating radiation following surgical excision for "Good Risk" DCIS: 12-year report from NRG/ RTOG 9804. Int J Radiat Oncol Biol Phys. 2018. ASTRO Annual Meeting Late-breaking Abstract Selection (LBA1).
33. Goodwin A, Parker S, Ghersi D, Wilcken N. Post-operative radiotherapy for ductal carcinoma in situ of the breast–a systematic review of the randomised trials. Breast. 2009;18(3):143–9.
34. Narod SA, Iqbal J, Giannakeas V, et al. Breast Cancer mortality after a diagnosis of ductal carcinoma in situ. JAMA Oncol. 2015;1:888.
35. Sagara Y, Freedman RA, Vaz-Luis I, Mallory MA, Wong SM, Aydogan F, et al. Patient prognostic score and associations with survival improvement offered by radiotherapy after breast-conserving surgery for ductal carcinoma in situ: a population-based longitudinal cohort study. J Clin Oncol. 2016;34(11):1190.
36. Moran MS, Zhao Y, Ma S, Kirova Y, Fourquet A, Chen P, et al. Association of radiotherapy boost for ductal carcinoma in situ with local control after whole-breast radiotherapy. JAMA Oncol. 2017;3(8):1060–8.
37. Gilleard O, Goodman A, Cooper M, Davies M, Dunn J. The significance of the Van Nuys prognostic index in the management of ductal carcinoma in situ. World J Surg Oncol. 2008;6(1):61.
38. Di Saverio S, Catena F, Santini D, Ansaloni L, Fogacci T, Mignani S, et al. 259 Patients with DCIS of the breast applying USC/Van Nuys prognostic index: a retrospective review with long term follow up. Breast Cancer Res Treat. 2008;109(3):405–16.
39. Hughes LL, Wang M, Page DL, Gray R, Solin LJ, Davidson NE, et al. Local excision alone without irradiation for ductal carcinoma in situ of the breast: a trial of the eastern cooperative oncology group. J Clin Oncol. 2009;27(32):5319.
40. Chao KK, Vicini FA, Wallace M, Mitchell C, Chen P, Ghilezan M, et al. Analysis of treatment efficacy, cosmesis, and toxicity using the MammoSite breast brachytherapy catheter to deliver

accelerated partial-breast irradiation: the William Beaumont Hospital experience. Int J Radiat Oncol Biol Phys. 2007;69(1):32–40.

41. Shah C, Vicini F, Shaitelman SF, Hepel J, Keisch M, Arthur D, Khan AJ, Kuske R, Patel R, Wazer DE. The American brachytherapy society consensus statement for accelerated partial-breast irradiation. Brachytherapy. 2018;17(1):154–70.

42. Ciervide R, Dhage S, Guth A, et al. Five year outcome of 145 patients with ductal carcinoma in situ (DCIS) after accelerated breast radiotherapy. Int J Radiat Oncol Biol Phys. 2012;83:e159.

43. Smith BD, Bellon JR, Blitzblau R, Freedman G, Haffty B, Hahn C, et al. Radiation therapy for the whole breast: executive summary of an American Society for Radiation Oncology (ASTRO) evidence-based guideline. Pract Radiat Oncol. 2018;8(3):145–52.

44. Selim AA, El-Ayat G, Wells CA. Androgen receptor expression in ductal carcinoma in situ of the breast: relation to oestrogen and progesterone receptors. J Clin Pathol. 2002;55(1):14–6.

45. National Comprehensive Cancer Network. NCCN clinical practice guidelines in oncology: breast cancer, version 1. 2018. http://www.nccn.org/professionals/physician_gls/f_guidelines. asp. Accessed Aug 2018.

46. Staley H, McCallum I, Bruce J. Postoperative tamoxifen for ductal carcinoma in situ. Cochrane Database Syst Rev. 2012(10).

47. Allred DC, Anderson SJ, Paik S, Wickerham DL, Nagtegaal ID, Swain SM, et al. Adjuvant tamoxifen reduces subsequent breast cancer in women with estrogen receptor–positive ductal carcinoma in situ: a study based on NSABP protocol B-24. J Clin Oncol. 2012;30(12):1268.

48. Margolese RG, Cecchini RS, Julian TB, Ganz PA, Costantino JP, Vallow LA, et al. Anastrozole versus tamoxifen in postmenopausal women with ductal carcinoma in situ undergoing lumpectomy plus radiotherapy (NSABP B-35): a randomised, double-blind, phase 3 clinical trial. Lancet. 2016;387(10021):849–56.

49. Forbes JF, Sestak I, Howell A, Bonanni B, Bundred N, Levy C, et al. Anastrozole versus tamoxifen for the prevention of locoregional and contralateral breast cancer in postmenopausal women with locally excised ductal carcinoma in situ (IBIS-II DCIS): a double-blind, randomised controlled trial. Lancet. 2016;387(10021):866–73.

Radiation Treatment in Early Breast Cancer: An Overview

14

Anand Radhakrishnan, Beena Kunheri, and Kurian Joseph

14.1 Introduction

The current gold standard of local treatment in early breast cancer (EBC) remains breast-conserving surgery (BCS) followed by whole breast irradiation (WBI). This approach evaluated by the Early Breast Cancer Trialists' Collaborative Group (EBCTCG) showed a 50% reduction in 10-year risk of first recurrence and reduction in risk of dying from breast cancer following radiotherapy (RT) [1]. For WBI, the long-term standard was conventional fractionation of 1.8–2 Gy per fraction up to a total dose of 45–50 Gy to whole breast and regional nodal irradiation if indicated. In patients who have undergone mastectomy, the indications for RT depend on the pathological factors. The definite indications are T3, T4, four or more node-positive or positive margins [2]. In the case of EBC, the recent EBCTCG meta-analysis proves improvement in both local control and overall survival; 1.5 locoregional recurrence prevented at 10 years is 1 breast cancer death prevented at 20 years [3].

WBI and post-mastectomy RT are associated with a few acute and late effects. Acute effects usually are self-limiting effects on skin and subcutaneous tissue and breast edema. The long-term effects are rare, but serious side effects are effects on lung, cardia, and second malignancy. Other rare side effects include brachial plexopathy and lymphoedema.

A. Radhakrishnan
Department of Radiation Oncology, Medical College, Thiruvananthapuram, Kerala, India

B. Kunheri (✉)
Department of Radiation Oncology, Amrita Institute of Medical Sciences and Research Centre, Amrita Vishwa Vidyapeetham University, Kochi, Kerala, India

K. Joseph
Cross Cancer Institute, University of Alberta, Edmonton, AB, Canada

© Springer Nature Singapore Pte Ltd. 2021
B. Kunheri, D. K. Vijaykumar (eds.), *Management of Early Stage Breast Cancer*,
https://doi.org/10.1007/978-981-15-6171-9_14

14.2 Timing of Radiotherapy

For patients who have been recommended to receive adjuvant chemotherapy, RT is generally administered following the completion of chemotherapy as no study has demonstrated an advantage of delivering RT immediately after surgery. For patients in whom adjuvant endocrine therapy alone is indicated, RT can be given concurrently or prior to its initiation.

For patients in whom adjuvant trastuzumab is indicated, it can be given concurrently.

14.3 Fractionation for Breast Radiation

Several investigators have attempted to examine whether a shorter fractionation, lesser total dose, or single doses would provide equivalent disease control with improved toxicities.

The UK Coordinating Committee for Cancer Research (now National Cancer Research Institute) based on pilot trial ran two combined parallel trials, the START A and START B, where shorter, hypofractionated regimens were tested against the conventional 50 Gy in a 25-fraction regimen [4]. The authors concluded that shorter regimens were equivalent to the conventional one in efficacy. Ten-year follow-up data while confirming the equivalence in efficacy noted that the 40 Gy in a 15-fraction arm in START B trial had better cosmetic outcomes [4, 5]. Radiobiological modeling predicted a low α/β ratio for breast cancer, thus providing a biological rationale for hypofractionation. The Canadian randomized study also confirmed that hypofractionation was equivalent to conventional RT in terms of local control and cosmetic outcome [6].

The ASTRO in its recent update noted that in spite of convincing evidence as to the equivalence, cost, and convienience advantages of hypofractionated whole breast radiotherapy (HF-WBI) compared to conventional fractionated radiotherapy (CF-WBI) in eligible patients, adoption of this technique remains low, and a majority of this variation is owing to physician decision rather than patient related [7, 8]. The ASTRO recommends WBI with or without the inclusion of the low axilla; the preferred dose-fractionation scheme is HF-WBI to a dose of 4000 cGy in 15 fractions or 4250 cGy in 16 fractions [7].

A few questions remain even at the end of such convincing evidence. It is unclear what would be the role and efficacy of hypofractionated RT in locally advanced node-positive patients. Similarly, the risk–benefit ratio of boost radiation in a breast that has already received higher dose per fraction could be elucidated only with results of large randomized mature data.

14.4 Radiation Boost to Tumor Bed

It is a common practice to further increase the primary tumor-bearing area dose by another 10–14 Gy at 1.8–2 Gy per fraction [9, 10]. Romestaing et al. observed a 3.6% relapse rate in those who received a 10 Gy boost vs 4.6% in those who did not. The rate of telangiectasia was higher in the boost group (12.4 vs 5.9%); however, the self-assessment scores were similar.

A large randomized trial by EORTC involving more than 5000 patients concluded that boost RT resulted in a significantly lower local recurrence rate, a lower mastectomy first salvage rate, and increased fibrosis with there being no difference in either DFS, OS, or death from breast cancer rates. As age advances, especially above 60 years, the gain in local control is small [9, 10].

It can therefore be reasonably concluded that RT boost of at least 10 Gy should be administered to the primary tumor bed. As age advances, the benefit is less. Boost may be omitted in patients under the following conditions: >60 years, low grade, or favorable biological profile [9].

14.5 Accelerated Partial Breast Irradiation (APBI)

Recurrences after primary surgery for carcinoma breast tend to occur in and around the excision site. APBI delivers focussed, higher dose per fraction to the index quadrant alone and therefore presents an exciting alternative in providing cure, and control rates do not suffer from acceptable cosmesis. APBI may be delivered by a variety of techniques, viz. multicatheter brachytherapy, intraoperative photons or electrons, or EBRT.

At this point in time, it is generally accepted that APBI should be used as a sole modality in selected low-risk patients until more mature data are available. ASTRO recommends APBI for patients under the following conditions: aged 50 years or older, less than 3 cm tumors, and node-negative disease with negative surgical margins with low-risk pathological features [11].

14.6 Multicatheter Brachytherapy

The GEC-ESTRO randomized phase III noninferiority trial on interstitial multicatheter brachytherapy conducted by the GEC-ESTRO group randomized 1184 patients who were randomized to APBI with multicatheter brachytherapy technique or WBI of 50 Gy in 2 Gy fractions with a sequential boost of 10 Gy. The primary endpoint was an ipsilateral local recurrence. The final analysis concluded a 5-year local recurrence rate of 0.9% for EBRT and 1.4% for APBI as sole RT modality ($p = 0.42$). Overall survival was not significantly different. Only this trial has 10-year follow-up data on APBI. GEC-ESTRO recommends guidelines for target contouring for APBI with multicatheter brachytherapy technique [12].

14.7   Intraoperative Radiotherapy

TARGIT – A trial randomized patients either to receive WBI with or without boost or IORT with a 50-KV spherical applicator. If additional risk factors were detected in the post-surgical pathological workup, further WBI was indicated. In its most recent report, the trial concluded that it established noninferiority as intended [13]. However, it was severely criticized in the scientific press for the short follow-up and statistical methods.

The ELIOT study examined the use of intraoperative electrons instead of low-KV X-rays. The trial reported a significantly higher local recurrence rate in the IOERT-arm with 4.4% compared to 0.4% in the WBI-arm ($p < 0.001$) [14].

APBI with external-beam radiotherapy should be cautiously offered with special attention to target volume definition and dose-fractionation schemes.

Much awaited results of trials such as RAPID, NSABP B-39/RTOG 0413, and IMPORT LOW are now published.

RAPID trial results indicate that external-beam APBI was noninferior to WBI in preventing IBTR, but the regimen used was associated with an increase in moderate late toxicity and adverse cosmesis, which might be related to the twice-per-day treatment [15]. Other approaches, such as treatment once per day, might not adversely affect cosmesis as in IMPORT LOW.

NSABP B-39/RTOG 0413 trial results failed to prove the equivalence in IBTR between WBI and APBI [16].

Future clinical adoption of APBI will depend on meta-analysis of all the APBI trials with different techniques and long-term follow-up reports.

14.8   Regional Nodal Irradiation

Most authorities agree that patients would merit regional nodal irradiation for four or more node-positive patients. This approach stems from the published data of EBCTCG analysis (2005), EBCTCG analysis (2014), British Columbia, and the Danish trials [2, 3]. The adjuvant radiation treatment of 1–3 lymph node positivity is controversial. A SEER observational study concluded that while RT improved mortality for patients with 3 or more nodes or T size more than 2 cm with 2 or more involved nodes, no benefit could be observed in patients having one node positive with T size less than 2 cm. However, the British Columbia and the Danish trials and few institutional review reports could demonstrate improved breast cancer-free survival in node-positive patients receiving PMRT, regardless of the number [17, 18].

The NCIC MA.20 trial demonstrated that while the addition of axillary nodal radiation to whole breast RT improved DFS in node-positive, high-risk disease, the OS was not improved. In this trial, 85% of patients had 1–3 lymph nodes removed. A similar trial, the EORTC 22922/10925, concluded that it significantly improved the DFS and mortality from breast cancer with a nonsignificant trend in the improvement of OS. In light of the mentioned trial results, it might be advisable to consider RT in 1–3 lymph node positivity as well [19–21].

The benefit may also depend on tumor biology, and hence, it may be reasonable to go for a risk-adapted approach.

Sentinel node technique has been accepted as the standard of care in clinically node-negative EBC.

The role of radiation/axillary surgery in clinically negative, but sentinel node-positive cases was addressed in ACOSOG Z-0011, IBCSG 23-01, and AMAROS trials [22, 23]. The detailed discussion is provided in the chapter on regional nodal irradiation.

14.9   Node-Negative, High-Risk Disease

For the purpose of discussion on node-negative, high-risk disease in early breast cancer, it is worthwhile to consider RT for T2 tumors with high-risk features of the primary disease such as ER negativity, high-grade differentiation, or lymphovascular invasion. As noted earlier, in both MA 20 and EORTC trials, these patients with node-negative, high-risk features had an improvement with RT compared to those who did not.

In the EORTC study, the DFS was 76% in those receiving RT versus 72% in those who did not, whereas the 10-year DFS was 84 versus 72, respectively, in the MA 20 trial [19, 20]. Outside clinical trials, there are no enough data to recommend RT in high-risk, node-negative cases.

14.10   Omission of RT in the Elderly

The Postoperative Radiotherapy in Minimum Risk Elderly (PRIME) 2 study found that RT in postmenopausal women aged more than 65 years, with node-negative, ER-positive small tumors (less than 3 cm), resulted in a lower chance of recurrence compared to the patients who did not receive RT without any difference in OS, distant metastasis, or new breast cancers [24]. A meta-analysis of 5 randomized trials published in 2014 also concluded that adjuvant RT in patients more than 65 years, with receptor-positive, T1 tumors, reduced locoregional recurrence without affecting survival. Therefore, it would seem reasonable to safely avoid RT in the elderly with less than 3-cm size tumors, who are receptor positive and node negative, avoiding the potential risks and toxicities albeit accepting a higher local recurrence rate, provided that the patients can take endocrine therapy for 5 years.

14.11 Conclusion

For women with nonmetastatic breast cancer, multidisciplinary care is the norm, incorporating inputs from breast radiologists, breast pathologists, onco surgeons, radiation oncologists, and medical oncologists. The objective of adjuvant radiotherapy is to sterilize the microscopic disease remaining after surgery to improve the locoregional control, disease-specific survival, and overall survival. The last two decades witnessed escalation as well as de-escalation in all aspects of breast cancer treatment, and the focus in the future will be on personalized treatment based on gene expression signatures and biological profile.

References

1. Early Breast Cancer Trialists' Collaborative Group (EBCTCG), Darby S, McGale P, Correa C, Taylor C, Arriagada R, Clarke M, Cutter D, Davies C, Ewertz M, Godwin J, Gray R, Pierce L, Whelan T, Wang Y, Peto R. Effect of radiotherapy after breast-conserving surgery on 10-year recurrence and 15-year breast cancer death: meta-analysis of individual patient data for 10 801 women in 17 randomised trials. Lancet. 2011;378(9804):1707–16.
2. Recht A, Comen EA, Fine RE, et al. Postmastectomy radiotherapy. An American Society of Clinical Oncology American Society for Radiation Oncology and Society of surgical oncology focused guideline update. Pract Radiat Oncol. 2016;6:e219.
3. McGale P, Taylor C, Correa C, Cutter D, Duane F, Ewertz M, et al. Effect of radiotherapy after mastectomy and axillary surgery on 10-year recurrence and 20-year breast cancer mortality: meta-analysis of individual patient data for 8135 women in 22 randomised trials. Lancet. 2014;383:2127–35.
4. Haviland JS, Owen JR, Dewar JA, et al. The UK standardisation of breast radiotherapy (START) trials of radiotherapy hypofractionation for treatment of early breast cancer: 10-year follow-up results of two randomised controlled trials. Lancet Oncol. 2013;14:1086–94.
5. START Trialists' Group. The UK standardisation of breast radiotherapy (START) trial B of radiotherapy hypofractionation for treatment of early breast cancer: a randomised trial. Lancet. 2008;371:1098–107.
6. Whelan TJ, Pignol JP, Levine MN, et al. Long-term results of hypofractionated radiation therapy for breast cancer. N Engl J Med. 2010;362:513–20.
7. Smith BD, Bellon JR, Blitzblau R, et al. Radiation therapy for the whole breast : executive summary of an American Society for Radiation Oncology (ASTRO) evidence-based guideline. Pract Radiat Oncol. 2018;81:59–68.
8. Jagsi R, Falchook AD, Hendrix LH, Curry H, Chen RC. Adoption of hypofractionated radiation therapy for breast cancer after publication of randomized trials. Int J Radiat Oncol Biol Phys. 2014;90:1001–9.
9. Vrieling C, van Werkhoven E, Maingon P, et al. Prognostic factors for local control in breast cancer after long-term follow-up in the EORTC boost vs no boost trial: a randomized clinical trial. JAMA Oncol. 2017;3:42–8.
10. Bartelink H, Maingon P, Poortmans P, et al. Whole-breast irradiation with or without a boost for patients treated with breast-conserving surgery for early breast cancer: 20-year follow-up of a randomised phase 3 trial. Lancet Oncol. 2015;16:47–56.
11. Correa C, Harris EE, Leonardi MC, et al. Accelerated partial breast irradiation: executive summary for the update of an ASTRO evidence-based consensus statement. Pract Radiat Oncol. 2017;7:73–9.
12. Major T, Gutierrez C, Guix B, van Limbergen E, Strnad V, Polgár C. Recommendations from GEC ESTRO Breast Cancer Working Group (II): target definition and target delineation for

accelerated or boost partial breast irradiation using multicatheter interstitial brachytherapy after breast conserving open cavity surgery. Radiother Oncol. 2016;118(1):199–204.

13. Vaidya JS, Bulsara M, Wenz F, et al. Pride, prejudice, or science: attitudes towards the results of the TARGIT-A trial of targeted intraoperative radiation therapy for breast cancer. Int J Radiat Oncol Biol Phys. 2015;92(3):491–7.

14. Veronesi U, Orecchia R, Maisonneuve P, et al. Intraoperative radiotherapy vs external radiotherapy for early breast cancer (ELIOT): a randomised controlled equivalence trial. Lancet Oncol. 2013;14(13):1269–77.

15. Whelan TJ, Julian JA, Berrang TS, Kim D-H, Germain I, Nichol AM, Akra M, Lavertu S, Germain F, Fyles A, et al. External beam accelerated partial breast irradiation versus whole breast irradiation after breast conserving surgery in women with ductal carcinoma in situ and node-negative breast cancer (RAPID): a randomised controlled trial. Lancet. 2019;394(10215):2165–72. https://doi.org/10.1016/S0140-6736(19)32515-2.

16. Vicini FA, Cecchini RS, White JR, Arthur DW, Julian TB, Rabinovitch RA, Kuske RR, Ganz PA, et al. Long-term primary results of accelerated partial breast irradiation after breast-conserving surgery for early-stage breast cancer: a randomized, phase 3, equivalence trial (NSABP B-39/RTOG 0413). Lancet. 2019;394(10215):2155–64. https://doi.org/10.1016/S0140-6736(19)32514-0.

17. Overgaard M, Nielsen HM, Overgaard J. Is the benefit of postmastectomy irradiation limited to patients with four or more positive nodes, as recommended in international consensus reports? A subgroup analysis of the DBCG 82 b&c randomized trials. Radiother Oncol. 2007;82:247–53.

18. Yang PS, Chen CM, Liu MC, Jian JM, Horng CF, Liu MJ, Yu BL, Lee MY, Chi CW. Radiotherapy can decrease locoregional recurrence and increase survival in mastectomy patients with T1 to T2 breast cancer and one to three positive nodes with negative estrogen receptor and positive lymphovascular invasion status. Int J Radiat Oncol Biol Phys. 2010;77:516–22.

19. Whelan TJ, Olivotto IA, Parulekar WR, Ackerman I, Chua BH, Nabid A, Vallis KA, White JR, Rousseau P, Fortin A, Pierce LJ, Manchul L, Chafe S, Nolan MC, Craighead P, Bowen J, McCready DR, Pritchard KI, Gelmon K, Murray Y, Chapman JA, Chen BE, Levine MN, MA.20 Study Investigators. Regional nodal irradiation in early-stage breast cancer. N Engl J Med. 2015;373(4):307.

20. Poortmans PM, Collette S, Kirkove C, Van Limbergen E, Budach V, Struikmans H, Collette L, Fourquet A, Maingon P, Valli M, De Winter K, Marnitz S, Barillot I, Scandolaro L, Vonk E, Rodenhuis C, Marsiglia H, Weidner N, van Tienhoven G, Glanzmann C, Kuten A, Arriagada R, Bartelink H, Van den Bogaert W. Internal mammary and medial supraclavicular irradiation in breast cancer. N Engl J Med. 2015;373(4):317.

21. Smith BD, Bellon JR, Blitzblau R, Freedman G, Haffty B, Hahn C, Halberg F, Hoffman K, Jagsi R, et al. Radiation therapy for the whole breast: executive summary of an American Society for Radiation Oncology (ASTRO)evidence-based guideline. Pract Radiat Oncol. 2018;8:145–52.

22. Giuliano AE, Ballman KV, McCall L, Beitsch PD, Brennan MB, Kelemen PR, Ollila DW, Hansen NM, Whitworth PW, Blumencranz PW, Leitch AM, Saha S, Hunt KK, Morrow M. Effect of axillary dissection vs no axillary dissection on 10-year overall survival among women with invasive breast cancer and sentinel node metastasis: the ACOSOG Z0011 (Alliance) randomized clinical trial. JAMA. 2017;318(10):918–26.

23. Donker M, van Tienhoven G, Straver ME, Meijnen P, van de Velde CJH, Mansel RE, et al. Radiotherapy or surgery of the axilla after a positive sentinel node in breast cancer (EORTC 10981-22023 AMAROS): a randomised, multicentre, open-label, phase 3 non-inferiority trial. Lancet Oncol. 2014;15(12):1303–10.

24. Kunkler IH, Williams LJ, Jack WJL, et al. Breast-conserving surgery with or without irradiation in women aged 65 years or older with early breast cancer (PRIME II). Lancet Oncol. 2015;16:266–73.

Breast Radiation Therapy Techniques

15

Vishnu R. Nambiar, Haridas M, Dinesh Makuny, and Beena Kunheri

15.1 Introduction

The radiation therapy planning has evolved over the decades from the surface anatomy and X-ray-based two-dimensional era to the current CT-based three-dimensional plans, which would in the future evolve to MRI- and PET-based planning, bringing with it newer challenges for the radiation oncology fraternity. Availability of higher quality image registration, and incorporation of newer motion management and respiratory gating techniques, allows for greater precision in treatment delivery, while improving local control and reducing long-term toxicity and thereby preventing many deaths.

This chapter, while acknowledging the continuing newer developments and techniques in breast cancer radiation therapy, will focus on the discussion of established treatment techniques, with respect to the present-day evidence.

Radiation treatment techniques in both post-mastectomy and post-breast conservation surgery scenarios will be dealt with.

V. R. Nambiar
Department of Radiation Oncology, Baby Memorial Hospital, Calicut, Kerala, India

H. M
Department of Radiation Oncology, Amrita Institute of Medical Sciences, Kochi, Kerala, India

D. Makuny
Department of Radiation Oncology, MVR Cancer Center, Kozhikode, Kerala, India

B. Kunheri (✉)
Department of Radiation Oncology, Amrita Institute of Medical Sciences and Research Centre, Amrita Vishwa Vidyapeetham University, Kochi, Kerala, India

© Springer Nature Singapore Pte Ltd. 2021
B. Kunheri, D. K. Vijaykumar (eds.), *Management of Early Stage Breast Cancer*,
https://doi.org/10.1007/978-981-15-6171-9_15

15.2 Patient Positioning and Immobilization

Appropriate patient positioning with adequate immobilization is essential to achieve reasonably good reproducibility while ensuring patient comfort—both are pre-requisites for accurate delivery of radiation therapy.

Several immobilzation devices are available, commercially, to help minimize day-to-day positioning errors.

15.2.1 Torso Position

Patients are simulated, most frequently, in the supine position on an angled breast board with the ipsilateral arm abducted, by an angle of 90° or more, and externally rotated (Fig. 15.1).

A slight angulation of the positioning board aligns the sternum and upper chest wall horizontally and more parallel to the treatment couch. This minimizes the curvature of the upper chest wall and allows, the beam, a more uniform enface entry into the chest wall, while reducing the need for larger angulations in the beam geometry.

The degree of angulation of the breast board is usually limited by the CT scanner bore size.

Alternatively, positioning the patient flat, without angulation, may allow the breast mound to migrate superiorly and reduce skin reactions in the infra-mammary fold during the course of treatment.

These boards have a number of fixed angle positions, arm supports, hand grips, and head and bottom/knee supports, which can be indexed and individualized for each patient so as to be able to reproduce the same position without major variations.

Fig. 15.1 Patient set-up with breast board in CT simulator

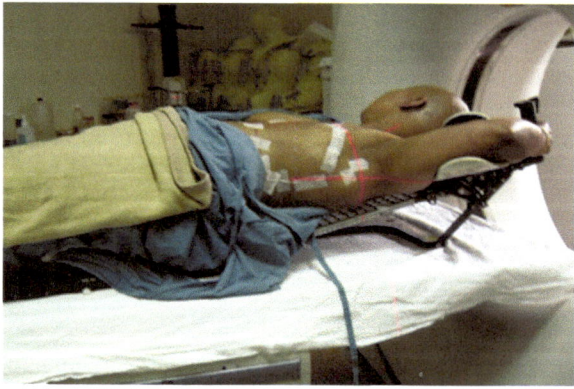

15.2.2   Arm Position

Elevation of the ipsilateral arm above the head helps expose the breast and axilla better, without creating significant skin folds, and helps avoid unwanted radiation to the upper arm in tangential fields.

Bilateral arms may be elevated, as per convenience, for better symmetry and also in the case of bilateral breast irradiation.

15.2.3   Head Position

A good headrest can be used to stabilize the head position. Mild elevation of the chin and turning the head to the opposite side helps reduce the neck skin folds within the SCF field.

Pendulous and large breasts pose a major problem because of increased field size and may be associated with significant variations in the daily set-up.

Remedial options, in this scenario, include the use of thermoplastic shells for immobilization of the breast, which, though, may result in a partial loss of skin sparing. Bra-type supports can raise the breast and reduce skin-fold reactions. Raising the breast also elevates the lateral field border anteriorly and thus reduces the volume of lung and heart (in left-sided cases) in the radiation field.

Simulation in the prone position is an alternative option, especially in larger, pendulous breasts. Patients are positioned prone over a board, with the arms resting over the head. The treated breast is allowed to hang through a hole in the breast board, while the other breast is pushed away to avoid the radiation beams.

In this position, the lung and heart doses are reduced [1], and also skin reactions in the infra-mammary fold are avoided. The limitation of this position is that it is subject to significant set-up errors and would not be suitable for patients requiring nodal irradiation [2–4].

15.2.3.1   Simulation

After the patient is positioned on the couch, the scar and drain sites are marked with radio-opaque wires. In post-mastectomy patients, wires are also placed along the mid-axillary line (lateral edge of the field) and midline (medial edge of the field), thus defining the posterior border or the entry/exit points of the tangent fields. In patients with intact breast, the palpable breast tissue limits are marked with radio-opaque wires to reduce the intra-observer variation. Radio-opaque external fiducial markers are placed on the skin anteriorly in the midline and on the right and left mid-axillary lines.

When a conventional simulator is used for simulation, the clinician has to rely upon the radiological bony landmarks and soft-tissue shadows for treatment planning. The fluoroscopic simulator reveals the extent of respiratory motion, the cardiac silhouette, and lung volume.

Computerized tomography (CT)-based simulation gives detailed, three-dimensional anatomical information of the breast tissue, nodal regions, and organs at risk (OARs). CT simulation is the preferred technique nowadays, since it offers better visualization and allows individualization of target coverage and OAR exposure.

Patients are usually scanned from the chin, superiorly, to the lower border of L1 vertebra, inferiorly. The objective is to include, in the scan, the planned treatment volume, along with adequate peripheral tissue margins, to allow for greater accuracy in computerized dose calculations. Images are acquired with a slice thickness of approximately 3–5 mm to ensure a high-quality digital image reconstruction.

If motion management techniques, such as deep-inspiration breath hold (DIBH) or active breathing control (ABC), are being employed for treatment of certain cases, it is expected that these techniques would be incorporated into the simulation protocol. Many of these techniques require patient compliance with active participation and, often, extra therapist participation. Appropriate patient preparation and training prior to the simulation procedure is needed to ensure reproducibility.

15.3   Target Localization and Contouring

The common target volumes in breast radiotherapy may involve the chest wall or the whole breast, with tumour bed and nodal stations (supraclavicular, axillary level 1–3, internal mammary) depending on the nature of surgery and stage of disease.

These targets may be localized using conventional 2D or CT-based 3D techniques.

- GTV—Radiation therapy is employed in breast cancer as an adjuvant therapy in the post-operative setting and consequently will not have a GTV usually. GTV may need to be delineated in rare scenarios involving neo-adjuvant chemo-radiation or palliative or primary breast radiation, where the tumour is intact.
- CTV_1—May be (a) the whole breast in a post-BCS setting, or
- (b) the ipsilateral chest wall CTV in post-mastectomy patients.
- CTV_2—(boost volume)—Tumour bed with margins.
- CTV_{Nodal}—May include the supraclavicular, axillary levels I–III, and/or internal mammary nodes.
- PTV—Institutionally defined (5 mm to 1 cm).

Historically, radiation fields to cover the targets were localized clinically by inspection, palpation, and with the help of bony or radiological landmarks. This form of target localization was subject to errors, and CT scanning led to the adjustment of conventionally set-up medial and lateral field borders [5].

15.4   Whole Breast or Chest Wall Irradiation

Palpable breast tissue is commonly marked with radio-opaque wires to minimize clinical underestimation of the posterior and lateral extent of breast tissue on imaging. The use of CT imaging improves the visualization of glandular breast tissue, but localizing the upper limit of the breast, using any technique, remains a difficult task nonetheless.

Delineating the whole breast is subject to inter-observer as well as intra-observer variation. While MRI gives excellent breast delineation, its use in breast radiotherapy planning is limited due to potential problems like image distortion and difficulty in co-registration.

Post-mastectomy chest wall localization, on the other hand, is simpler and requires only a proper inspection with marking of the scar. CT imaging may be useful to determine the chest wall depth and volume of lung/heart in the treatment volume.

Standard whole breast irradiation technique involves two opposed tangential beams: a medial and a lateral tangent beam. The beams are usually angulated such that the posterior edges of both beams are aligned to avoid beam divergence into the lung. Alternatively, half-beam fields can also be employed to eliminate divergence into the lung, by defining the posterior border of tangent fields as the central axis of the beams. Commonly, beams of energy 4–6 MV are used, but higher energy photon beams may, occasionally, be used if separation is >20 cm.

15.5   Traditional Field Borders for the Tangent Fields
   (Fig. 15.2)

- *Superior border* is defined as the upper limit of the breast with 1 cm margin, and this usually corresponds to the inferior edge of the clavicular head. If the SCF field is present, the upper border is matched with the inferior border of the SCF field.

Fig. 15.2 Standard medial and lateral tangent beams

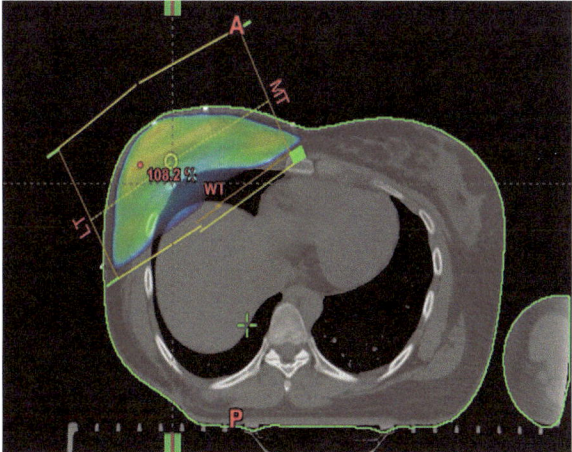

- *Inferior border* is defined as 2 cm below the infra-mammary fold or 1–2 cm below the lower limit of the breast.
- *Medial border* is usually at the midline for most patients. This border is extended across the midline when IMN nodes are to be included.
- *Lateral border* is defined such that it adequately covers the whole breast tissue with 1 cm margin and usually corresponds to the mid-axillary line.
- *Posterior border* or the deep edges of the tangents must be coincident, and this is determined by the medial and lateral borders.
- *Anterior border* is flashed by a 2 cm margin beyond the anterior-most aspect of the breast.

To achieve better dose homogeneity, modulation with multiple field-in-fields may be utilized. This is usually required when inter-field separation of tangents is >15–20 cm (Fig. 15.3). Inner borders (medial borders) of the tangential field may be matched or to avoid divergence to the deeper structures, especially the lung and heart. Another method is to use a half-beam technique (Fig. 15.4).

The post-mastectomy chest wall may be treated by utilizing a similar opposed beam field arrangement. Alternatively, an en face electron field (Fig. 15.5) may be used to treat the chest wall, while ensuring better sparing of the heart and lung. Beams of suitable energy with appropriate re-scaling, along with an appropriate

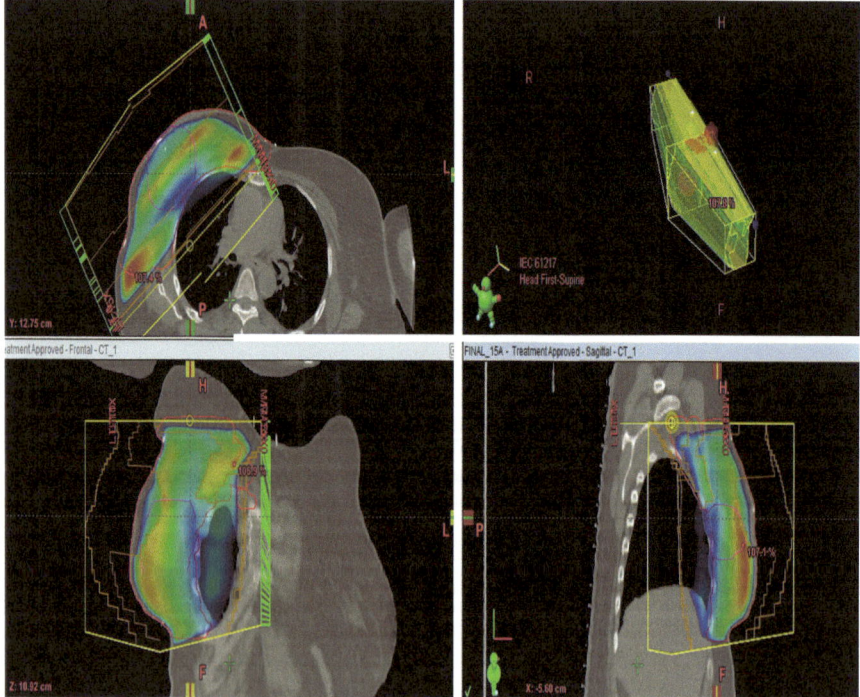

Fig. 15.3 Multiple sub-fields in the medial and lateral tangential orientation

Fig. 15.4 Matching the medial edges of the tangential beams

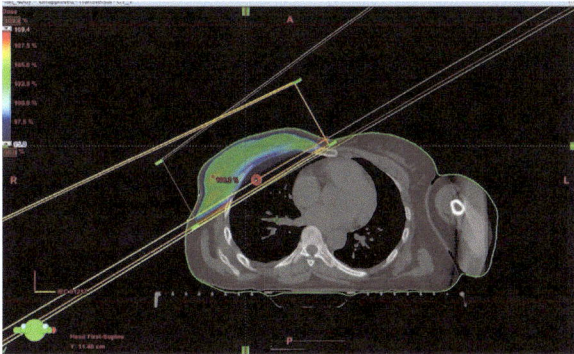

Fig. 15.5 Chest wall enface electron beam

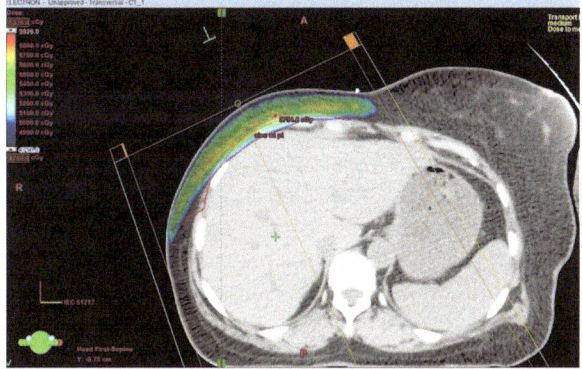

beam angle, are chosen based on the thickness and curvature of the chest wall. The target depth for chest wall treatment is to cover up to the ventral side of pectoralis major muscle, or, if defining that is difficult, up to the ribs.

15.6 Tumour Bed Irradiation

Accurate tumour bed delineation is essential to deliver a boost dose, which is required in most cases, in addition to the whole breast irradiation.

The surgical bed needs to be marked with surgical clips or fiducial markers, which are placed in situ, by the surgeon, prior to closure. These surgical clips allow a more accurate localization of tumour bed than the traditional methods of tumour bed delineation based on the information from pre-operative imaging, clinical examination, and seroma collection within the surgical cavity, if present.

Errors with traditional methods lead to either an underestimation of the tumour cavity resulting in under-dosing or overestimation resulting in unwanted irradiation of normal tissue. Standardizing the method of surgical clip placement is also important to minimize misinterpretation. An appropriate technique, commonly practiced, would be to place five clips, with each one marking the medial, lateral, superior, inferior, and deepest extents of the tumour bed.

Tumour bed localization is much more challenging in patients undergoing onco-plastic or reconstructive breast surgery, where tumour bed relocation is common. Pre- and post-surgery image registrations, marking of the surgical cavity with an adequate number of clips, and placement of these clips, following tumour resection, and prior to oncoplastic reconstruction, would help improve accuracy in tumour bed localization [6, 7].

The optimal boost volume is not known. Usually, a 0.5-mm margin expansion in all directions, from the tumour bed, defines the boost CTV which is clipped anteriorly from the skin and posteriorly from the chest wall [8].

The delineated tumour bed or 'boost volume' is usually irradiated using two photon fields oriented tangentially to the breast/chest wall, with reduced field borders. Electron beams are also commonly employed for a superficial tumour bed/low volume breast, using an appropriate electron energy that covers the target volume depth (usual 8–12 MeV). Some centres also employ interstitial brachytherapy to deliver the tumour bed boost, where brachytherapy catheters are either placed intra-operatively or post-operatively under ultrasound guidance.

Tumour boost irradiation is delivered sequentially either before or after the whole breast irradiation or as a simultaneous integrated treatment.

Partial breast irradiation is increasingly being explored as an alternative to whole breast irradiation. Prominent bodies such as ASTRO, ABS, and ASBS have formulated criteria for selecting suitable patients for accelerated partial breast irradiation. Various techniques being used include interstitial brachytherapy, intra-operative radiation therapy (IORT), and external-beam radiation therapy.

The lumpectomy cavity is delineated based on surgical changes, seroma, and clips. CTV is defined as including a 1.5–2-cm margin around the lumpectomy cavity.

15.7 Nodal Irradiation

CT-based planning is recommended for accurate delineation of the regional nodal stations—supraclavicular, axillary levels I–III, and internal mammary nodes.

Some of the most commonly used, and validated, anatomical contouring guidelines for nodal volumes include the RTOG Breast Contouring Atlas (2009), Danish Breast Co-operative Group (DBCG) Breast Contouring Guidelines (2013), and the ESTRO Breast Contouring Guidelines (2015) [9–11].

Supraclavicular and axillary nodal irradiation is delivered with an anterior oblique field. The lower border of this field is matched with the upper border of tangential fields. This field is usually angulated medially by approximately 15–20° to avoid treating the anterior central structures and cervical spinal cord.

The supraclavicular field includes the true supraclavicular nodal station and level III axillary nodes. This region is commonly treated in all node-positive or T3/T4 cases. Photon beam, usually of 6 MV energy, is prescribed conventionally to a depth

Fig. 15.6 Supraclavicular field

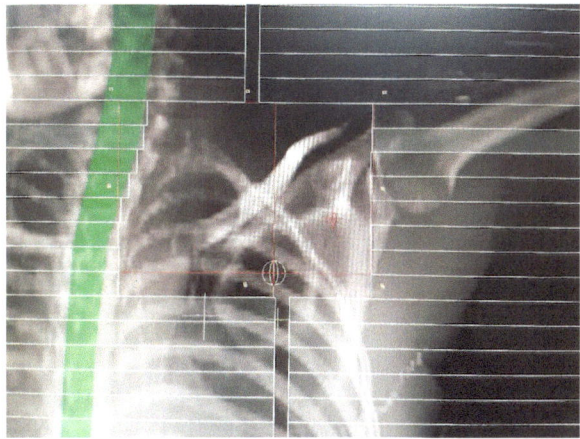

of 3 cm below the skin surface. Nodal depths vary, and ideally CT-based planning should be used to define the prescription depth.

Field borders of supraclavicular (SCF) field alone (Fig. 15.6):

- *Superior border* is usually placed at the lower border of the cricoid cartilage.
- *Inferior border* is matched with the upper border of tangential fields, usually at the level of the inferior edge of the clavicular head.
- *Medial border* is usually 1 cm across the midline from the centre of suprasternal notch following the medial border of SCM.
- *Lateral border* is a vertical line at the level of the coracoid process, medial to the humeral head.

Supraclavicular + axillary field has the same borders as the SCF field except for the lateral border, which is usually at the junction of medial two-thirds and lateral one-third of the humeral head. This anterior SCF field is extended laterally in situations that require axillary nodal stations to be fully covered. All axillary nodal stations must be adequately covered in cases with extensive extranodal extension or inadequate axillary nodal dissection or undissected axilla. The field flashes the skin laterally to adequately cover the axilla completely, and blocks are used to shield the humeral head. The standard tangent fields usually, inadvertently, cover the axillary levels I and part of level II nodal stations. While using electrons for chest wall radiation, the lower border of the 'SCF + axilla' field have to be lowered if full axillary coverage is warranted.

When adequate coverage is not achieved in the mid-axillary region with only an anterior field, a posterior axillary field may be added.

Field borders of this posterior axillary field are as follows:

- *Superomedial border* splits the clavicle.
- *Inferomedial border* is drawn to permit 1.5–2 cm of the lung.
- *Superolateral border* shields or splits the humeral head.

- *Inferolateral border* flashes the skin to completely cover the axilla.
- *Inferior border* is at the same level as inferior border of 'SCF + axilla' field.

15.8   Internal Mammary Nodal Irradiation

Evidence for using routine internal mammary nodal (IMN) irradiation is lacking, but some high-risk patient groups may benefit from this. Achieving adequate coverage without irradiating higher volumes of normal tissue is a challenge in IMN irradiation.

Two common techniques have been employed, which are as follows:

1. Using a direct anterior field matched to the tangential fields [12]. Field borders of the IMN field: Medial border is 1 cm across the midline and lateral border is approximately 5 cm lateral to the midline, corresponding to the parasternal region. Superior border matches the inferior border of the SCF field, and inferior border is usually at the level of the inferior border of fourth costochondral junction. The disadvantage of this method is that it is practically difficult to match this field with the medial tangent field without some degree of overlap or miss.
2. Using modified wide tangents which covers the whole breast/chest wall and IMN region. In this technique, the medial border of the tangent field is placed 3 cm across the midline to cover the IMN CTV [13]. A major drawback of this technique is the increase in the volume of cardiac and lung irradiation. Appropriate shielding of the heart and ipsilateral lung is advised below the third intercostal space.

IMRT techniques would help to achieve adequate coverage and a homogeneous dose distribution in the IMN CTV. The high-dose region to the heart and lung can be significantly reduced, but it may result in an increased low-dose spill, the long-term effect of which is not known.

15.9   Matching the Tangential and Supraclavicular Fields

Different methods exist to adjust for the divergence of the tangential/SCF fields, thereby avoiding overlap/under-dosing.

- A collimator and couch rotation can be given so that the superior edges of both tangents align with the inferior edge of the SCF field.
- Half-beam blocking may be used to eliminate the inferior divergence of the SCF field and superior divergence of tangential fields.
- Mono-isocentre technique may be used to match the fields. This method employs a single isocentre at the SCF and tangent field junction so that the non-diverging central axes of all beams match perfectly.

15.10 Delineation of Organs at Risk (OARs)

The organs at risk in breast cancer radiation therapy include the heart, lungs, spinal cord, trachea, oesophagus, contralateral breast, and brachial plexus and need to be delineated for dose assessment.

With improved patient survival following treatment for breast cancer and increased understanding of the long-term complications of cardiac exposure to radiation, the contouring of the heart has evolved into identifying and documenting radiation doses to critical subunits or substructures of the heart. Cardiac contouring atlases have been developed for consistently delineating the chambers and coronary arteries [14, 15].

15.11 Dose Schedules

15.11.1 Whole Breast/Chest Wall/Regional Nodes

The most widely practiced conventional dose schedule for adjuvant radiation therapy in breast cancer is 50 Gy in 25 fractions, 200 cGy/fraction, 5 fractions/week over 5 weeks.

Hypofractionated radiation therapy in breast cancer is, increasingly, being adopted in many centres across the world with long-term mature data from the UK and Canadian Phase III trials becoming available [16, 17]. ASTRO recently updated its recommendations (2018), encouraging wider use of hypofractionated regimes in localized as well as locally advanced breast cancer [18].

The common hypofractionated regimens are the following:

1. 40 Gy in 15 fractions, 2.67 Gy/fraction, over 3 weeks.
2. 42.5 Gy in 16 fractions, 2.66 cGy/fraction, over 3 weeks.

15.11.2 Tumour Bed Boost

Generally, boost dose to the tumour bed is delivered sequentially after whole breast/chest wall/regional node radiation. A wide range of doses for tumour bed boost is in use. The commonly practiced boost dose schedules are 16 Gy in 8 fractions or 10 Gy in 5 fractions [19].

15.12 Conclusion

Adjuvant radiotherapy in breast cancer is associated with significant improvement in locoregional control and survival. Newer techniques of radiation and careful radiation planning have undoubtedly improved the cosmetic outcome and morbidity.

Personalized treatment based on tumour biology would be the norm for future.

References

1. Kirby AM, Evans PM, Donovan EM, et al. Prone versus supine positioning for whole and partial-breast radiotherapy: a comparison of non-target tissue dosimetry. Radiother Oncol. 2010;96:178–84.
2. Varga Z, Hideghety K, Mezo T, et al. Individual positioning: a comparative study of adjuvant breast radiotherapy in the prone versus supine position. Int J Radiat Oncol Biol Phys. 2009;75:94–100.
3. Morrow NV, Stepaniak C, White J, et al. Intra- and interfractional variations for prone breast irradiation: an indication for image-guided radiotherapy. Int J Radiat Oncol Biol Phys. 2007;69:910–7.
4. Kirby AM, Evans PM, Helyer SJ, et al. A randomised trial of supine versus prone breast radiotherapy (SuPr study): comparing set-up errors and respiratory motion. Radiother Oncol. 2011;100(2):221–6.
5. Bentel G, Marks LB, Hardenbergh P, Prosnitz L. Variability of the location of internal mammary vessels and glandular breast tissue in breast cancer patients undergoing routine CT-based treatment planning. Int J Radiat Oncol Biol Phys. 1999;44(5):1017–25.
6. Pezner RD, et al. Radiation therapy for breast cancer patients who undergo oncoplastic surgery: localization of the tumor bed for the local boost. Am J Clin Oncol. 2013;36(6):535–9.
7. Alco G, et al. Replacement of the tumor bed following oncoplastic breast-conserving surgery with immediate latissimus dorsi mini-flap. Mol Clin Oncol. 2016;5(4):365–71.
8. Nielsen MH, Berg M, Pedersen AN, Andersen K, et al. Delineation of target volumes and organs at risk in adjuvant radiotherapy of early breast cancer: national guidelines and contouring atlas by the Danish breast cancer cooperative group. Acta Oncol. 2013;52(4):703–10.
9. RTOG Breast Cancer Contouring Atlas. http://www.rtog.org/CoreLab/ContouringAtlases/BreastCancerAtlas.aspx. Accessed July 29, 2012.
10. Nielsen MH, et al.; on behalf of the Danish Breast Cancer Cooperative Group Radiotherapy Committee. Delineation of target volumes and organs at risk in adjuvant radiotherapy of early breast cancer: national guidelines and contouring atlas by the Danish breast cancer cooperative group. Acta Oncol. 2013;52(4):703–710.
11. Offersen BV, et al. ESTRO consensus guideline on target volume delineation for elective radiation therapy of early stage breast cancer. Radiother Oncol. 2015;114(1):3–10. https://doi.org/10.1016/j.radonc.2014.11.030.
12. Lievens Y, Poortmans P, Van den Bogaert W. A glance on quality assurance in EORTC study 22922 evaluating techniques for internal mammary and medial supraclavicular lymph node chain irradiation in breast cancer. Radiother Oncol. 2001;60(3):257–65.
13. Nielsen HM, et al. A simple method to test if the internal mammary lymph nodes are covered by the wide tangent technique in radiotherapy for high-risk breast cancer. Clin Oncol (R Coll Radiol). 2003;15(1):17–24.
14. Feng M, et al. Development and validation of a heart atlas to study cardiac exposure to radiation following treatment for breast cancer. Int J Radiat Oncol Biol Phys. 2011;79(1):10–8.
15. Duane F, et al. A cardiac contouring atlas for radiotherapy. Radiother Oncol. 2017;122(3):416–22.
16. Whelan TJ, Pignol JP, Levine MN, et al. Long-term results of hypofractionated radiation therapy for breast cancer. N Engl J Med. 2010;362:513–20.
17. START Trialists' Group, Bentzen SM, Agrawal RK, et al. The UK standardisation of breast radiotherapy (START) trial B of radiotherapy hypofractionation for treatment of early breast

cancer: a randomised trial. Lancet. 2008;371(9618):1098–1107. https://doi.org/10.1016/S0140-6736(08)60348-7.

18. Smith BD, Bellon JR, Blitzblau R, Freedman G, Haffty B, Hahn C, Halberg F, Hoffman K, Jagsi R, et al. Radiation therapy for the whole breast: executive summary of an American Society for Radiation Oncology (ASTRO) evidence-based guideline. Pract Radiat Oncol. 2018;8:145–52.

19. Bartelink H, Maingon P, et al. Whole-breast irradiation with or without a boost for patients treated with breast-conserving surgery for early breast cancer: 20-year follow-up of a randomised phase 3 trial. Lancet Oncol. 2015;16(1):47–56. https://doi.org/10.1016/S1470-2045(14)71156-8.

Role of Radiation Therapy in Early Breast Cancer Patients with One to Three Pathological Nodes

16

Vishnu R. Nambiar, Ram Madhavan, and Beena Kunheri

In early-stage, operable breast cancer, clinically node-negative axilla harbors microscopic nodal disease in up to 40% of patients [1]. Hence, it is necessary to address the axilla either by dissection or by nodal irradiation even in clinically node-negative, early-stage breast cancers. If adequate axillary dissection has been done and the nodes are pathologically negative, the role of regional nodal irradiation is limited. There is considerable variation in the irradiation of regional lymphatics in patients with pathological node-positive disease. In patients with four or more nodes positive, most radiation oncologists favour supraclavicular nodal irradiation based on the potential disease-free and overall survival advantage [2]. However, there is a difference of opinion among radiation oncologists in irradiating regional lymphatics, in addition to breast, in patients with one to three positive nodes.

16.1 Early Breast Cancers (EBCs) Undergoing Breast Conservation Surgery (BCS) with Axillary Lymph Node Dissection (ALND)

Breast-conserving surgery followed by radiotherapy (BCS + RT) has been shown to produce survival rates similar to total mastectomy alone (TM) in early-stage breast cancer in two important, prospective, randomized controlled trials with long-term

V. R. Nambiar (✉)
Department of Radiation Oncology, Baby Memorial Hospital, Calicut, Kerala, India

R. Madhavan
Department of Radiation Oncology, Amrita Institute of Medical Sciences, Kochi, Kerala, India

B. Kunheri
Department of Radiation Oncology, Amrita Institute of Medical Sciences and Research Centre, Amrita Vishwa Vidyapeetham University, Kochi, Kerala, India

© Springer Nature Singapore Pte Ltd. 2021
B. Kunheri, D. K. Vijaykumar (eds.), *Management of Early Stage Breast Cancer*,
https://doi.org/10.1007/978-981-15-6171-9_16

follow-up [3, 4]. The evident, additional cosmetic advantage offered by this breast conservation therapy (BCT), as shown in these studies, resulted in a paradigm shift from TM to BCT in the treatment of early-stage breast cancer.

The EBCTCG 2011 meta-analysis of 17 trials, which included 10,800 women, conclusively demonstrated the benefit of adding adjuvant radiation therapy, following BCS [5].

Adjuvant breast irradiation, following breast conservation surgery, with directed nodal radiation in patients having four or more pathologically involved nodes, has now become the accepted standard of care in EBCs [2]. However, the addition of directed nodal radiation, to breast irradiation, in EBCs with only one to three pathologically positive nodes remains a contentious issue.

The two most important contemporary trials that address this issue and could assist in decision making are the MA-20 trial and the EORTC 22922/10925 trial, which are briefly discussed below.

The 2015 MA-20 trial [6], which included 1832 patients, evaluated the role of adding regional nodal radiation (treatment included internal mammary and supraclavicular and axillary nodes) to whole breast radiation in node-positive EBCs and high-risk node-negative patients. In this trial, 99% of patients had T1–2 tumours and 85% of patients had one to three positive nodes (T4 and N2–3 cases were excluded). The trial showed a significantly improved disease-free survival (DFS), though improved overall survival (OS) could not be demonstrated.

Similarly, a large EORTC trial, EORTC 22922/10925 [7, 8], involving 4004 women, was conducted to evaluate the role of adding directed regional nodal radiation (treatment included internal mammary and medial supraclavicular nodes) in EBCs, irrespective of nodal status (44% of patients were node negative, while 43% had one to three nodes). At 15-year follow-up, there was a significant reduction in breast cancer mortality (15.8 vs 19.7%) and breast cancer recurrence (24.5 vs 27.1%), with the addition of regional nodal irradiation.

Both of these major trials had 85%, or more, of the patient population, consisting of women having three or fewer positive nodes, suggesting that the addition of directed nodal radiation to breast irradiation may have a beneficial role in EBCs with one to three pathologically involved nodes.

Selection of nodal groups to be included in the radiation therapy would require additional dedicated studies to be more specifically defined.

16.2 Early Breast Cancers (EBC) Undergoing Sentinel Lymph Node Biopsy (SLNB)

Recently, with the advent of sentinel lymph node biopsy (SLNB), further axillary dissection and directed nodal irradiation may be omitted based on the pathological findings of the SLNB. Major studies have shown a very low probability of microscopic nodal disease if the sentinel lymph node, dissected by an experienced surgeon, turned out to be negative [9, 10].

Defining the role of nodal irradiation, in EBC patients undergoing a breast conservation surgery (BCS), with an SLNB, would require further studies, but the results of two major trials—the ACOSOG Z-0011 [11] and the AMAROS trial [12]—may be helpful in this regard.

The ACOSOG Z-0011 trial demonstrated that patients with T1–2 tumours, with a clinically node-negative axilla, and having less than three positive sentinel lymph nodes (SLN), need not be subjected to further axillary lymph node dissection (ALND). Eighty-nine percentage of patients in this trial had received whole breast irradiation, and a radiation field design review [13] revealed that 50% of evaluable patients in the trial had high tangents and would have received at least partial nodal irradiation, and 18.9% of the total patients had also received directed nodal radiation.

The EORTC-AMAROS trial showed that both ALND, as well as axillary nodal radiation, resulted in comparable axillary control in EBCs having positive sentinel nodes, with significantly lower rates of lymphedema in the radiation therapy arm.

We may, therefore, reasonably surmise the following in patients with EBCs undergoing BCS with SLNB alone:

1. Patients with T1–2 tumours, with a clinically node-negative axilla, and having one or two positive sentinel nodes, may not require directed nodal irradiation, if whole breast radiation is being administered. This, though, is based on the supposition of a 'spillover' nodal irradiation and needs to be specifically investigated further. It may not be prudent, therefore, to extrapolate these results to avoid nodal irradiation, in the same group of patients, if they are being treated with partial breast irradiation.
2. Patients with T1–2 tumours, with a clinically negative axilla, having three or more positive SLNs, would require directed nodal radiation, along with breast irradiation, if ALND is not being performed.

Further evidence is required to define, more precisely, the role of radiation therapy in EBCs undergoing SLNB.

16.3 Early Breast Cancers (EBCs) Undergoing Total Mastectomy (TM) with ALND

A significant percentage of patients, with early-stage breast cancer, still undergo mastectomy for a whole host of reasons, which include multifocal or multicentric tumours, diffusely scattered microcalcifications, persistent positive margin after repeated attempts at BCS, or patient preference.

While most clinicians agree on the negligible benefit of post-mastectomy radiation therapy (PMRT), in node-negative early-stage breast cancer, the use of PMRT has been controversial for patients with T1–2 primary breast cancer having one to three pathologically involved nodes (T1–2/N1) with a 10-year risk of locoregional recurrence less than 15%.

A survey of European and North American radiation oncologists regarding the use of post-mastectomy radiation therapy [PMRT], in women with one to three positive nodes, has shown significant variations in practice between American and European respondents and between academic and non-academic institutions [14]. This may reflect the absence of definitive data from randomized trials, assessing the value of adjuvant irradiation in this group of patients.

Various prospective randomized trials, evaluating PMRT for axillary node-positive patients, receiving adjuvant systemic therapy, have shown the ability of radiation to reduce locoregional recurrence [LRR]. The absolute reduction in risk ranged from 10% to 28% for patients with four or more nodes involved and from 3% to 23% for patients with one to three involved nodes. Locoregional failure following mastectomy and systemic therapy alone commonly occurs on the chest wall and is considerably less common in the axilla or supraclavicular fossa, and it is rarer still in the internal mammary nodes. Most of the survival benefit is thought to be a contribution of the chest wall irradiation.

Among the studies, which have suggested a beneficial role of PMRT in T1–2 breast patients with one to three positive axillary lymph nodes, a subgroup analysis of the Danish Breast Cancer Cooperative Group (DBCG) 82 trial [15] showed a significant reduction in the 15-year LRR from 27% to 4% ($p < 0.001$) and increase in the 15-year OS from 48% to 57% in the patient group with one to three positive ALNs ($p = 0.03$).

While all the subgroups of patients showed a survival benefit, those patients with one to three involved nodes and patients with a tumour size of 2 cm or less showed maximum benefit. This appears to suggest that, while locoregional radiotherapy may confer the most benefit in locoregional control of larger tumours, a greater survival benefit might be conferred on patients with smaller tumours and having fewer numbers of involved nodes [15]. A retrospective analysis of three European Organisation for Research and Treatment of Cancer (EORTC) adjuvant breast cancer trials [16] appears to support this hypothesis. It has shown that patients having one to three involved nodes had maximum gains in terms of survival (RR 0.48, 99% CI 0.31–0.75, $p = 0.001$). This analysis was retrospective, and caution has to be exercised while interpreting the same.

A meta-analysis of 22 randomized control trials [17], involving 8135 women, by the Early Breast Cancer Trialists' Collaborative Group – EBCTCG (2014), of cases treated between 1964 and 1986, included trials where patients underwent total mastectomy with axillary dissection, and radiation, if administered, included treatment of chest wall, supraclavicular fossa and/or axilla, and internal mammary chain. Among these women, 1314 women had axillary dissection with only one to three positive nodes, and addition of radiation therapy reduced locoregional recurrence ($2p < 0.00001$), overall recurrence (RR 0.68, 95% CI 0.57–0.82, $2p = 0.00006$), and breast cancer mortality (RR 0.80, 95% CI 0.67–0.95, $2p = 0.01$) in this group. While these results seem to put forward a strong case for adjuvant radiotherapy following mastectomy, in early breast cancers, having one to three positive nodes, it must be kept in mind that there has been significant improvement in systemic chemotherapy and addition of targeted therapy, in the following decades, and the risk of locoregional recurrence in a similar group of patients may be lesser today.

A more recent Korean study (2016) compared the treatment outcomes of patients with T1–2 primary breast cancer and one to three positive ALNs, who underwent either breast-conserving surgery (BCS) followed by radiotherapy (BCS + RT) or total mastectomy alone (TM), in the modern era of adjuvant systemic therapy [18]. The BCS + RT group had a decreased 5-year cumulative incidence rate of locoregional recurrence from 9.5% to 2.5% ($p = 0.016$), and TM was a relative risk for LRR ($p = 0.003$). The study design inherently suggests a benefit for adjuvant radiation therapy in patients with one to three pathologically positive nodes.

Whether PMRT can increase the DFS and OS of T1–2 breast cancer patients with one to three positive ALNs is still debatable. In a recent analysis of data from the Breast International Group (BIG) 02-98 trial, Zeidan et al. found that addition of post-mastectomy radiation therapy (PMRT) was associated with a significantly reduced risk of locoregional recurrence in women with T1–T2 breast cancer and one to three positive nodes, but no difference in 10-year cancer-specific or overall survival could be demonstrated [19].

The results of the trials discussed above, and many others, represent a growing pool of data, which appear to tilt the scales in favour of post-mastectomy radiation therapy in EBCs having one to three pathologically positive nodes. However, most of these trials are plagued by one or more shortcomings, in that they may not represent a modern early breast cancer patient, with access to the most advanced screening and evaluation, systemic chemotherapy and targeted therapies, and also modern advanced radiotherapy techniques. The results of the SUPREMO trial, in which patients with one to three positive lymph nodes have been included and randomized to adjuvant radiotherapy or no radiotherapy, will probably provide definitive answers to this controversial scenario in future [20]. However, the results will not be available for a number of years due to a minimum 10-year follow-up.

16.4   Selecting Early Breast Cancers (EBC) for PMRT: Can We Identify Additional High-Risk Factors?

The incessant debates and controversies, surrounding adjuvant therapy, arise from the desire to minimize treatment-induced morbidity. Symptoms in the arm are quite common after locoregional treatment, and late effects of radiotherapy such as cardiac morbidity, brachial plexus neuropathy, arm lymphedema, and impaired shoulder motion can progress decades after treatment. It is therefore important to carefully consider radiotherapy target volumes and indications for radiotherapy.

At present, we are not able to clearly define the risk factors for local failure in T1–2 breast cancer patients with one to three positive ALNs.

Many studies are including young age, tumour size, pre-menopausal status, the number of lymph nodes, molecular subtype, lymphovascular invasion (LVI), and lymph nodal ratio (LNR).

Hamamoto et al. found that the risk factors for locoregional failure in patients who underwent mastectomy without radiotherapy included four or more positive axillary lymph nodes [ALN], pT4, primary tumour larger than 5 cm, lymphatic invasion, and negative hormone receptor status on multivariate analysis. 'Four or more ALNs' was the main risk factor, while the others were minor risk factors [21].

Five National Surgical Adjuvant Breast and Bowel Project (NSABP) Randomized Clinical Trials reported age, tumour size, pre-menopausal status, and the number of lymph nodes to be risk factors of LRFS [22].

Yang et al. reported ER-negative status and presence of LVI to be statistically significant risk factors for locoregional failure [23], while Truong et al. found that the lymph node ratio (LNR) >0.20 was closely related to locoregional failure [24].

According to a recent study by Cihan YB et al., the significant risk factors were found to be an invasive ductal carcinoma histology, tumour diameter > 2 cm, three lymph nodes, and stage 2b in patients with one to three ALNs, and patients with these risk factors benefit from PMRT [25].

Quantification of the estrogen receptor (ER), progesterone receptor (PR), human epidermal growth factor receptor 2 (HER2), and Ki-67 protein expression have been helpful in making clinical decisions and predicting the outcome [26].

In a recent report from China, 1369 patients with T1–2 tumours, having one to three positive ALNs, were studied to evaluate the role of molecular subtype as a factor affecting LRR. Among the patients, the luminal A, luminal B, HER2-positive, and triple-negative subgroups accounted for 33.0%, 42.9%, 11.9%, and 12.2%, respectively. The molecular subtype was associated with LRR by single and multiple variable analyses ($p < 0.001$). The rate of LRR in HER2-positive and triple-negative subtypes were higher (23.3% and 22.2%) than the luminal A and luminal B subtypes (11.5% and 15.0%) [27].

Another report from Europe showed ER-positive breast cancer patients to have a lower local recurrence rate than ER-negative patients (9.9% vs. 11.5%, $p = 0.01$) in the first 5 years. After 5 years, ER-positive patients showed a higher local recurrence rate ($p < 0.001$) [28]. Furthermore, Shih-Fan Lai et al. reported that triple-negative breast cancer patients had a higher rate of LRR [29].

Since the molecular subtype is closely associated with the patient's therapeutic results, survival, and prognosis, treatments may be tailored accordingly for the different molecular subtypes. Nonetheless, the quantitative influence of the subtype on LRR is still disputed and needs large-scale randomized studies to be appropriately quantified.

Many potential 'high-risk factors' have been identified, and their possible role in contributing to decision making, while selecting EBCs with one to three pathological nodes for PMRT, needs to be further examined in randomized trials.

16.5 Conclusion

To summarize, PMRT in women with breast cancer having one to three positive lymph nodes is associated with a significant decrease in locoregional recurrence (LRR) while having a relatively smaller overall survival benefit.

Despite the growing body of evidence, in favour of adding PMRT, in patients with intermediate risk of local recurrence, the following questions still remain: Is the benefit due to the prevention of local recurrence (and hence would local chest wall irradiation alone suffice?) or adjuvant nodal regional treatment? Is the expected benefit annulled by the late (cardiac) toxicity?

In their routine clinical practice, radiation oncologists are frequently confronted by patients with one to three positive lymph nodes following mastectomy, and arriving at a decision as to whether a patient should receive radiation therapy to the chest wall, with or without regional lymphatic irradiation, is often difficult, with a dilemma of selecting the most appropriate prognostic risk factors.

In view of the relatively small OS benefit and acknowledging the risk of late toxicity, especially cardiac morbidity, it would be reasonable to recommend the addition of PMRT to a selected group of patients, having other additional risk factors such as young age, oestrogen receptor-negative status, HER2-positive status, large tumours, poorly differentiated tumours, and lymphovascular invasion, following a detailed multidisciplinary discussion, until the results of ongoing large-scale randomized controlled trials become available.

References

1. Fisher B, Jeong JH, Anderson S, et al. Twenty-five-year follow-up of a randomized trial comparing radical mastectomy, total mastectomy, and total mastectomy followed by irradiation. N Engl J Med. 2002;347(8):567–75.
2. Mehta K, Haffty BG. Long-term outcome in patients with four or more positive lymph nodes treated with conservative surgery and radiation therapy. Int J Radiat Oncol Biol Phys. 1996;35(4):679–85.
3. Veronesi U, Cascinelli N, Mariani L, Greco M, Saccozzi R, Luini A, et al. Twenty-year follow-up of a randomized study comparing breast-conserving surgery with radical mastectomy for early breast cancer. N Engl J Med. 2002;347(16):1227–32.
4. Fisher B, Anderson S, Bryant J, Margolese RG, Deutsch M, Fisher ER, et al. Twenty-year follow-up of a randomized trial comparing total mastectomy, lumpectomy, and lumpectomy plus irradiation for the treatment of invasive breast cancer. N Engl J Med. 2002;347(16): 1233–41.
5. Darby S, McGale P, Correa C, Taylor C, Arriagada R, Clarke M, Cutter D, Davies C, Ewertz M, Godwin J, Gray R, Pierce L, Whelan T, Wang Y, Peto R, Early breast cancer trialists' collaborative group (EBCTCG). Effect of radiotherapy after breast-conserving surgery on 10-year recurrence and 15-year breast cancer death: meta-analysis of individual patient data for 10,801 women in 17 randomised trials. Lancet. 2011;378(9804):1707–16.
6. Whelan TJ, Olivotto IA, Parulekar WR, Ackerman I, Chua BH, Nabid A, Vallis KA, White JR, Rousseau P, Fortin A, Pierce LJ, Manchul L, Chafe S, Nolan MC, Craighead P, Bowen J, McCready DR, Pritchard KI, Gelmon K, Murray Y, Chapman JA, Chen BE, Levine MN, MA.20 Study Investigators. Regional nodal irradiation in early-stage breast cancer. N Engl J Med. 2015;373(4):307.
7. Poortmans PM, Collette S, Kirkove C, Van Limbergen E, Budach V, Struikmans H, Collette L, Fourquet A, Maingon P, Valli M, De Winter K, Marnitz S, Barillot I, Scandolaro L, Vonk E, Rodenhuis C, Marsiglia H, Weidner N, van Tienhoven G, Glanzmann C, Kuten A, Arriagada R, Bartelink H, Van den Bogaert W. Internal mammary and medial supraclavicular irradiation in breast cancer. N Engl J Med. 2015;373(4):317.
8. Poortmans P, Collette S, Struikmans H, De Winter K, Van Limbergen E, Kirkove C, et al. Fifteen-year results of the randomised EORTC trial 22922/10925 investigating internal mam-

mary and medial supraclavicular (IM-MS) lymph node irradiation in stage I-III breast cancer. J Clin Oncol. 2018;36(15_suppl):504.

9. Krag D, Harlow S, Julian T. Breast cancer and the NSABP-B32 sentinel node trial. Breast Cancer. 2004;11(3):221–6.

10. Mansel RE, Fallowfield L, Kissin M, et al. Randomized multicenter trial of sentinel node biopsy versus standard axillary treatment in operable breast cancer: the ALMANAC trial. J Natl Cancer Inst. 2006;98(9):599–609.

11. Giuliano AE, Ballman KV, McCall L, Beitsch PD, Brennan MB, Kelemen PR, Ollila DW, Hansen NM, Whitworth PW, Blumencranz PW, Leitch AM, Saha S, Hunt KK, Morrow M. Effect of axillary dissection vs no axillary dissection on 10-year overall survival among women with invasive breast cancer and sentinel node metastasis: the ACOSOG Z0011 (Alliance) randomized clinical trial. JAMA. 2017;318(10):918–26.

12. Donker M, van Tienhoven G, Straver ME, Meijnen P, van de Velde CJ, Mansel RE, Cataliotti L, Westenberg AH, Klinkenbijl JH, Orzalesi L, Bouma WH, van der Mijle HC, Nieuwenhuijzen GA, Veltkamp SC, Slaets L, Duez NJ, de Graaf PW, van Dalen T, Marinelli A, Rijna H, Snoj M, Bundred NJ, Merkus JW, Belkacemi Y, Petignat P, Schinagl DA, Coens C, Messina CG, Bogaerts J, Rutgers EJ. Radiotherapy or surgery of the axilla after a positive sentinel node in breast cancer (EORTC 10981–22023 AMAROS): a randomised, multicentre, open-label, phase 3 non-inferiority trial. Lancet Oncol. 2014;15(12):1303.

13. Jagsi R, Chadha M, Moni J, Ballman K, Laurie F, Buchholz TA, Giuliano A, Haffty BG. Radiation field design in the ACOSOG Z0011 (Alliance) trial. J Clin Oncol. 2014;32(32):3600.

14. Ceilley E, Jagsi R, Goldberg S, et al. Radiotherapy for invasive breast cancer in North America and Europe: results of a survey. Int J Radiat Oncol Biol Phys. 2005;61(2):365–73. https://doi.org/10.1016/j.ijrobp.2004.05.069.

15. Overgaard M, Nielsen HM, Overgaard J. Is the benefit of postmastectomy irradiation limited to patients with four or more positive nodes, as recommended in international consensus reports? A subgroup analysis of the DBCG 82 b&c randomized trials. Radiother Oncol. 2007;82:247–53.

16. van der Hage JA, Putter H, Bonnema J, Bartelink H, Therasse P, van de Velde CJH. Impact of locoregional treatment on the early-stage breast cancer patients. Eur. J. Cancer. 2003;39(15):2192–199.

17. McGale P, Taylor C, Correa C, Cutter D, Duane F, Ewertz M, Gray R, Mannu G, Peto R, Whelan T, Wang Y, Wang Z, Darby S. EBCTCG (early breast Cancer Trialists' collaborative group) effect of radiotherapy after mastectomy and axillary surgery on 10-year recurrence and 20-year breast cancer mortality: meta-analysis of individual patient data for 8135 women in 22 randomised trials. Lancet. 2014;383:2127–35.

18. Kim SW, Chun M, Han S, Jung YS, Choi JH, Kang SY, Jang H, Jo S. Comparison of treatment outcomes between breast conserving surgery followed by radiotherapy and mastectomy alone in patients with T1-2 stage and 1-3 axillary lymph nodes in the era of modern adjuvant systemic treatments. PLoS One. 2016;11:e0163748.

19. Zeidan YH, Habib JG, Ameye L, Paesmans M, de Azambuja E, Gelber RD, Campbell I, Nordenskjöld B, Gutiérez J, Anderson M, Lluch A. Postmastectomy radiation therapy in women with T1-T2 tumors and 1 to 3 positive lymph nodes: analysis of the breast international group 02-98 trial. Int J Radiat Oncol Biol Phys. 2018;101(2):316–24.

20. Kunkler IH, Canney P, van Tienhoven G, et al. Elucidating the role of chest wall irradiation in 'intermediate-risk' breast cancer: the MRC/EORTC SUPREMO trial. Clin Oncol (R Coll Radiol). 2008;20:31–4.

21. Hamamoto Y, Ohsumi S, Aogi K, Shinohara S, Nakajima N, Kataoka M, Takashima S. Are there high-risk subgroups for isolated locoregional failure in patients who had T1/2 breast cancer with one to three positive lymph nodes and received mastectomy without radiotherapy? Breast Cancer. 2014;21:177–82.

22. Taghian A, Jeong JH, Mamounas E, Anderson S, Bryant J, Deutsch M, Wolmark N. Patterns of locoregional failure in patients with operable breast cancer treated by mastectomy and adjuvant chemotherapy with or without tamoxifen and without radiotherapy: results from five

National Surgical Adjuvant Breast and bowel project randomized clinical trials. J Clin Oncol. 2004;22:4247–54.

23. Yang PS, Chen CM, Liu MC, Jian JM, Horng CF, Liu MJ, Yu BL, Lee MY, Chi CW. Radiotherapy can decrease locoregional recurrence and increase survival in mastectomy patients with T1 to T2 breast cancer and one to three positive nodes with negative estrogen receptor and positive lymphovascular invasion status. Int J Radiat Oncol Biol Phys. 2010;77:516–22.

24. Truong PT, Woodward WA, Thames HD, Ragaz J, Olivotto IA, Buchholz TA. The ratio of positive to excised nodes identifies high-risk subsets and reduces inter-institutional differences in locoregional recurrence risk estimates in breast cancer patients with 1-3 positive nodes: an analysis of prospective data from British Columbia and the M. D. Anderson Cancer center. Int J Radiat Oncol Biol Phys. 2007;68:59–65.

25. Cihan YB, Sarigoz T. Role of postmastectomy radiation therapy in breast cancer patients with T1-2 and 1-3 positive lymph nodes. Onco Targets Ther. 2016;9:5587–95.

26. Voduc KD, Cheang MC, Tyldesley S, Gelmon K, Nielsen TO, Kennecke H. Breast cancer subtypes and the risk of local and regional relapse. J Clin Oncol. 2010;28:1684–91.

27. Shen H, Zhao L, Wang L, Liu X, Liu X, Liu J, Niu F, Lv S, Niu Y. Postmastectomy radiotherapy benefit in Chinese breast cancer patients with T1-T2 tumor and 1-3 positive axillary lymph nodes by molecular subtypes: an analysis of 1369 cases. Tumour Biol. 2016;37:6465–75.

28. Colleoni M, Sun Z, Price KN, Karlsson P, Forbes JF, Thürlimann B, Gianni L, Castiglione M, Gelber RD, Coates AS, Goldhirsch A. Annual hazard rates of recurrence for breast cancer during 24 years of follow-up: results from the international breast Cancer study group trials I to V. J Clin Oncol. 2016;34:927–35.

29. Lai SF, Chen YH, Kuo WH, Lien HC, Wang MY, Lu YS, Lo C, Kuo SH, Cheng AL, Huang CS. Locoregional recurrence risk for Postmastectomy breast Cancer patients with T1-2 and one to three positive lymph nodes receiving modern systemic treatment without radiotherapy. Ann Surg Oncol. 2016;23:3860–9.

Regional Nodal Irradiation in Early Breast Cancer

Shyama Sudha Prem, Shiva Kumar Siripuram, and Pragna Sagar Rapole

17.1 Introduction

Early-stage breast cancer [EBC] is described as those with stage I, IIA, or IIB. A subset of stage IIB is cT3N0, which is included as an early stage by some investigators. The standard treatment of early-stage breast cancer is breast-conserving surgery followed by whole-breast irradiation. The term regional nodal irradiation refers to irradiation of the regional nodes, which include axillary nodes (levels I–III), supraclavicular nodes, and internal mammary nodes. Irradiation of the chest wall and the regional nodes is indicated after mastectomy in women with positive nodes. In this scenario, the benefit of RNI is indisputable. RNI reduces the incidence of locoregional and distant recurrence and also improves overall survival [1–3]. However, regional nodal irradiation makes the technique of radiotherapy more complex since it involves irradiation of the axillary and supraclavicular nodes and sometimes the internal mammary nodes.

RNI also increases the risk of complications such as lymphedema, brachial plexopathy, pneumonitis, cardiac disease, and secondary malignancies. Whether the inclusion of regional nodes along with whole breast in adjuvant radiation after breast-conserving surgery in early breast cancer is beneficial is debatable. In this chapter, we attempt to throw light on this controversial topic.

For the purpose of easy understanding, we have broadly categorized patients with early breast cancer into two groups: those with and without clinically palpable axillary nodes. These groups are further subdivided into the following subgroups: (1) patients without clinically palpable nodes and those who undergo sentinel lymph node biopsy [SLNB], (2) patients without clinically palpable nodes and those who

S. S. Prem (✉) · S. K. Siripuram · P. S. Rapole
JIPMER, Pondicherry, PY, India

© Springer Nature Singapore Pte Ltd. 2021
B. Kunheri, D. K. Vijaykumar (eds.), *Management of Early Stage Breast Cancer*,
https://doi.org/10.1007/978-981-15-6171-9_17

undergo axillary lymph node dissection [ALND], and (3) patients with clinically palpable nodes or more than two positive sentinel lymph nodes and those who undergo axillary dissection.

17.2   Role of RNI in Patients Without Clinically Palpable Nodes Who Undergo Sentinel Lymph Node Biopsy

17.2.1 SLNB-Negative Patients

Patients who undergo breast conservation in early-stage breast cancer have two surgical options regarding a clinically negative axilla. They can be offered SLNB or a complete axillary dissection upfront. If a patient undergoes SLNB and the result is a negative SLNB, no further management of axilla is required. There is no rationale for nodal irradiation in patients with negative axillary nodes because nodal recurrence rates after a negative sentinel lymph node biopsy are less than 1%. In the meta-analysis conducted by Van der Ploeg, the recurrence in the axilla in sentinel node-negative patients was 0.3%. Even internal mammary node recurrences in medial tumors are rare if SLNB is negative [4]. Hence, there is uniform consensus regarding management of an SLNB-negative axilla, which is no further treatment to the axilla: neither axillary nodal radiation nor completion axillary dissection.

17.2.2 Patients with One to Two Positive Sentinel Lymph Nodes

Women with early-stage breast cancer with clinically negative axilla who have undergone breast conservation treatment and SLNB, the SLNB shows one to two positive sentinel nodes, also do not require any further treatment to axilla (either RNI or completion of axillary dissection) if breast is treated with tangentials and patient receives 5 years of harmonal therapy.

If the SLNB shows one to two positive nodes, the two options that can be employed are either to go ahead with completion of axillary dissection or axillary irradiation. Various trials were conducted using either of the two modalities. However, none of the trials, addressing the axilla either by surgery or radiation, showed any improvement in either decreasing locoregional recurrence or overall survival in patients receiving whole-breast radiation by tangential fields and systemic therapy. Hence, there is uniform consensus regarding the management of an SLNB with one to two nodes-positive axilla in patients who undergo breast conservation treatment that there is no further treatment to the axilla—either axillary nodal radiation or completion of axillary dissection.

The ACOSOG Z-OO11 trial studied the role of axillary dissection in addition to sentinel lymph node dissection in patients with pathologically positive one to two sentinel nodes. All patients underwent SLNB with breast conservation and received whole-breast irradiation using tangential fields with adjuvant systemic therapy. RNI was prohibited. Patients with one to two positive SLNs were randomized to two-arm completion of axillary dissection or no further axillary treatment. There was no significant difference in 5-year locoregional recurrence rates, disease-free survival, or overall survival between the two arms. The frequency and severity of surgery-related toxicity were more in the axillary dissection arm. Update on overall survival at 10-year follow-up also confirmed the above findings. The overall survival of patients who underwent sentinel lymph node dissection alone was noninferior to those who underwent axillary lymph node dissection. The main limitation of this study was the low event rates and accrual rates. The possible explanations for low event rates are (a) the use of tangential fields that must have inadvertently irradiated the lower axilla eradicating the disease and (b) the use of systemic therapy. The authors concluded that they do not advocate the routine use of axillary lymph node dissection in patients with one to two positive SLNs [5, 6].

The IBCSG 23-01 trial has also studied the role of axillary dissection in addition to sentinel lymph node biopsy in patients who had one or more micro-metastatic (≤ 2 mm) sentinel lymph nodes [sn pN1mi] and a primary tumor with a size of <5 cm. Results of the trial were identical to those of the ACOSOG trial with the outcomes in the SLND arm being noninferior to the AD arm. The complications were routinely observed more in the axillary dissection group. The authors concluded that axillary dissection should be avoided in patients with early breast cancer who underwent breast conservation treatment and received adjuvant systemic therapy when the sentinel lymph nodes are minimally involved. This could preclude the complications of axillary surgery without compromising on survival [7].

Before the advent of sentinel node biopsy, axillary radiotherapy was considered as an alternative for axillary lymph node dissection in clinically node-negative patients. In a randomized trial from Institute Curie by Christine Louis-Sylvestre et al., patients with carcinoma of the breast ≤ 3 cm in diameter and clinically negative lymph nodes were randomized to axillary dissection or axillary radiotherapy. All patients had a lumpectomy and whole-breast RT. A 15-year follow-up revealed no difference in survival, recurrence rates in the breast or supraclavicular fossa, or distant metastasis even though axillary control was better in the dissection group (axillary recurrence was 1% vs 3% in the axillary dissection and RT arms, respectively). However, axillary radiotherapy was associated with lesser side-effects when compared to axillary dissection [8].

The choice of an ideal axillary treatment, axillary radiation, or completion of axillary lymph node dissection in patients with positive sentinel lymph nodes was first addressed by the AMAROS and the OTOASOR trials.

The AMAROS (After Mapping of Axilla, Radiotherapy or Surgery) trial has evaluated the noninferiority of axillary radiation over axillary dissection in clinically T1/T2 lesions with positive nodes on sentinel lymph node biopsy. The noninferiority studied was a 5-year local recurrence in the axilla. It was hypothesized that the risk of axillary recurrence was determined by the presence of a positive sentinel lymph node. Patients with clinically T1/T2, node-negative lesions underwent either BCS or mastectomy. Four-fifths of the patients underwent breast conservation surgery, and one-fifth underwent mastectomy. All patients underwent SLNB. While 95% of the patients had one to two positive sentinel lymph nodes, 4% had three positive LNs and 1% had four or more axillary lymph nodes. In the case of a positive sentinel lymph node, patients were randomized to two arms—axillary dissection and axillary radiotherapy. There was no significant difference in the 5-year recurrence rate in the axilla—0.43% [95% CI 0.00–0.92] vs 1.2% [95% CI 0.31–2.08] in axillary dissection and radiotherapy arms, respectively. The morbidity was significantly less in the radiotherapy arm. Even though the planned noninferiority was underpowered since the number of events with respect to axillary recurrence did not occur, the results revealed the very low recurrence rates in the axilla even in the presence of one to two positive SLNs. The results of AMARAOS confirm that in the method of management of the axilla in patients with positive lymph nodes, radiation or surgery has no impact on survival. However, the complications are much lesser after radiation [9].

OTOASOR (Optimal Treatment of the Axilla—Surgery or Radiotherapy?) was a randomized noninferiority trial similar to the AMAROS trial. They also studied the noninferiority of RNI to axillary dissection in early breast cancer patients (cN0, T size <3 cm) with positive sentinel lymph nodes with respect to axillary recurrence rate, disease-free survival, and overall survival. There was no difference in axillary recurrence in the two arms (2.0% in the ALND arm vs. 1.7% in RNI arm; $p = 1.00$). There was also no difference in OS and DFS. The authors concluded that axillary radiation provides excellent axillary control comparable to axillary dissection in patients with early-stage breast cancer with one to two positive sentinel lymph nodes. Also, axillary radiation results in significantly less morbidity [10].

For patients with T1/T2 lesions with one to two positive lymph nodes on SLNB who receive whole-breast radiation and adjuvant systemic therapy, there is uniform consensus that there is no need for further axillary management in the form of either completion of axillary dissection or axillary radiation. In others (i.e., patients who do not receive any adjuvant systemic therapy or whole-breast radiation and who undergo partial breast irradiation, irradiation of the breast in prone position, or intraoperative irradiation), axillary nodal radiation can be considered as an acceptable alternative to axillary nodal dissection with significantly less morbidity.

17.3 Role of RNI in Patients with Early Breast Cancer Who Undergo Axillary Lymph Node Dissection (with Clinically Palpable Nodes or More than Two Positive Sentinel Lymph Nodes)

Patients with early-stage breast cancer with clinically palpable lymph nodes or more than two positive sentinel lymph nodes should undergo axillary lymph node dissection. They can be subdivided into three groups.

The first group comprises patients with early-stage breast cancer with clinically palpable axillary nodes but pathologically negative axilla with low-risk features after axillary dissection. This includes tumor <5 cm, with adequate axillary dissection, ER-positive tumors, Grade 1 or 2, and no lymphovascular space invasion. There is no role for RNI in this group of patients since the risk of regional failure is low [11].

The second group comprises patients with early-stage breast cancer with pathologically negative axilla with high-risk features after axillary dissection. This includes tumor measuring 5 cm or more [T3] or T > 2 cm with inadequate axillary dissection with any one of the following high-risk features: ER-negative tumors, Grade 3, and lymphovascular space invasion.

The third group comprises patients with early-stage breast cancer with pathologically positive nodes in the axilla.

There is a definitive role of RNI in these two groups of patients since the risk of locoregional failure is high [11–15].

Two major trials evaluated the use of RNI in early breast cancer patients with positive nodes or pathologically negative axilla with high-risk features: the NCIC Group MA.20 trial and EORTC 22922 trial.

In the NCIC Group MA.20 trial, Whelan et al. studied the effect of RNI in clinically T1/T2 lesions with pathologically positive nodes or patients with pathologically negative axillary nodes with high-risk features. High-risk features included tumor measuring 5 cm or more or T more than 2 cm with inadequate axillary dissection with any one of the following high-risk features: ER-negative tumors, Grade 3 tumors, and lymphovascular space invasion. All the patients underwent BCS with whole-breast radiation. At the 10-year follow-up, there was no significant difference in overall survival [82.8% and 81.8% ($p = 0.38$) in the nodal-irradiation and control group, respectively]. However, the disease-free survival was higher in the nodal-irradiation group (82% vs 77.0%; $p = 0.01$). The incidence of Grade 2 or greater acute pneumonitis (1.2% vs. 0.2%, $p = 0.01$) and lymphedema (8.4% vs. 4.5%, $p = 0.001$) were higher in the nodal-irradiation group. The authors concluded that the addition of RNI to whole-breast radiotherapy did not improve the overall survival in women with positive nodes or negative nodes with high-risk features of breast cancer. However, RNI was associated with a reduced rate of breast cancer recurrence [16].

Poortmans et al. (EORTC 22922/10925) studied the effect of RNI (internal mammary and medial supraclavicular lymph-node irradiation) in patients with stage I–III breast cancer, either with central or medial tumors irrespective of axillary nodal involvement or with lateral tumors with axillary nodal involvement. In this study, 76% underwent BCS and 24% had mastectomy, followed by radiation to breast or chest wall with or without regional nodal irradiation, 60% had T1 tumors, 35% had T2 tumors, 44% were node negative, 43% had one to three positive nodes, and only 12% of the patients had more than four positive axillary nodes. RNI significantly improved the rates of disease-free survival, distant DFS, and breast cancer mortality. The authors concluded that RNI was beneficial to women with early-stage breast cancer. The authors also emphasized that their findings are not to be generalized to patients with node-negative tumors in the outer quadrant [17].

Budach et al. conducted a meta-analysis and studied the contribution of the addition of radiotherapy of regional nodes to whole-breast irradiation to improve overall survival in early breast cancer. Three trials (NCIC Group MA.20, EORTC 22922/10925, and French trial) were included in the analysis as per the inclusion criteria. Regional nodal RT had a significant effect on improvement in overall survival [HR 0.90 (95% CL 0.82–0.99)], though the effect on OS was not significant in individual trials. There was a significant improvement in disease-free survival (DFS) and distant metastasis-free survival (DMFS), consistent with the MA 20 and EORTC 22922/10925 trials [15].

As regional lymph nodes do not have a different likelihood of harboring disease in patients who undergo either mastectomy or lumpectomy [16, 18], the management of axilla post-axillary dissection can be extrapolated from post-mastectomy studies. EBCTCG meta-analysis (2014 update) also favors the addition of regional nodal irradiation in one to three positive nodes in axillary dissection. In these women, radiotherapy reduced locoregional recurrence (3.8% vs 20.3% in the RT and no RT groups, respectively; $2p < 0.00001$). The overall recurrence was also reduced in the RT arm (RR 0.68, 95% CI 0.57–0.82, $2p = 0.00006$), and breast cancer mortality was reduced in the RT arm (RR 0.80, 95% CI 0.67–0.95, $2p = 0.01$). This was similar to the established benefit in patients with more than four positive nodes [12].

17.4 Controversies

So, do all node-positive patients require radiotherapy? What about T1N1? Or what about T2N0 with high-risk features like Grade 3 and or LVSI positivity (the so-called intermediate risk)? Ongoing trials such as the SUPREMO trial [Selective Use of Postoperative Radiotherapy AftEr MastectOmy] addresses these issues.

The MA.20 and EORTC 22922/10925 trials demonstrated that aggressive regional treatment improved disease-free survival in the node-positive or high-risk breast cancer. However, these trials were conducted in the pre-trastuzumab era. The applicability of these results to HER2-positive breast cancer patients treated with anti-HER2 therapy was studied by retrospectively analyzing the patients with node-positive breast cancer who were enrolled in the Adjuvant Lapatinib and/or Trastuzumab Treatment Optimization [ALTTO] adjuvant trial. There was no benefit in disease-free survival with the addition of RNI in HER2-positive, node-positive patients treated with adjuvant HER2-targeted therapy. The authors concluded that the benefit of RNI in HER2-positive breast cancer needs further evaluation.

There is also controversy regarding RNI in patients who received neoadjuvant chemotherapy. In a study that used the data from the National Cancer Database (NCDB), the ACSOG evaluated the impact of radiotherapy in women with clinically node-positive breast cancer who received neoadjuvant chemotherapy. The patients had cT1–3 disease and underwent either mastectomy or breast conservation after neoadjuvant chemotherapy. PMRT was associated with improved OS for all pathologic nodal subgroups [ypN0-ypN+]. However, there was no difference in overall survival with the addition of RNI to whole-breast radiation after breast-conserving surgery [ypN0-ypN+] [19].

17.5 How Do We Decide on Taking a Decision Regarding RNI?

Various nomograms are available to assist in decision making in cases of regional nodal irradiation. The breast cancer nomogram (BCN) is an online tool developed by the Memorial Sloan-Kettering Cancer Center (MSKCC), which is used to predict the risk of positive non-SLN in SLN-positive patients [20]. The nomogram uses nine parameters. After entering the details into the nomogram, it calculates the probability of having metastatic spread to the additional nonsentinel lymph nodes. The values are given in %. These nomograms can aid the clinician in deciding whether to opt for RNI. The MSKCC model was validated by many centers [21, 22]. At the Institut Curie, the validation did not reliably predict positive non-sentinel lymphnodes in cases with micro-metastatic (<2 mm) positive SLN, although it predicted accurately for macro-metastasis [23].

17.6 Fields of Regional Nodal Irradiation

Fields of RNI are individualized based on the level of regional nodes being treated.

17.6.1   Immobilization and Position of the Patient

The patient lies supine on a breast board with the arm abducted to 90 using an arm-rest with immobilization. The head is turned to the opposite side.

17.7   Fields Borders for Level 1–3 Axilla and Supraclavicular Nodes (Fig. 17.1)

Level 1–3 axilla and supraclavicular nodes are treated using one large AP field and a small PA field.

Large AP beam: The medial border is kept at the middle of the sternum; the lateral border is kept at the interpectoral groove of the humerus. This region corresponds to the insertion of the pectoralis major muscle in the humerus.

The cranial border is 3 cm above sternoclavicular joint, and the caudal border is at the level of the sternal insertion of the second rib, medially and at the level of the fourth rib, laterally.

PA beam: The medial border is placed at the coracoid process; the lateral, cranial, and caudal borders are the same as for the large AP beam.

17.8   Field Borders for Level 3 Axilla and Supraclavicular Nodes (Fig. 17.2)

Level 3 axilla and supraclavicular nodes are treated using one small AP field.

Single AP beam: The medial border is placed at the midline of sternum, the lateral border is placed medial to the coracoid process, the cranial border is kept 3 cm

Fig. 17.1 Field borders for nodes of SCF and axilla I–III

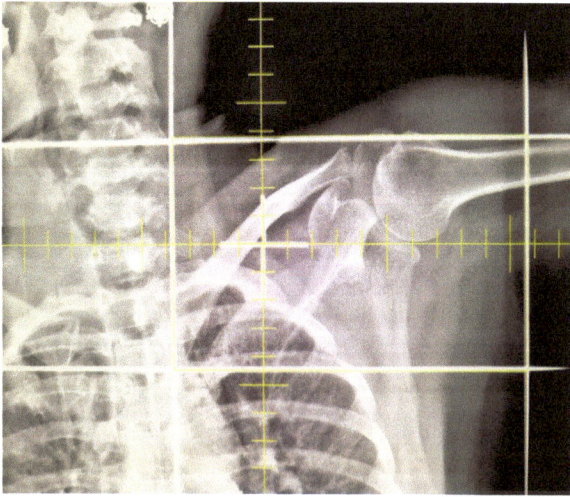

Fig. 17.2 Field borders
for nodes of SCF and axilla
I–III

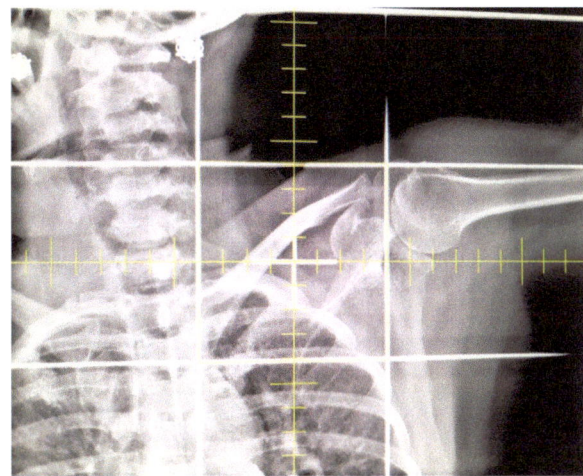

above sternoclavicular joint, with at least 1 cm skin sparing, and the caudal border
is placed at the level of the sternal insertion of the second rib.

17.9   Dose Specification

The prescribed dose is 50 Gy in 25 fractions, 1 fraction a day, 5 fractions a week for 5
and a half weeks. The dose is prescribed at a depth of half patient thickness for level
1 and 2 nodes and at 3 cm for level 3 and supraclavicular nodes. The dose should not
vary by more than ±5–7% across the target volume. Accepted beam energies include
4–10 MV. Shoulder joint should be shielded using blocks, ensuring that the block does
not go beyond more than half the thickness of the shaft of the humerus into the axilla.
The block should not extend beyond the acromioclavicular joint medially.

17.10   Field Borders for Internal Mammary Nodes (Fig. 17.3)

The internal mammary chain lies adjacent to the sternum, usually from the first to
the third intercostal spaces with few nodes extending to the fourth and fifth intercostal spaces. Only the ipsilateral internal mammary chain is irradiated. Internal
mammary nodes are ideally treated by mixed photon and electron beams in order to
achieve maximum sparing of the heart and lungs.

- Cranial border: Head of the clavicle.
- Medial border: 1 cm lateral to the midline.
- Lateral border: 5 cm lateral from the midline. The lower border of the fourth rib
  defines the inferior border. It may be extended to include the fifth intercostal
  space in medial and lower quadrant tumors.

Fig. 17.3 Field borders
for internal
mammary nodes

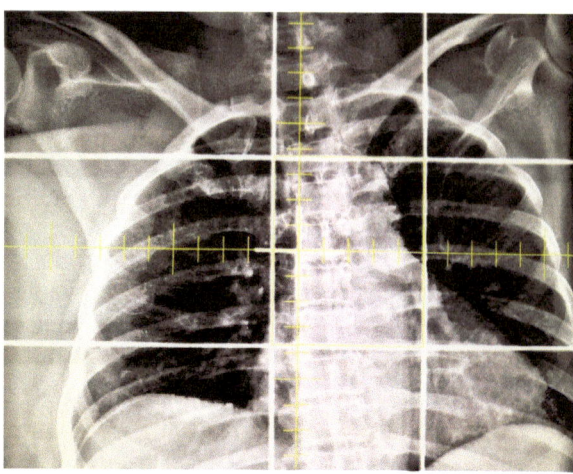

17.11 Dose Specification

The prescribed dose for the photon field is 26 Gy in 13 fractions, 2 Gy per fraction, 1 fraction a day, 5 fractions a week for 2 and a half weeks. The prescribed dose for the electron field is 24 Gy in 12 fractions, 2 Gy per fraction, 1 fraction a day, 5 fractions a week for 2 weeks. The dose is prescribed at a depth of 3 cm for photons and at for electrons at a depth of D-max. Accepted beam energies include 4–10 MV for photons and 12–14 MeV for electrons.

17.12 Complications of Regional Nodal Irradiation

Complications of regional nodal irradiation include lymphedema, skin and soft tissue fibrosis and necrosis, restriction of movements at shoulder, brachial plexopathy, and pulmonary and cardiac toxicity.

17.12.1 Lymphedema

RNI is an additive risk factor for those who have undergone axillary node dissection. Lymphedema usually develops at a median interval of 10–12 months after radiation. In the AMAROS trial, the proportion of patients with lymphedema and those with >10% increase in circumference of the arm was more in patients who underwent axillary dissection. At 5 years, the proportion of patients with lymphedema was 23% in the axillary dissection arm versus 11% in the RNI arm ($p < 0.00001$) [9].

17.12.2 Skin and Soft Tissue Fibrosis and Necrosis

This risk of skin and soft tissue fibrosis and necrosis is low, with the use of skin-sparing megavoltage beams. With the addition of RNI, although uncommonly seen, fibrosis due to radiation is more often because of overlapping treatment fields. It typically presents 4–12 months after radiation and progresses over years. Signs and symptoms can include skin retraction and induration, pain, necrosis, and ulceration, especially at the junction of the two fields. Management includes early initiation of active and passive physical therapy measures, pentoxifylline alone or in combination with tocopherol. Soft tissue necrosis is extremely rare with an estimated incidence of 0.2% of patients undergoing RT for early breast cancer [24].

17.12.3 Brachial Plexopathy

This risk of brachial plexopathy is low. With the addition of RNI, although uncommonly seen, this complication is more often because of overlapping treatment fields. It manifests as paresthesia or weakness in the arm or hand and pain. The incidence of brachial plexopathy is less than 1% in women receiving ≤50 Gy in 2 Gy fractions to the supraclavicular field [24]; it increases to around 5% in patients receiving 45 Gy in 15 fractions [25]. The incidence of plexopathy is significantly higher with higher doses of radiation to axilla (>50 Gy), concomitant chemotherapy, and increased dose per fraction (>2.0Gy/#). In the MA.20 trial, the rates of brachial plexopathy was not significantly different with the addition of RNI to whole-breast irradiation: 1.8% vs 2.5% ($p = 0.42$) without and with RNI arms, respectively [16].

17.12.4 Radiation-Induced Lung Injury

Radiation-induced lung injury usually presents as acute radiation pneumonitis, which is seen usually within 4–12 weeks following radiation. Pulmonary fibrosis is a late complication usually seen 6–12 months following RT. Symptoms and signs include nonproductive cough, dyspnea, low-grade fever, pleuritic or substernal pain, crackles, or a pleural rub. In more severe cases, patients can develop tachypnea, cyanosis, or pulmonary hypertension. In the EORTC 22992 trial, the rate of pulmonary fibrosis was significantly higher with RNI if internal mammary nodes were irradiated, but still less (<5%); it is acceptable keeping in mind the risk–benefit ratio. The rates of pneumonitis of Grade 2 or more were common with RNI, especially if internal mammary nodes were also irradiated [17].

17.12.5 Cardiac Morbidity

Injury to the heart due to radiation is mostly encountered after chest wall or whole-breast irradiation. In the MA20 trial, there was no significant difference in cardiac morbidity with addition of RNI (including internal mammary nodes) with the morbidity being <1% [0.4% vs 0.9%; $p = 0.26$] [16].

17.12.6 Shoulder Joint Dysfunction

Shoulder joint dysfunction is mainly due to axillary treatment, presenting as a restriction in movements of the shoulder joint, sometimes associated with pain. Type of surgery plays a more important role as patients undergoing mastectomy are more prone than those undergoing conservation surgery [26]. In early breast cancer patients post-BCT with or without RNI, there was no significant difference in arm mobility [9, 16].

17.12.7 Secondary Neoplasms

Radiation is associated with an increase in secondary neoplasms. Solid tumors (contralateral breast cancer, esophageal cancer, and lung cancer), leukemia, and angiosarcomas have been reported. Increased risk of contralateral breast cancer, lung cancer (RR = 2.10; 95% CI, 1.48 to 2.98; $p = 001$), and nonbreast/nonlung cancers (RR = 1.19; 95% CI, 1.07 to 1.32) was increased [27]. The risk of a secondary malignancy varies with time post-treatment. Leukemias occur 5–7 years, esophageal cancer 10 years, and angiosarcoma 5–8 years post-radiation. However, in the EORTC 22992 trial, there was no increase in second neoplasms post-RNI (the median follow-up duration was not sufficient to comment on this).

17.13 Conclusion

The decision to treat the regional lymph nodes in early breast cancer is still a topic of debate. There are nomograms that can aid the physician in decision making. The treatment decisions should be individualized and should be based only after a detailed discussion of the potential benefits and risks in a multidisciplinary team and with each patient. We have summarized our recommendations below that could aid the oncologist in decision making for regional nodal irradiation in early breast cancer (Table 17.1).

Table 17.1 Recommendation for the approach to a patient with early breast cancer

RNI in early breast cancer

Early breast cancer						
	cN− (Negative)	Sentinel lymph node biopsy (SLNB)	SLNB negative	No further treatment to axilla		
			SLNB positive	1 or 2 nodes	WBRT with tangential fields + systemic therapy	No further Rx to axilla	ACOSOGZ-OO11, IBCSG 23-01
					No systemic therapy, PBI, RT in prone, Intra op RT	RNI	ACOSOGZ-OO11, AMAROS, OTOASOR
				≥3 Nodes	Axillary nodal dissection		
	cN+ (Positive)	Axillary nodal dissection (level I & II)	pN0, LRF	No RNI		
			pN0, HRF	RNI (SCF, IM, axilla)	M.A. 20 EORTC 22922/10925	
			pN+	ECE−	RNI	Decision regarding the inclusion of axilla I and II in cases of ECE taken according to the departmental protocol
				ECE+	RNI	

cN− clinically node negative, *cN+* clinically node positive, *pN0* pathologically node negative, *pN+* pathologically node positive, *LRF* low risk features (tumor <5 cm, with adequate axillary dissection, ER positive tumors, Grade 1 or 2 and no lymphovascular space invasion), *HRF* high risk features (tumor measuring 5 cm or more [T3] or T > 2 cm with inadequate axillary dissection with any one of the following high risk features-ER negative tumors, Grade 3 and lymphovascular space invasion), *ECE−* no extra capsular extension, *ECE+* extra capsular extension positive, *SCF* supra clavicular fossa, *IM* internal mammary

References

1. Ragaz J, Jackson SM, Le N, Plenderleith IH, Spinelli JJ, Basco VE, et al. Adjuvant radio-therapy and chemotherapy in node-positive premenopausal women with breast cancer. N Engl J Med. 1997;337(14):956–62.
2. Overgaard M, Hansen PS, Overgaard J, Rose C, Andersson M, Bach F, et al. Postoperative radiotherapy in high-risk premenopausal women with breast cancer who receive adjuvant che-motherapy. N Engl J Med. 1997;337(14):949–55.
3. Overgaard M, Jensen M-B, Overgaard J, Hansen PS, Rose C, Andersson M, et al. Postoperative radiotherapy in high-risk postmenopausal breast-cancer patients given adju-vant tamoxifen: Danish breast cancer cooperative group DBCG 82c randomised trial. Lancet. 1999;353(9165):1641–8.
4. van der Ploeg IMC, Nieweg OE, van Rijk MC, Valdés Olmos RA, Kroon BBR. Axillary recur-rence after a tumour-negative sentinel node biopsy in breast cancer patients: a systematic review and meta-analysis of the literature. Eur J Surg Oncol. 2008;34(12):1277–84.
5. Giuliano AE, McCall L, Beitsch P, Whitworth PW, Blumencranz P, Leitch AM, et al. Locoregional recurrence after sentinel lymph node dissection with or without axillary dis-section in patients with sentinel lymph node metastases: the American College of Surgeons Oncology group Z0011 randomized trial. Trans Meet Am Surg Assoc. 2010;128:12–21.
6. Lucci A, McCall LM, Beitsch PD, Whitworth PW, Reintgen DS, Blumencranz PW, et al. Surgical complications associated with sentinel lymph node dissection (SLND) plus axil-lary lymph node dissection compared with SLND alone in the American College of Surgeons oncology group trial Z0011. J Clin Oncol. 2007;25(24):3657–63.
7. Galimberti V, Cole BF, Zurrida S, Viale G, Luini A, Veronesi P, et al. Axillary dissection versus no axillary dissection in patients with sentinel-node micrometastases (IBCSG 23-01): a phase 3 randomised controlled trial. Lancet Oncol. 2013;14(4):297–305.
8. Louis-Sylvestre C, Clough K, Asselain B, Vilcoq JR, Salmon RJ, Campana F, et al. Axillary treatment in conservative management of operable breast cancer: dissection or radiotherapy? Results of a randomized study with 15 years of follow-up. J Clin Oncol. 2004;22(1):97–101.
9. Donker M, van Tienhoven G, Straver ME, Meijnen P, van de Velde CJH, Mansel RE, et al. Radiotherapy or surgery of the axilla after a positive sentinel node in breast cancer (EORTC 10981-22023 AMAROS): a randomised, multicentre, open-label, phase 3 non-inferiority trial. Lancet Oncol. 2014;15(12):1303–10.
10. Sávolt Á, Péley G, Polgár C, Udvarhely N, Rubovszky G, Kovács E, et al. Eight-year follow up result of the OTOASOR trial: the optimal treatment of the axilla—surgery or radiother-apy after positive sentinel lymph node biopsy in early-stage breast cancer. Eur J Surg Oncol. 2017;43(4):672–9.
11. Effect of radiotherapy after breast-conserving surgery on 10-year recurrence and 15-year breast cancer death: meta-analysis of individual patient data for 10 801 women in 17 ran-domised trials. Lancet. 2011;378(9804):1707–16.
12. McGale P, Taylor C, Correa C, Cutter D, Duane F, Ewertz M, et al. Effect of radiotherapy after mastectomy and axillary surgery on 10-year recurrence and 20-year breast cancer mortal-ity: meta-analysis of individual patient data for 8135 women in 22 randomised trials. Lancet. 2014;383(9935):2127–35.
13. Moreno AC, Shaitelman SF, Buchholz TA. A clinical perspective on regional nodal irradiation for breast cancer. Breast. 2017;34:S85–90.
14. Moreno AC, Lin YH, Bedrosian I, Shen Y, Stauder MC, Smith BD, et al. Use of regional nodal irradiation and its association with survival for women with high-risk, early stage breast can-cer: a National Cancer Database analysis. Adv Radiat Oncol. 2017;2(3):291–300.
15. Budach W, Bölke E, Kammers K, Gerber PA, Nestle-Krämling C, Matuschek C. Adjuvant radiation therapy of regional lymph nodes in breast cancer—a meta-analysis of randomized trials—an update. Radiat Oncol. 2015;10:258.

16. Whelan TJ, Olivotto IA, Parulekar WR, Ackerman I, Chua BH, Nabid A, et al. Regional nodal irradiation in early-stage breast cancer. N Engl J Med. 2015;373(4):307–16.
17. Poortmans PM, Collette S, Kirkove C, Van Limbergen E, Budach V, Struikmans H, et al. Internal mammary and medial supraclavicular irradiation in breast cancer. N Engl J Med. 2015;373(4):317–27.
18. Jagsi R. Postmastectomy radiation therapy: an overview for the practicing surgeon. ISRN Surg. 2013;2013:1–16.
19. Rusthoven CG, Rabinovitch RA, Jones BL, Koshy M, Amini A, Yeh N, et al. The impact of postmastectomy and regional nodal radiation after neoadjuvant chemotherapy for clinically lymph node-positive breast cancer: a National Cancer Database (NCDB) analysis. Ann Oncol. 2016;27(5):818–27.
20. Breast Cancer Nomogram: Breast Additional Non SLN Metastases | Memorial Sloan Kettering Cancer Center. 2018. http://nomograms.mskcc.org/breast/BreastAdditionalNonSLNMetastasesPage.aspx
21. Van Zee KJ, Manasseh D-ME, Bevilacqua JLB, Boolbol SK, Fey JV, Tan LK, et al. A nomogram for predicting the likelihood of additional nodal metastases in breast cancer patients with a positive sentinel node biopsy. Ann Surg Oncol. 2003;10(10):1140–51.
22. Specht MC, Kattan MW, Gonen M, Fey J, Van Zee KJ. Predicting nonsentinel node status after positive sentinel lymph biopsy for breast cancer: clinicians versus nomogram. Ann Surg Oncol. 2005;12(8):654–9.
23. Alran S, De Rycke Y, Fourchotte V, Charitansky H, Laki F, Falcou MC, et al. Validation and limitations of use of a breast cancer nomogram predicting the likelihood of non-sentinel node involvement after positive sentinel node biopsy. Ann Surg Oncol. 2007;14(8):2195–201.
24. Pierce SM, Recht A, Lingos TI, Abner A, Vicini F, Silver B, et al. Long-term radiation complications following conservative surgery (CS) and radiation therapy (RT) in patients with early stage breast cancer. Int J Radiat Oncol. 1992;23(5):915–23.
25. Powell S, Cooke J, Parsons C. Radiation-induced brachial plexus injury: follow-up of two different fractionation schedules. Radiother Oncol J Eur Soc Ther Radiol Oncol. 1990;18(3):213–20.
26. Sugden EM, Rezvani M, Harrison JM, Hughes LK. Shoulder movement after the treatment of early stage breast cancer. Clin Oncol R Coll Radiol G B. 1998;10(3):173–81.
27. Taylor C, Correa C, Duane FK, Aznar MC, Anderson SJ, Bergh J, et al. Estimating the risks of breast cancer radiotherapy: evidence from modern radiation doses to the lungs and heart and from previous randomized trials. J Clin Oncol. 2017;35(15):1641–9.

Sanjiv Sharma

Hypofractionation represents the most important recent advance in breast cancer radiotherapy, supported by robust level I evidence [1–10]. Despite its well-documented benefits, clinical adoption has been slow.

18.1 Biologic Rationale

For breast irradiation, an ideal fractionation schedule should respect the delicate balance between the probability of local recurrence and the possibility of side effects, both early as well as late. Conventionally fractionated radiotherapy (CFRT) employing dose per fraction of 1.8–2.0 Gy delivering 50 Gy is one such schedule. Long clinical experience with this schedule has shown low rates of local recurrence and morbidity, due to which it represents the contemporary standard of care.

Clinical experience and radiobiological modeling have shown that the therapeutic ratio is a function of fraction size as well as the total dose of radiation. Initial efforts at hypofractionated radiotherapy (HFRT) in the 1960s led to considerable toxicity, including severe fibrosis, brachial plexopathy, and rib fractures, as the need to reduce the total dose was not recognized at that time [11]. This fear has led to the slow adoption of HFRT in clinical practice and continues to do so.

Investigators realized in the 1990s that HFRT employing less number of fractions (around 15) using higher dose per fraction but to decreased total doses appeared comparable to CFRT regarding local recurrence and complication rates. Modern radiobiology has provided a firm scientific rationale to this clinical experience so that different variables that impact the therapeutic ratio can be modified to improve it. Decades of clinical experience and laboratory experiments have led to the development of the linear-quadratic (LQ) model [12] based on the following equation:

S. Sharma (✉)
Department of Radiation Oncology, Manipal Hospital, Bangalore, India

© Springer Nature Singapore Pte Ltd. 2021
B. Kunheri, D. K. Vijaykumar (eds.), *Management of Early Stage Breast Cancer*,
https://doi.org/10.1007/978-981-15-6171-9_18

$$\text{Biological effective dose}\,(\text{BED}) = \text{total dose}\,(\text{TD}) \left[1 + \frac{\text{Fraction size}}{\alpha/\beta} \right].$$

This model incorporates a dual theory, considering a nonrepairable (α) and repairable (β) damage. The sensitivity of various tissues to different fraction sizes can be represented as a ratio of alpha and beta (α/β). The model suggests that the biological effect of radiation can be predicted by a combination of total dose and fraction size and that the α/β ratio representing the intrinsic radiosensitivity of the tissues will modify the effect of the fraction size. As per this model, if the α/β ratio of the tumor is the same or less than that of critical normal tissue, then a higher fractional dose with a modest reduction in total dose is likely to be equieffective to CFRT or potentially more effective.

It has been suggested by previous investigators [13] that the dose–response curve of normal tissue complication probability is likely to be steeper than that for subclinical breast tumor control since it is known that local control without radiation is approximately 70% without any morbidity. Thus, a modest reduction in total dose will result in a considerable decrease in normal tissue toxicity without any significant impact on tumor control.

18.2 Clinical Rationale

Hypofractionation is an attractive proposition, since the treatment is delivered with lesser number of fractions in a shorter overall time, resulting in patient convenience, reduced cost to the patient as well as the health care system, and reduced resource utilization. Additionally, due to the lower total doses being utilized, it results in less skin toxicity, thus leading to improved patient care.

18.3 Evidence

The first landmark study conducted in Canada involved 1234 women with early-stage node-negative breast cancer and negative surgical margins after breast-conserving surgery (BCS) and axillary dissection. They were randomized to WBI either by HFRT of 42.5 Gy in 16 fractions over 22 days or a CFRT of 50 Gy in 25 fractions over 35 days [1, 2]. Because of the concerns about dose inhomogeneity potentially leading to more normal tissue morbidity, a breast width of more than 25 cm at the posterior edge of the tangential portals was an exclusion criterion. Contemporary megavoltage radiation techniques were employed. Tumor bed boost was not permitted, and adjuvant systemic therapy was advised as per standard guidelines prevalent at that time. At a median follow-up of 12 years, there was no statistically significant difference in the 10-year risk of local recurrence (6.7% with CFRT versus 6.2% with HFRT) and the good or excellent cosmetic outcome at 10 years (71.3% versus 69.8%). Age, tumor size, estrogen receptor status, or use of systemic therapy had no impact on local recurrence. In the initial analysis, the HFRT regimen had a higher local recurrence (15.6% versus 4.7% with CFRT, p = 0.01) in patients with high-grade tumors, but this effect was not found in a subsequent analysis of 989 patients that incorporated a central review of pathology [3]. Cosmetic outcome was affected by the time from randomization (odds ratio per year 0.93 {range 0.90–0.95}, $p < 0.001$), the patients' age, and tumor size, but the fractionation schedule had no impact. No difference was observed in overall survival and cardiac mortality.

The START PILOT trial randomized 1410 patients to either 50 Gy of CFRT delivered in 25 fractions over a period of 5 weeks or two HFRT schedules of 39 or 42.9 Gy in 13 fractions over the same duration [4]. The overall treatment time was kept the same so that the effect of fractionation on late breast tissue morbidity could be evaluated. Completely resected patients with invasive breast cancer stage pT1–3, N0–1 treated with BCS were included. Local guidelines determined axillary treatment (surgery and/or radiation), tumor bed boost, and adjuvant systemic therapy. Standard wedged tangential portals using 4–10 MV photons or telecobalt radiation were used for treatment. Late radiation effects were assessed, employing clinical photographs to assess breast appearance and clinical examination for induration. Breast appearance was found to be unchanged at 10 years in 46.6%, 42.0%, and 43.9% of patients treated with 50 Gy, 42.9 Gy, and 39 Gy, respectively. Both HFRT schedules resulted in less change than patients treated with CFRT ($p = 0.01$ and 0.05, respectively). At 10 years, statistically significant differences were found for the absence of moderate or marked breast induration (63.7%, 48.9%, and 72.3% of patients treated with 50, 42.9, and 39 Gy, respectively). Local recurrence results published later [5] did not show any statistical difference between any of the arms, which, at 10 years, was 12.1% for 50 Gy, 9.6% for 42.9 Gy, and 14.8% for 39 Gy. This study yielded an α/β ratio of 3.6 Gy for breast appearance and 4.0 Gy for local recurrence.

This study provided robust clinical evidence in support of the hypothesis that the α/β ratio is low for normal breast tissue (3–3.5 Gy) as well as breast cancer (around 4 Gy). It also validated the radiobiological rationale of HFRT, which, along with a modest reduction in total dose, would have efficacy similar to CFRT regarding local control and delayed normal tissue morbidity.

Standardization of Radiotherapy (START) trials A and B [6, 7] were subsequently initiated based upon the observations of this trial. These trials included patients with invasive breast cancer (pT1–3, pN0–1, M0), treated with BCS or mastectomy, whose tumors had been excised completely. Immediate surgical reconstruction was not permitted. Local practice determined the boost (10 Gy in 5 fractions), lymphatic radiation, and adjuvant systemic therapy. Patient self-assessment, evaluation by a physician, and clinical photographs were employed to compare the late effects of radiation on various normal tissues such as breast, arm, and shoulder.

The START-A trial, similar to START PILOT, again compared the standard schedule of CFRT (50 Gy in 25 fractions over 5 weeks) with two slightly different HFRT schedules of 41.6 or 39 Gy in 13 fractions over 5 weeks. Again, overall treatment time was kept the same to eliminate its impact on the determination of the effect of fractionation so that more data could be generated about the α/β ratio for breast cancer and an optimal HFRT schedule could be determined. The START B trial employed the same CFRT schedule of 50 Gy in 25 fractions over 5 weeks, but the HFRT schedule chosen was an accelerated one using 40 Gy in 15 fractions over 3 weeks. An individual patient data meta-analysis was also conducted combining all the three trials.

The 10-year results of both the trials have been reported [8]. A total of 2236 patients were enrolled in the START-A trial. At a median follow-up of 9.3 years, no significant difference in 10-year locoregional relapse could be detected between the three arms (7.4% for 50 Gy, 6.3% for 41.6 Gy, and 8.8% for 39 Gy). Late normal tissue effects such as induration, telangiectasia, and edema of breast were significantly less with 39 Gy as compared to 50 Gy, whereas they were similar for 41·6 Gy and 50 Gy cohorts. No significant difference could be detected among various dose schedules regarding distant metastases, disease-free survival, and overall survival. The α/β value for local-regional relapse was estimated to be 4 Gy.

The START B trial recruited 2215 patients who were followed for a median of 9.9 years. The 10-year locoregional relapse rates were similar between the two groups (4·3% for 40 Gy versus 5.5% for 50 Gy, p = 0·21). The 40 Gy schedule caused significantly less normal tissue morbidity (shrinkage, telangiectasia, and edema of breast) than the 50 Gy schedule. Surprisingly though, distant metastases, disease-free survival, and overall survival were significantly better with the HFRT schedule.

18.4 Summary of Evidence

A meta-analysis [9], conducted using pooled data from all four trials, demonstrated the HFRT and CFRT after breast-conserving surgery to be equally effective, with a hazard ratio of 1.00. No impact of any of the patient-, tumor-, or treatment-related factors was observed. The HFRT schedule of 40 Gy in 15 fractions over 3 weeks was the only one associated with a significant survival benefit. HFRT produced less acute as well as late normal tissue morbidity related to skin and breast, whereas the incidence of toxicity in other tissues of concern such as the heart, lungs, ribs, and brachial plexus was similar.

A Cochrane systematic review [10] was performed to evaluate the quality of the trials. It concluded that the conduct of the trials and the reporting of results was of good quality and that the trials lacked any significant bias.

18.5 Barriers to Adoption

This robust evidence (Table 18.1) has led to the widespread adoption of the schedule of 40 Gy in 15 fractions over 3 weeks, which represents the current standard of care. Using the α/β value derived from the START trials, this is equivalent to 45 Gy in 2 Gy fractions (E_qD_2), if a value of 3.5 Gy is applied for late normal tissue effects.

Table 18.1 Patient characteristics of four randomized trials

	ONTARIO (1–3)	START PILOT (4, 5)	START A (6, 8)	START B (7, 8)
No. of patients	1234	1410	2236	2215
Age < 50 (years)	25%	30.3%	23%	21%
Stage	pT1–2, N0–1	pT1–3, N0–1	pT1–3, N0–1	pT1–3, N0–1
Dose per fraction (Gy)	2.0 vs 2.7	2.0 vs 3.0 vs 3.3	2.0 vs 3.0 vs 3.2	2.0 vs 2.6
Mastectomy	0%	0%	15%	8%
Node positive	0%	32.7%	28.8%	22.8%
Boost	0%	74.5%	60.6%	42.6%
Boost dose	0%	14 Gy/7 fr	10 Gy/5 fr	10 Gy/5 fr
Nodal radiation	0% -	20.6%	14.2%	7.3%
Adjuvant chemotherapy	11.0%	13.9%	35.5%	22.2%
Grade III	–	28.1%	23%	19%

Thus, this regimen is less damaging to the normal tissues while being effective for treatment of cancer. The incidence of pulmonary toxicity, cardiac events, rib fractures, and brachial plexopathy at 10 years with this schedule is as low as that with the CFRT schedules, making it the regime of choice.

Despite the fact that adoption has been very slow in many parts of the world, notably the United States, it is prudent to discuss the concerns responsible for this. Lots of physicians feel uncomfortable about using HFRT for many patient groups having clinical characteristics similar to the patients enrolled for these trials. In an attempt to alleviate these concerns and fears, a post hoc meta-analysis of all the START trials was performed to evaluate the impact of HFRT schedules on various patient subgroups. Within the constraints of its post hoc nature, locoregional relapse was independent of various patient-, tumor- and treatment-related factors such as age of the patient, size of the breast, nature of surgery, axillary nodal status, grade of the tumor, use of adjuvant systemic chemotherapy, tumor bed boost, and nodal irradiation. Similarly, no correlation with any of these factors was observed for late normal tissue morbidity in the breast.

There is concern whether these results can be extrapolated to the patient groups that were either not included or had poor representation in these trials. Age less than 50 years, histology of ductal carcinoma in situ, locally advanced breast cancer, neoadjuvant chemotherapy usage, mastectomy (5%), immediate breast reconstruction, and regional nodal irradiation (8%) are some of these patient groups. It is felt that further data are needed before routine use of HFRT in these patient groups. Radiobiologically, it is unlikely for the effects of HFRT in these patient groups to be substantially different. Contemporary prospective data [14] have shown that age is no bar for HFRT, and recent ASTRO guidelines [15] also recommend the same.

Targeted agents such as trastuzumab were not available at the time these trials were conducted, and hence, there is no data about the use of HFRT in these patients. Since trastuzumab has been shown to be safe after or concurrently with CFRT after

BCS or mastectomy [16], especially in the absence of the internal mammary nodal irradiation, results are unlikely to be any different with HFRT. Until the availability of long-term safety data, judicious use would be appropriate but with caution.

Since only 8% of the patients in the trials received nodal irradiation, fear of injury to the brachial plexus has emerged as a major concern while employing HFRT for such patients. Only one case of brachial plexopathy was reported in the 41.6 Gy arm in the START A trial. It is well known that this devastating complication can appear as late as 30 years after radiotherapy. What is also well understood is the fact that around 75% of the cases would have appeared by 10 years [17]. Thus, it can be safely concluded with reasonable certainty that this complication would never be a cause for concern. Additional confidence can be gained from the fact that the E_qD_2 of 40 Gy in 15 fractions is lower than 50 Gy in 25 fractions, even with α/β values lower than the one commonly accepted for neural tissues (E_qD_2 of 49.0 Gy, 47.7 Gy, and 46.8 Gy, assuming α/β values of 1.0 Gy, 1.5 Gy, and 2.0 Gy). The dose is expected to be even lower at the depth at which the brachial plexus is normally located. Thus, 40 Gy in 15 fractions is expected to be safer for the brachial plexus than is 50 Gy in 25 fractions. The British Columbia randomized trial of post-mastectomy radiotherapy [18] employed HFRT for regional sites including internal mammary chain, and the 20-year results showed no incidence of brachial plexus injury, thus providing an additional level of reassurance. Nevertheless, HFRT for the nodal irradiation should be applied with extra caution; the 40 Gy in 15 fractions schedule would be optimal and meticulous attention in planning is needed to avoid overdosing of the brachial plexus.

Dose likely to be delivered to the heart with HFRT has been another major reason for its suboptimal utilization. Cardiotoxicity associated with most of the commonly used chemotherapy drugs adds to the concern. Contemporary radiobiological research suggests that for HFRT to be more toxic to the heart than the CFRT, the α/β value of the heart would have to be below 0.75 Gy, while employing the dose schedule of 40 Gy in 15 fractions (E_qD_2 of 50.0 Gy with α/β values of 0.75 Gy). Most investigators agree that the α/β ratio for the heart is much higher [18], thus suggesting that HFRT might be safer for the heart than CFRT [19]. Regardless, all efforts should be directed toward minimizing the dose to the heart, as this radiobiological observation needs clinical validation with longer follow-up. There is a paucity of long-term data for internal mammary nodal irradiation using HFRT. Though potentially feasible, caution is advised until more data are available, and the use of modern conformal radiation techniques is highly recommended.

HFRT in large breasts has always been a cause of concern due to larger dose inhomogeneity leading to a possible overdose. The ONTARIO trial explicitly excluded patients with a breast width greater than 25 cm at the posterior edge of the tangential portals. The presumption has been that this overdose would lead to increased toxicity with HFRT. However, using the same logic as was employed for brachial plexus and heart, it has been suggested that 40 Gy in 15 fractions would be less deleterious as long as the α/β ratio of the normal breast tissue is >1 Gy. Again, the value derived from the START trial data is higher than that, thus suggesting that HFRT would not increase the toxicity to normal breast tissue and that the patients with large breast size should be offered HFRT. Regardless, advanced radiation techniques such as field-in-field, also known as forward intensity-modulated radiotherapy, should be routinely applied to minimize hot spots.

A retrospective analysis of prospectively collected data of all START trials revealed low incidence of physician-assessed and patient-reported moderate and marked arm and/or shoulder symptoms with no significant difference detected between the two arms [20].

Although the randomized trials included patients only with invasive cancer, enough prospective data exist to support its efficacy and safety in ductal carcinoma in situ [21]. There appears to be no logical reason to presume that the normal tissue response to HFRT would be different in these patients. One ongoing Australian randomized trial is addressing this issue [22].

Poor representation of high-risk patients having undergone mastectomy and requiring regional irradiation has been a stumbling block in offering HFRT to these patients. A Chinese phase 3 trial [23] randomized 820 patients of age 18–75 years with invasive breast carcinoma, who had undergone mastectomy for T3–4 and/ or N2–3 disease, to the CFRT or HFRT schedule of 43.5 Gy in 15 fractions. At a median follow-up of 58.5 months, no significant difference in the locoregional relapse and acute or chronic toxicity could be observed, except for acute grade 3 skin toxicity, which was significantly less with HFRT (3% versus 8%, $p < 0.0001$). A recent meta-analysis and systematic review, involving 25 randomized control trials having 3871 patients undergoing post-mastectomy radiotherapy, confirmed these results [24].

18.6 Which Schedule to Follow

The accelerated HFRT schedule used in the START B regimen, delivering 40 Gy in 15 fractions of 2.67 Gy over a period of 3 weeks, appears most promising. This regimen had the optimal therapeutic ratio with significantly less early and delayed morbidity as well as significantly reduced distant metastasis rate and better overall survival. That has led to the widespread adoption of this schedule across the world and has emerged as the current standard of care and regimen of choice. Tumor bed boost can be incorporated as clinically indicated.

Many societies, including the American Society for Radiation Oncology (ASTRO), National Institute for Health and Care Excellence (NICE), have incorporated the evidence generated by the HFRT trials into their national treatment guidelines [14, 25–27].

18.7 Future Direction

Various trials are in progress to investigate extreme fractionation, with a focus on 5-fraction schedules. The FAST trial [28], conducted by the UK National Cancer Research Network (NCRN), recently reported its 10-year outcome data of 915 patients of stage pT1–2 N0 invasive breast cancer, randomized between 5 weekly fractions of 5.7 Gy or 6.0 Gy (total dose of 28.5 Gy and 30 Gy, respectively) versus CFRT. Nodal irradiation, tumor bed boost, and neoadjuvant chemotherapy were not permitted. At a median follow-up of 9.9 years, the 10-year incidence of marked normal tissue effects and local recurrence was low across all schedules, with the 30 Gy schedule having significantly higher adverse effects, and hence not recommended. The investigators suggest such a schedule to be considered for patients unable to visit hospital daily for 3–5 weeks. Efforts to test the limits of hypofractionation further have led to the development of a 5-fraction schedule delivered in 5 consecutive days, considered feasible with modern radiation techniques ensuring homogeneous dose distribution and cardiac sparing. FAST-Forward [29], a phase 3 multicenter trial, randomized 4096 early-stage (pT1–3 N0–1 M0) patients with invasive carcinoma, after breast conservation surgery or mastectomy (reconstruction allowed), to receive radiation to whole breast (sequential tumor bed boost permitted) or chest wall alone, to two dose levels of 27 Gy and 26 Gy of a 5-fraction regimen delivered in 1 week against 40 Gy in 15 fractions over 3 weeks. At a median follow-up of 71.5 months, the 5-year local tumor control was noninferior in the 5 fraction arm as compared to the standard HFRT arm. Clinician-assessed, patient-reported, and photographically evaluated moderate to marked normal tissue adverse effects related to breast and chest wall were not significantly different between the 40 Gy arm and the 26 Gy arm, whereas the 27 Gy arm had significantly more incidence. These results take hypofractionation one step forward, and the schedule of 26 Gy delivered in five fractions over 1 week is potentially the new standard of care. A substudy of this trial is currently evaluating this protocol for patients requiring nodal irradiation. An ongoing trial, NRG Oncology RTOG 1005, is testing new paradigms in the field of HFRT by incorporating concurrent boost while comparing it with CFRT.

As part of ongoing research, HFRT and CFRT are being compared in patients undergoing immediate breast reconstruction after mastectomy, and two trials by the Alliance for Clinical Trials in Oncology cooperative group (A221505) and Dana-Farber Cancer Institute (NCT03422003), are currently recruiting patients. Future studies will also need to focus on determining if all molecular subtypes of breast cancer are equally well controlled with hypofractionation.

References

1. Whelan T, MacKenzie R, Julian J, et al. Randomized trial of breast irradiation schedules after lumpectomy for women with lymph node-negative breast cancer. J Natl Cancer Inst. 2002;94:1143–50.
2. Whelan TJ, Pignol JP, Levine MN, et al. Long-term results of hypofractionated radiation therapy for breast cancer. N Engl J Med. 2010;362:513–20.
3. Bane AL, Whelan TJ, Pond GR, et al. Tumor factors predictive of response to hypofractionated radiotherapy in a randomized trial following breast conserving therapy. Ann Oncol. 2014;25:992–8.
4. Yarnold J, Ashton A, Bliss J, et al. Fractionation sensitivity and dose response of late adverse effects in the breast after radiotherapy for early breast cancer: long-term results of a randomised trial. Radiother Oncol. 2005;75:9–17.

5. Owen JR, Ashton A, Bliss JM, et al. Effect of radiotherapy fraction size on tumour control in patients with early-stage breast cancer after local tumour excision: long-term results of a randomised trial. Lancet Oncol. 2006;7:467–71.
6. START Trialists'Group. The UK standardisation of breast radiotherapy (START) trial a of radiotherapy hypofractionation for treatment of early breast cancer: a randomised trial. Lancet Oncol. 2008;9:331–41.
7. START Trialists' Group. The UK standardisation of breast radiotherapy (START) trial B of radiotherapy hypofractionation for treatment of early breast cancer: a randomised trial. Lancet. 2008;371:1098–107.
8. Haviland JS, Owen JR, Dewar JA, et al. The UK standardisation of breast radiotherapy (START) trials of radiotherapy hypofractionation for treatment of early breast cancer: 10-year follow-up results of two randomised controlled trials. Lancet Oncol. 2013;14:1086–94.
9. Budach W, Bölke E, Matuschek C. Hypofractionated radiotherapy as adjuvant treatment in early breast cancer. A review and meta-analysis of randomized controlled trials. Breast Care. 2015;10:240–5.
10. James ML, Lehman M, Hider PN, Jeffery M, Hickey BE, Francis DP. Fraction size in radiation treatment for breast conservation in early breast cancer. Cochrane Database Syst Rev. 2010;11:CD003860.
11. Fletcher GH. Hypofractionation: lessons from complications. Radiother Oncol. 1991;20:10–5.
12. Fowler JF. The linear-quadratic formula and progress in fractionated radiotherapy. Br J Radiol. 1989;62:679–94.
13. Yarnold J, Bentzen SM, Coles C, et al. Hypofractionated whole-breast radiotherapy for women with early breast cancer: myths and realities. Int J Radiat Oncol Biol Phys. 2011;79:1–9.
14. Shaikh F, Chew J, Hochman T, et al. Hypofractionated whole breast irradiation in women less than 50 years old treated on four prospective protocols. Int J Radiat Oncol Biol Phys. 101(5):1159–67.
15. Smith BD, Bellon JR, Blitzblau R, et al. Radiation therapy for the whole breast : executive summary of an American Society for Radiation Oncology(ASTRO) evidence-based guideline. Pract Radiat Oncol. 2018;81:59–68.
16. Halyard MY, Pisansky TM, Dueck AC, et al. Radiotherapy and adjuvant trastuzumab in operable breast cancer: tolerability and adverse event data from theNCCTG phase III trial N9831. J Clin Oncol. 2009;27:2638–44.
17. Galecki J, Hicer-Grzenkowicz J, Grudzien-Kowalska M, et al. Radiation-induced brachial plexopathy and hypofractionated regimens in adjuvant irradiation of patients with breast cancer—a review. Acta Oncol. 2006;45:280–4.
18. Gagliardi G, Constine LS, Moiseenko V, et al. Radiation dose-volume effects in the heart. Int J Radiat Oncol Biol Phys. 2010;76(3 suppl):S77–85.
19. Appelt AL, Vogelius IR, Bentzen SM. Modern hypofractionation schedules for tangential whole breast irradiation decrease the fraction size-corrected dose to the heart. Clin Oncol (R Coll Radiol). 2013;25:147–52.
20. Haviland JS, Mannino M, Griffin C, et al. Late normal tissue effects in the arm and shoulder following lymphaticradiotherapy: results from the UK START (standardisation of breast radiotherapy) trials. Radiother Oncol. 2018;126:155–62.
21. Nilsson C, Valachis A. The role of boost and hypofractionation as adjuvant radiotherapy in patients with DCIS: a meta-analysis of observational studies. Radiother Oncol. 2015;114:50–5.
22. Trans-Tasman Radiation Oncology Group (TROG). Radiation doses and fractionation schedules in non-low risk Ductal carcinoma in situ (DCIS) of the breast. https://clinicaltrials.gov/ct2/show/NCT00470236?term=ductal+carcinoma+in+situ&rank=24.
23. Wang SL, Fang H, Song YW, et al. Hypofractionated versus conventional fractionated postmastectomy radiotherapy for patients with high-risk breast cancer: a randomised, non-inferiority, open-label, phase 3 trial. Lancet Oncol. 2019;20(3):352–60.
24. Liu L, Yang Y, Guo Q, et al. Comparing hypofractionated to conventional fractionated radiotherapy in postmastectomy breast cancer: a meta-analysis and systematic review. Radiat Oncol. 2020;17:1–15.

25. National Institute for Health and Clinical Excellence. NICE clinical guideline 80: early and locally advanced breast cancer: diagnosis and treatment. 2009.
26. Sedlmayer F, Sautter-Bihl ML, Budach W, et al. DEGRO practical guidelines: radiotherapy of breast cancer I: radiotherapy following breast conserving therapy for invasive breast cancer. Strahlenther Onkol. 2013;189:825–33.
27. Senkus E, Kyriakides S, Penault-Llorca F, et al. Primary breast cancer: ESMO clinical practice guidelines for diagnosis, treatment and follow-up. Ann Oncol. 2013;24(suppl 6):7–23.
28. Brunt AM, Haviland J, Sydenham M, et al. FAST phase III RCT of radiotherapy hypofractionation for treatment of early breast cancer: 10 year results (CRUKE/04/015). Int J Radiat Oncol Biol Phys. 2018;102:1603–4.
29. Brunt AM, Haviland JS, Wheatley DA, et al. Hypofractionated breast radiotherapy for 1 week versus 3 weeks (FAST-forward): 5 year efficacy and late normal tissue effects results from a multicenter, non-inferiority, randomized, phase 3 trial. Lancet. 2020;120:114–8.

Accelerated Partial-Breast Irradiation: Current Evidence and Techniques

19

Sruthi Kalavagunta and Beena Kunheri

19.1 Rationale for APBI

By definition, early breast cancer (EBC) includes all the breast cancers that are stage II or less [2]. As awareness of breast cancer is increasing and also with a widespread availability of screening techniques such as mammography, the diagnosis of early breast cancer is on the rise. Breast conservation therapy (BCT) is being increasingly used and has become the standard of care surgery in EBC. Radiation therapy forms a core component in the breast conservation therapy.

Traditionally, whole-breast radiation to a total dose of 45–50 Gy in 1.8 Gy to 2 Gy fractions is delivered over 5–6 weeks followed by a tumour bed boost of 10–15 Gy. The NSABP B-06 studies have established equivalent local control and survival rates between BCT and mastectomy [3].

The Early Breast Cancer Trialists' Collaborative Group (EBCTCG) in their meta-analysis of individual patient data for 10,801 women in 17 randomized trials showed that after breast-conserving surgery, radiotherapy to the conserved breast halves the rate at which the disease recurs and reduces the breast cancer death rate by about a sixth. Overall, radiotherapy reduced the 10-year risk of any (i.e. locoregional or distant) first recurrence from 35% to 19.3% and reduced the 15-year risk of breast cancer death from 25.2% to 21.4% [4]. The National Institutes of Health, United States issued a consensus statement that breast-conserving treatment is the preferable option for women with early-stage breast cancer [5].

S. Kalavagunta
Department of Radiation Oncology, Amrita Institute of Medical Sciences, Kochi, Kerala, India

B. Kunheri (✉)
Department of Radiation Oncology, Amrita Institute of Medical Sciences and Research Centre, Amrita Vishwa Vidyapeetham University, Kochi, Kerala, India

© Springer Nature Singapore Pte Ltd. 2021
B. Kunheri, D. K. Vijaykumar (eds.), *Management of Early Stage Breast Cancer*,
https://doi.org/10.1007/978-981-15-6171-9_19

In the Groupe Européen de Curiethérapie of the European Society for Radiotherapy and Oncology (GEC-ESTRO) trial, 1184 patients were enrolled in a phase 3, non-inferiority trial and were randomized to WBI plus a tumour bed boost or APBI delivered with multi-catheter interstitial brachytherapy [1]. The 5-year risk of ipsilateral breast tumour recurrence (IBTR) was less than 2% in both treatment arms, and the study concluded that APBI was not inferior to WBI. In addition, there were no differences in toxicity over 5 years [6].

IMPORT LOW is a multicentre, randomized, controlled, phase 3, non-inferiority trial done in 30 radiotherapy centres in the UK and is the first phase 3 trial reporting 5-year outcome data for local relapse and adverse effects after partial-breast radiotherapy delivered using standard external-beam radiotherapy techniques. At 5 years, partial-breast radiotherapy delivered using a simple and standard technique showed no increase in local relapse rates compared with whole-breast radiotherapy and produced equivalent or reduced late adverse effects [7].

Radiobiological rationale behind APBI is that a higher dose can be delivered over a smaller target area in a shorter treatment time and simultaneously not compromising on the tumour control. The linear quadratic model (LQM) may not be accurately showing the cell kill at higher doses and hence may not be appropriate for APBI as it overestimates cell killing at high single doses [8, 9].

Radiobiological models are needed to know the optimal dose and fractionation for the different APBI techniques. Dose selection is based on the concept of equivalent uniform biologically effective dose (EUBED) and use actual patient dose matrix data that the maximum fraction size needed to deliver a biologically equivalent dose using 3D-CRT is 3.82 Gy with an equivalent total prescription dose of 38.2 Gy, supporting the continued use of 3.85 Gy BID [10].

Though the BCT has been stated as the preferable option, there has been underutilization of the technique as some women are not ready to undergo the protracted 6–7-week radiation therapy after BCS. Many contributing factors such as prolonged treatment time, convenience of treatment, the need to go for daily treatments, accessibility, cost of treatment, distance from the treatment centre, lack of social support and fear of radiation are associated with this underutilization of BCT [11].

Thus, the need to shorten the treatment time and achieve similar control rates by delivering radiation to the area at the highest risk of recurrence keeping in mind the radiobiology and the physics involved enabling the BCT to be made available to more women led to the development of APBI in early-stage breast cancer.

Several studies have supported the evolution of APBI based on the fact that the local recurrences occur close to the tumour bed. Recurrences outside the tumour bed occur in less than 4% of the cases. In APBI, only the portion of the breast at the greatest risk of recurrence is irradiated, and the 6 weeks of therapy is 5 days of twice-daily fractionation. This is especially important in patients with limited access to transportation, thereby enabling treatment adherence in all eligible patients. In addition to improved convenience, APBI allows sparing of normal tissues from irradiation, such as breast tissue at less risk, adjacent ribs, lung and (for left-sided lesions) the heart. Rare effects of whole-breast irradiation include pulmonary fibrosis, pneumonitis or rib fractures [12].

19.2   Techniques of APBI

In APBI, the lumpectomy bed plus a margin of 1–2 cm is treated. The radiation dose per fraction is increased, and the target volume is decreased, allowing shorter over-all treatment time. APBI is delivered using techniques like multicatheter interstitial brachytherapy, balloon catheter brachytherapy, 3D-CRT (conformal radiation therapy) and intraoperative radiation therapy (IORT) [13]. APBI can be done intraoperatively or shortly after the surgery. The intraoperative techniques include photon or electron irradiation and interstitial high dose rate (HDR) brachytherapy, whereas the postoperative techniques comprise interstitial brachytherapy, be it HDR, pulse dose rate (PDR) or low dose rate (LDR), intracavitary brachytherapy and external-beam radiotherapy using electrons, photons or protons [14].

19.3   Intraoperative Techniques

A single, high dose of radiation is given with electrons or photons with special applicators. Intraoperative radiation therapy was first used in 1998 with a device called the Intrabeam that generated photons. Subsequently, two other mobile linear accelerators generating megavoltage electrons called the Mobetron and Novac-7 systems were introduced.

IORT has the advantage of delivering radiation before tumour proliferation. Also, tissues under surgical intervention have a rich vascularization, with aerobic metabolism, which makes them more sensitive to the action of the radiation (oxygen effect). As it is given under direct visualization, it could minimize toxicity to the skin, subcutaneous tissue, lung and the heart [15]. IORT enables treatment adherence as there is no delay and allows radiotherapy to be given without delaying the administration of chemotherapy or hormonal therapy [16]. Due to patient movement, difficulty in identifying the tumour site weeks or months postoperatively can occur in up to 70% of patients receiving conventional breast boost radiotherapy [17].

19.3.1 Intraoperative Techniques with Photons

Intrabeam is a miniature X-ray source that gives 30–50 KVp photons with a steep dose fall-off and uses spherical applicators of diameters ranging from 1.5 to 5 cm based on the size of the surgical cavity to ensure homogeneous dose distribution on the surface of the applicator and consequently on the surface of the tumour cavity [16]. The 3.5-cm applicator, which is commonly used, delivers 20 Gy at a radius of 1 mm from the surface, 5 Gy at 10 mm and 1 Gy at 27 mm in about 20 min. The treatment time is about 20–45 min, depending on the size of the lumpectomy cavity, the size of the selected applicator and the prescribed dose [18].

A phase III, prospective randomized non-inferiority trial called TARGIT (targeted intraoperative radiation therapy) comparing single-dose intraoperative radiation therapy targeted to the tumour bed to conventional whole-breast external-beam radiation therapy in early breast cancer showed that at 4-year follow-up the Kaplan–Meier estimate of local recurrence in the conserved breast was 1.20% (95% CI 0.53–2.71) in the targeted intraoperative radiotherapy and 0.95% (0.39–2.31) in the external-beam radiotherapy group. The rate of recurrence between the two groups was not statistically significant. Similarly, the total rate of major toxicities was similar in the two groups [19].

19.3.2 Intraoperative Techniques with Electrons

Mobetron can produce electrons of varying energies such as 4 MeV, 6 MeV, 9 MeV and 12 MeV with therapeutic ranges up to 4 cm. It can deliver a very large uniform dose of 10–25 Gy in a single fraction at a dose rate of 10 Gy/min while the NOVAC-7 system delivers electron beams of energies 3, 5, 7 and 9 MeV with a mobile linear accelerator.

In Electron Beam Intraoperative Radiotherapy (ELIOT), a phase III prospective randomized study, electrons with energies up to 9 MeV biologically equivalent to 58–60 Gy in standard fractionation were used to deliver a dose of 21 Gy to the 90% isodose at a depth of 1.5–3 cm over 15–20 min. A systematic review by Cuncins-Hearn et al. concluded that the short-term results were similar for both BCT and IORT in terms of local recurrence and disease-free and overall survival [20].

The demerit with IORT is the delay in the final histopathology report, which has been circumvented with a novel handheld probe (Dune Medical Devices, Caesarea, Israel) developed for intraoperative detection of positive margins that decreases the re-excision rate [21]. Also, prolonged time under general anaesthesia in the operation theatre and the possibility of delayed complications due to the high radiation dose are a cause for concern.

19.4   Postoperative Techniques

19.4.1 Interstitial Brachytherapy

Interstitial brachytherapy is a technique in which flexible catheters after loading are placed into the tumour bed at 1–1.5 cm intervals in several planes to include the tumour bed with a 1–2-cm margin and achieve homogeneous dose distribution avoiding hot or cold spots. After loading, brachytherapy technique is used and could be HDR (high dose rate)/LDR (low dose rate)/PDR (pulse dose rate).

With Iridium 192 HDR brachytherapy, a dose of 34 Gy in 10 fractions over 5 days is given (twice daily with a minimum interfraction interval of 6 h). This technique allows a good control of dose delivery to the skin and enables the shape of a reference isodose to be adjusted to the shape of the tumour bed and can be done as an outpatient procedure [22]. In the LDR brachytherapy technique, sources of Ir-192 sources are implanted for approximately 2–5 days while the patient is admitted as an inpatient.

The GEC-ESTRO Breast Cancer Working Group (II) recommended that while defining the target for APBI using multi-catheter interstitial brachytherapy after breast-conserving open cavity surgery, only the homogeneous part of the postoperative seroma has to be included in the contours and protrusions or sharp irregularities have to be excluded. When surgical clips are present, they have to be surrounded by the contour with close contact. CTV is created from the outlined surgical cavity with a non-isotropic geometrical extension, and a safety margin of 20 mm must be ensured. CTV is limited to chest wall/pectoral muscles and 5 mm below the skin surface [23].

Interstitial brachytherapy requires high skills and experience from the radiation oncologist. Also, inhomogeneous dose distribution in the implant can arise due to the presence of 'hot spots'. Several clinical studies of APBI using interstitial brachytherapy with more than 5-year follow-up showed 5-year local recurrence rate comparable to that of WBI and excellent cosmetic results [24, 25].

19.4.1.1 Intracavitary Brachytherapy

The balloon-based brachytherapy devices such as Mammosite, Axxent electronic brachytherapy and Contura are used, or the hybrid brachytherapy systems, which utilize the versatility and dosimetric conformity of multi-catheter interstitial brachytherapy with the convenience and aesthetics of single-entry devices such as Struts Adjusted Volume Implant (SAVI) and the ClearPath are used for intracavitary brachytherapy to deliver APBI.

19.4.1.2 Mammosite

Mammosite applicator has a silicone balloon with a 15-cm double lumen catheter with a small inflation channel and a channel for the passage of an Ir-192 HDR source. The balloon is inserted into the tumour bed intraoperatively or under USG guidance a few days after the surgery. Once inserted, the balloon is inflated with a saline solution with contrast [26, 27].

The minimum acceptable balloon to skin distance is 5 mm, and at least 7-mm threshold is recommended [28]. A symmetric implant in relation to the source channel is essential as non-symmetrical implant results in dose inhomogeneity as a single central source channel does not allow for shaping of the radiation isodose curves in the direction perpendicular to the central channel [27]. The Mammosite balloon (MSB) may not be suitable for upper inner quadrant tumours or in patients with smaller breasts as the skin to cavity distance criteria may not be met. To eliminate the drawback of a single lumen device, a multi-lumen Mammosite has been introduced by Hologic. The MSB was approved by the US Food and Drug Administration (FDA) in May 2002, and in September 2009, the multi-lumen device was also approved.

The Mammosite delivers 34 Gy over 10 fractions (3.4 Gy per fraction twice daily and a minimum 6-h interfraction interval) with a prescription point of 1 cm from the balloon surface. The data published about MSB with long-term follow-up are limited. MSB was used in 43 patients and had a median follow-up of 65 months with no locoregional recurrences and good-to-excellent cosmesis in 81.3% [29].

The American Society of Breast Surgeon (ASBS) registry trial reported 1440 patients treated, with a median follow-up of 30.1 months. There have been 23 cases (1.6%) of ipsilateral breast tumour recurrence for a 2-year actuarial rate of 1.04%. The cosmetic outcome of good to excellent was 95% at 12 months [30].

The MSB technique is simple, reproducible and can be planned easily. It is less invasive, but dose redistribution cannot be done to fit the tumour bed irregularities or to account for the adjacent skin and chest wall. High cost is a limitation. Most common adverse effects include erythema, dry and moist desquamation, telangiectasias, fat necrosis and development of seroma.

19.4.2 Axxent Electronic Brachytherapy

It has a balloon catheter similar to Mammosite inserted into the lumpectomy cavity by a percutaneous approach. It has a central lumen for source insertion, a second port for saline inflation and a third port for draining the serum fluid or air around the lumpectomy cavity. It does not need contrast for radiographic visualization as the wall of the balloon is covered in radiolucent material. It uses an electronic 50-KV HDR source in the form of a miniature X-ray tube, thereby obviating the need for a specifically shielded room or an HDR after loader unit. It can also be used for intraoperative radiation therapy. In 2006, it has received FDA clearance to treat breast cancer [27, 31, 32]. However, further clinical studies and long-term results of the use are still awaited.

19.4.3 Contura

Contura differs from the other balloon-based brachytherapy devices as it has multiple lumens for the HDR source to pass through, thereby enabling more dose flexibility and to reduce normal tissue toxicity. It was approved by the FDA in May 2007 [27, 33].

19.4.3.1 Hybrid Brachytherapy Devices

Strut-Adjusted Volume Implant (SAVI)
The SAVI device has a central strut surrounded by 6, 8 or 10 peripheral struts that can be differentially loaded with an HDR source. It is surgically implanted under ultrasound guidance in a collapsed form and later expanded to fit the lumpectomy cavity by clockwise rotation of a knob. A CT scan after positioning is needed for verifying the device deployment and treatment plan.

ClearPath (CP)
CP has inner and outer catheters which are expandable. In the centre of the expandable tubes is a central catheter surrounded by six additional catheters that allow the passage of an HDR Iridium-192 source, which is not in direct contact with the

breast tissue. Though clinical studies are limited, a phantom study has shown better skin-sparing effect with CP than MSB (median maximum skin dose: 113% vs 161%, respectively) [34].

19.4.4 External-Beam Radiotherapy

APBI can be delivered with external-beam radiotherapy by 3D CRT (conformal radiation therapy) with multiple photons, and/or electron fields, intensity-modulated radiation therapy (IMRT) or with protons. The tumour bed is defined by the computed tomography visualized seroma cavity, postoperative changes and surgical clips, when available. The clinical target volume (CTV) is defined as the tumour bed with a 1.5-cm margin limited by 0.5 cm from the skin and chest wall. The planning tumour volume (PTV) is defined as the CTV with a 1.0-cm margin. The prescription dose used for the NSABP/RTOG protocol is 3.85 Gy twice daily (separated by at least 6 h) to a total dose of 38.5 Gy delivered within 1 week [35].

EBRT is non-invasive, has widespread availability, is technically easier than brachytherapy and has simpler QA (quality assurance) procedures and a better uniformity between radiation oncologists [36]. However, delineation of lumpectomy cavity, appropriate dose and fractional scheme, intra- and interfraction motion, treatment set-up variation, higher integral dose and more normal tissue toxicity are the fallacies which need to be tackled while treating with external-beam radiation.

19.4.4.1 Which Patients Can be Taken up for APBI?

Improper selection criteria can lead to suboptimal results and skews the results of the procedure. The selection criteria for APBI have been given by many societies such as the American Society of Breast Surgeons (ASBS), the American Brachytherapy Society (ABS), the American Society for Radiation Oncology (ASTRO) and the European Society for Therapeutic Radiology and Oncology (ESTRO).

According to the American Brachytherapy Society, after evaluating multiple clinical studies of different APBI modalities, patient selection needs to be done based on the age ($\geq$50 years old), tumour size ($\leq$3 cm), histology (all invasive subtypes and ductal carcinoma in situ), surgical margins (negative), lymphovascular space invasion (not present) and nodal status (negative). The guidelines will enable clinicians to use APBI in a manner to optimize clinical outcomes and patient satisfaction [37].

The ASTRO consensus statement determines patients 'suitable' for APBI as those $\geq$50 years, surgical margins negative by at least 2 mm and a T stage of Tis or T1. Previously, DCIS was not taken up for APBI, but the present consensus states that DCIS which is screen-detected, of low to intermediate nuclear grade, size $\leq$2.5 cm and resected with margins negative at $\geq$3 mm is suitable for APBI.

The patients in the 'cautionary' group are those who are 40–49 years and if all other criteria for "suitable" are met or those who are $\geq$50 years and the patients have at least one of the following pathologic factors: size 2.1–3.0 cm, T2, close margins

(<2 mm), limited/focal LVSI, ER (−), clinically unifocal with total size 2.1–3.0 cm, invasive lobular histology, pure DCIS ≤3 cm if criteria for 'suitable' not fully met, EIC ≤3 cm and does not have any 'unsuitable factors'. With close surgical margins <2 mm or DCIS ≤3 cm and not meeting the criteria for 'suitable' group are also included with the cautionary group.

Patients who are <40 years or 40–49 years and do not meet the criteria for 'cautionary group' and patients with positive margins or with DCIS >3 cm are 'unsuitable' for APBI [1].

19.4.4.2 Toxicity of APBI

The toxicity profile of APBI is different with different techniques. Fat necrosis was increased with IORT, while skin side effects were lower [38].

In 1822 cases treated at the European Institute of Milan with electron intraoperative therapy, fat necrosis was seen in 4.2% and fibrosis in 1.8% of patients. After the median follow-up of 36.1 months, the rates of local recurrence, new primary cancer foci in the irradiated breast and distant metastases were 2.3%, 1.3% and 1.4%, respectively. The rates of 5- and 10-year overall survival were 97.4% and 89.7%, respectively [39].

IORT techniques have lower lung fibrosis and deaths from cardiovascular events than seen in the ELIOT and TARGIT trials, respectively [40].

In TARGIT A trial, patients were randomized to risk-adapted single-dose intraoperative radiation therapy (TARGIT-IORT) versus external-beam radiation therapy (EBRT). Those treated with IORT have similar self-reported cosmetic outcome but better breast-related QOL outcomes than patients treated with EBRT. EBRT patients experienced moderately higher levels of treatment-related symptoms, including breast and arm pain, swelling, oversensitivity, and skin problems [41].

The cosmetic outcomes of APBI delivered with external-beam radiotherapy are varied across several studies. A randomized trial of accelerated partial-breast irradiation trial (RAPID) randomized 2135 patients to WBI or 3D-CRT APBI. The cosmetic outcome, as assessed separately by patients, nurses and physician panels, was consistently worse at 3 and 5 years in patients randomized to 3D-CRT APBI [42]. Patients treated with APBI had a significantly higher proportion of adverse cosmesis than those treated with WBI at 3 years (29.0% vs. 16.5%) and at 5 years (32.8% vs. 13.4%). Telangiectasia, breast induration and grade 1 breast pain were more common in the APBI arm [43].

The University Florence phase 3 trial reported that IMRT APBI resulted in improved physician-rated cosmetic outcome compared with WBI [44].

APBI with external-beam radiotherapy should be cautiously offered with special attention to target volume definition and dose fractionation schemes. Much awaited updated results of trials such as RAPID, NSABP B-39/RTOG 0413, and IMPORT LOW are now published.

RAPID trial results indicate that external-beam APBI was non-inferior to WBI in preventing IBTR, but the regimen used was associated with an increase in moderate late toxicity and adverse cosmesis, which might be related to the twice per day treatment [46]. Other approaches, such as treatment once per day, might not adversely affect cosmesis as in IMPORT LOW.

NSABP B-39/RTOG 0413 trial results failed to prove the equivalence in IBTR between WBI and APBI [45].

19.5 Conclusion

APBI has evolved to be a convenient, cost-effective, acceptable treatment option in patients appropriately selected for the technique. Further long-term studies will provide more information on the safety, efficacy and toxicity of the different APBI techniques. Also, the different dosing schedules need to be radio biologically evaluated, and a consensus on the appropriate dosing schedule according to the treatment technique needs to be given.

References

1. Correa C, Harris EE, Leonardi MC, Smith BD, Taghian AG, Thompson AM, et al. Accelerated partial breast irradiation: executive summary for the update of an ASTRO evidence-based consensus statement. Pract Radiat Oncol. 2017;7:73–9.
2. Suzuki T, Toi M, Saji S, Horiguchi K, Aruga T, Suzuki E, et al. Early breast cancer. Int J Clin Oncol. 2006;11:108–19.
3. Fisher B, Anderson S, Bryant J, Margolese RG, Deutsch M, Fisher ER, et al. Twenty-year follow-up of a randomized trial comparing total mastectomy, lumpectomy, and lumpectomy plus irradiation for the treatment of invasive breast cancer. N Engl J Med. 2002;347:1233–41.
4. Early Breast Cancer Trialists' Collaborative Group (EBCTCG), Darby S, McGale P, Correa C, Taylor C, Arriagada R, et al. Effect of radiotherapy after breast conserving surgery on 10 year recurrence and 15 year breast cancer death:meta analysis of individual patient data for 10,801 women in 17 randomised trials. Lancet. 2011(378):1707–16.
5. Consensus statement: treatment of early-stage breast cancer. National Institutes of Health Consensus Development Panel. J Natl Cancer Inst Monogr. 1992;1–5.
6. Strnad V, Ott OJ, Hildebrandt G, et al. 5-year results of accelerated partial breast irradiation using sole interstitial multicatheter brachytherapy versus whole-breast irradiation with boost after breast-conserving surgery for low-risk invasive and in-situ carcinoma of the female breast: a randomised, phase 3, non-inferiority trial. Lancet. 2016;387(10015):229–38.
7. Coles CE, Griffin CL, Kirby AM, Titley J, Agrawal RK, Alhasso A, et al. Partial-breast radiotherapy after breast conservation surgery for patients with early breast cancer (UK IMPORT LOW trial): 5-year results from a multicentre, randomised, controlled, phase 3, non-inferiority trial. Lancet. 2017;390:1048–60.
8. Brown JM, Koong AC. High-dose single-fraction radiotherapy: exploiting a new biology? Int J Radiat Oncol Biol Phys. 2008;71:324–5.
9. Kirkpatrick JP, Brenner DJ, Orton CG. Point/counterpoint. The linear-quadratic model is inappropriate to model high dose per fraction effects in radiosurgery. Med Phys. 2009;36:3381–4.
10. Cuttino LW, Todor D, Pacyna L, Lin P-S, Arthur DW. Three-dimensional conformal external beam radiotherapy (3D-CRT) for accelerated partial breast irradiation(APBI): what is the correct prescription dose? Am J Clin Oncol. 2006;29(5):474–8.
11. Lazovich DA, White E, Thomas DB, Moe RE. Underutilization of breast-conserving surgery and radiation therapy among women with stage I or II breast cancer. JAMA. 1991;266:3433–8.

12. Sanders ME, Scroggins T, Ampil FL, Li BD. Accelerated partial breast irradiation in early-stage breast cancer. J Clin Oncol. 2007;25(8):996–1002.
13. Njeh CF, Saunders MW, Langton CM. Accelerated Partial Breast Irradiation (APBI): a review of the available techniques. Radiat Oncol. 2010;5:90. https://doi.org/10.1186/1748-717X-5-90.
14. Kacprowska A, Jassem J. Partial breast irradiation techniques in early breast cancer. Rep Pract Oncol Radiother. 2011;16:213–20.
15. Orecchia R, Luini A, Veronesi P, Ciocca M, Franzetti S, Gatti G, Veronesi U. Electron intraoperative treatment in patients with early-stage breast cancer: data update. Expert Rev Anticancer Ther. 2006;6:605–11.
16. Holmes DR, Baum M, Joseph D. The TARGIT trial: targeted intraoperative radiation therapy versus conventional postoperative whole-breast radiotherapy after breast-conserving surgery for the management of early-stage invasive breast cancer (a trial update). Am J Surg. 2007;194:507–10.
17. Benda RK, Yasuda G, Sethi A, Gabram SG, Hinerman RW, Mendenhall NP. Breast boost: are we missing the target? Cancer. 2003;97:905–9.
18. Vaidya JS, Tobias JS, Baum M, Keshtgar M, Joseph D, Wenz F, et al. Intraoperative radiotherapy for breast cancer. Lancet Oncol. 2004;5:165–73.
19. Vaidya JS, Joseph DJ, Tobias JS, Bulsara M, Wenz F, Saunders C, et al. Targeted intraoperative radiotherapy versus whole breast radiotherapy for breast cancer (TARGIT-A trial): an international, prospective, randomised, non-inferiority phase 3 trial. Lancet. 2010;376:91–102.
20. Cuncins-Hearn A, Saunders C, Walsh D, Borg M, Buckingham J, Frizelle F, Maddern G. A systematic review of intraoperative radiotherapy in early breast cancer. Breast Cancer Res Treat. 2004;85:271–80.
21. Karni T, Pappo I, Sandbank J, Lavon O, Kent V, Spector R, et al. A device for real-time, intraoperative margin assessment in breast-conservation surgery. Am J Surg. 2007;194:467–73.
22. Wazer DE. Point: brachytherapy for accelerated partial breast irradiation. Brachytherapy. 2009;8:181–3.
23. Major T, Gutierrez C, Guix B, van Limbergen E, Strnad V, Polgar C. Recommendations from GEC ESTRO Breast Cancer Working Group (II): target definition and target delineation for accelerated or boost partial breast irradiation using multicatheter interstitial brachytherapy after breast conserving open cavity surgery. Radiother Oncol. 2016;118(1):199–204.
24. Arthur DW, Winter K, Kuske RR, Bolton J, Rabinovitch R, White J, et al. A phase II trial of brachytherapy alone after lumpectomy for select breast cancer: tumour control and survival outcomes of RTOG 95-17. Int J Radiat Oncol Biol Phys. 2008;72:467–73.
25. Polgar C, Fodor J, Major T, Nemeth G, Lovey K, Orosz Z, et al. Breast-conserving treatment with partial or whole breast irradiation for low-risk invasive breast carcinoma–5-year results of a randomized trial. Int J Radiat Oncol Biol Phys. 2007;69:694–702.
26. Edmundson GK, Vicini FA, Chen PY, Mitchell C, Martinez AA. Dosimetric characteristics of the MammoSite RTS, a new breast brachytherapy applicator. Int J Radiat Oncol Biol Phys. 2002;52:1132–9.
27. Dickler A, Patel RR, Wazer D. Breast brachytherapy devices. Expert Rev Med Devices. 2009;6:325–33.
28. Niehoff P, Polgar C, Ostertag H, Major T, Sulyok Z, Kimmig B, Kovacs G. Clinical experience with the MammoSite radiation therapy system for brachytherapy of breast cancer: results from an international phase II trial. Radiother Oncol. 2006;79:316–20.
29. Benitez PR, Keisch ME, Vicini F, Stolier A, Scroggins T, Walker A, et al. Five-year results: the initial clinical trial of MammoSite balloon brachytherapy for partial breast irradiation in early-stage breast cancer. Am J Surg. 2007;194:456–62.
30. Vicini F, Beitsch PD, Quiet CA, Keleher AJ, Garcia D, Snider HC Jr, Gittleman MA, et al. Three-year analysis of treatment efficacy, cosmesis, and toxicity by the American Society of Breast Surgeons MammoSite breast brachytherapy registry trial in patients treated with accelerated partial breast irradiation (APBI). Cancer. 2008;112:758–66.

31. Dickler A, Ivanov O, Francescatti D. Intraoperative radiation therapy in the treatment of early-stage breast cancer utilizing xoftaxxent electronic brachytherapy. World J Surg Oncol. 2009;7:24.

32. Ivanov O, Dickler A, Lum BY, Pellicane JV, Francescatti DS. Twelve-month follow-up results of a trial utilizing Axxent electronic brachytherapy to deliver intraoperative radiation therapy for early-stage breast Cancer. Ann Surg Oncol. 2011;18(2):453–8.

33. Wilder RB, Curcio LD, Khanijou RK, Eisner ME, Kakkis JL, Chittenden L, et al. A contura catheter offers dosimetric advantages over a MammoSite catheter that increase the applicability of accelerated partial breast irradiation. Brachytherapy. 2009;8:373–8.

34. Beriwal S, Coon D, Kim H, Haley M, Patel R, Das R. Multicatheter hybrid breast brachytherapy: a potential alternative for patients with inadequate skin distance. Brachytherapy. 2008;7:301–4.

35. Hepel JT, Tokita M, MacAusland SG, Evans SB, Hiatt JR, Price LL, DiPetrillo T, Wazer DE. Toxicity of three-dimensional conformal radiotherapy for accelerated partial breast irradiation. Int J Radiat Oncol Biol Phys. 2009;75:1290–6.

36. Formenti SC. External-beam partial-breast irradiation. Semin Radiat Oncol. 2005;15:92–9.

37. Shah C, Vicini F, Wazer DE, Arthur D, Patel RR. The American Brachytherapy Society consensus statement on Accelerated partial breast irradiation. Brachytherapy. 2013;12:267–77.

38. Vaidya JS, Bulsara M, Wenz F, et al. Pride, prejudice, or science: attitudes towards the results of the TARGIT-A trial of targeted intraoperative radiation therapy for breast cancer. Int J Radiat Oncol Biol Phys. 2015;92(3):491–7.

39. Veronesi U, Orecchia R, Luini A, et al. Intraoperative radiotherapy during breast conserving surgery: a study on 1,822 cases treated with electrons. Breast Cancer Res Treat. 2010;124:141–51.

40. Sperk E, Welzel G, Keller A, et al. Late radiation toxicity after intraoperative radiotherapy (IORT) for breast cancer: results from the randomized phase III trial TARGIT a. Breast Cancer Res Treat. 2012;135(1):253–60.

41. Corica T, Nowak AK, Saunders CM, Bulsara M, Vaidya JS, Baum M, Joseph DJ. Cosmesis and breast-related quality of life outcomes after intraoperative radiation therapy for early breast cancer: a substudy of the TARGIT-A trial. Int J Radiat Oncol Biol Phys. 2016;96(1):55–64.

42. Jeruss JS, Kuerer HM, Beitsch PD, Vicini FA, Keisch M. Update on DCIS outcomes from the American Society of Breast Surgeons accelerated partial breast irradiation registry trial. Ann Surg Oncol. 2011;18(1):65–71.

43. Olivotto IA, Whelan TJ, Parpia S, Kim D-H, Berrang T, Truong PT, et al. Interim cosmetic and toxicity results from RAPID: a randomized trial of accelerated partial breast irradiation using three-dimensional conformal external beam radiation therapy. J Clin Oncol. 2013;31(32):4038–45.

44. Livi L, Meattini I, Marrazzo L, et al. Accelerated partial breast irradiation using intensity-modulated radiotherapy versus whole breast irradiation: 5-year survival analysis of a phase 3 randomised controlled trial. Eur J Cancer. 2015;51(4):451–63.

45. Vicini FA, Cecchini RS, White JR, Arthur DW, Julian TB, Rabinovitch RA, Kuske RR, Ganz PA, et al. Long-term primary results of accelerated partial breast irradiation after breast-conserving surgery for early-stage breast cancer: a randomized, phase 3, equivalence trial (NSABP B-39/RTOG 0413). Lancet. 2019;394(10215):2155–64. https://doi.org/10.1016/S0140-6736(19)32514-0.

46. Whelan TJ, Julian JA, Berrang TS, Kim D-H, Germain I, Nichol AM, Akra M, Lavertu S, Germain F, Fyles A, et al. External beam accelerated partial breast irradiation versus whole breast irradiation after breast conserving surgery in women with ductal carcinoma in situ and node-negative breast cancer (RAPID): a randomised controlled trial. Lancet. 2019;394(10215):2165–72. https://doi.org/10.1016/S0140-6736(19)32515-2.

Psychological Impact of Breast Cancer Diagnosis and Treatment: The Role of Psychooncology

Gilsa K. Gopinadhan, Koravangattu Valsraj, and Beena Kunheri

20.1 Introduction

The diagnosis of cancer is often followed by feelings of uncertainty for the affected individual and family regarding the course, prognosis, survival, burden to family and overall quality of life. This can in turn result in significant emotional distress [1]. In chronic illnesses such as cancer, various factors such as lifestyle, stress, social support, doctor–patient relationship, expectations and the ability to cope with pain and discomfort and various other psychosocial factors and stressors affect the psychological well-being. Even well-adjusted individuals are often shaken by the shock and stress inflicted upon their lives by cancer and its treatment. There is a significant reduction in quality of life, and even routine daily tasks become difficult [2]. Research has demonstrated that such a level of psychological distress can lead to poorer survival and higher mortality rates in cancer patients [3]. Hence, thorough knowledge of psychological and social context within which health and illnesses are experienced is essential for a better understanding of what keeps people healthy and what makes them recover.

The diagnosis of cancer causes severe emotional distress to the majority of the people, which in turn can have serious adverse effects on their personal, occupational and social functioning. In the long run, these problems could also affect their capacity to cope with the illness and can diminish their adherence to treatment [4].

G. K. Gopinadhan
Psycho-Oncology Division, Department of Clinical Psychology, Amrita Institute of Medical Sciences, Kochi, Kerala, India

K. Valsraj (✉)
South London and Maudsley NHS Foundation Trust, London, UK

Amrita Institute of Medical Sciences, Kochi, Kerala, India
e-mail: k.valsraj@nhs.net

B. Kunheri
Department of Radiation Oncology, Amrita Institute of Medical Sciences and Research Centre, Amrita Vishwa Vidyapeetham University, Kochi, Kerala, India

© Springer Nature Singapore Pte Ltd. 2021
B. Kunheri, D. K. Vijaykumar (eds.), *Management of Early Stage Breast Cancer*,
https://doi.org/10.1007/978-981-15-6171-9_20

Moreover, the treatment for cancer itself can be very distress inducing and plays a role in bringing about poor mental health outcomes in cancer patients [5, 6].

Hence, in the past few decades, there has been a significant focus on the psychosocial components of cancer and its treatment. *Psychooncology* is the discipline which aims to explore the psychological and sociocultural factors affecting the quality of life of cancer patients and their caregivers. *Psychooncology* plays a crucial role in the holistic approach towards cancer care and helps with better outcomes. Psychooncology studies the impact of cancer on the psychological function of the patient, carers and health care staff and also the role that various psychological and behavioural factors may have in cancer risk and survival [7].

Among the types of cancers studied for psychological impact, there is a wide range of literature indicating the impact of breast cancer on the mental health of an individual.

As per the 2018 Lancet oncology publication, the estimated number of incident breast cancer cases in India in 2016 was 118,000 (95% UI 107,000–130,000), 98·1% of which were in females, and the prevalent cases were 526,000 (474,000–574,000). Breast cancer is the leading cancer in Indian females, accounting for the largest crude incidence rate and prevalence of any cancer type [8]. Being an illness with high prevalence rate and requiring complex treatment procedures, breast cancer poses a preponderance of psychological morbidity.

20.2 Psychosocial Impact of Breast Cancer

There are numerous factors affecting patients' response to the diagnosis of breast cancer and accepting the diagnosis, such as medical factors (stage of disease, type of treatment, availability of rehabilitation services), psychosocial factors (coping skills, prior history of psychiatric illness, availability of social support) and current sociocultural context, treatment options and decision making [9].

According to Meyerowitz, three kinds of possible psychosocial responses to breast cancer are psychological discomfort, behavioural changes and concerns related to body image, recurrence, or death [10]. These responses are, however, usually dependent on various medical factors (severity of illness/stage at which the disease is diagnosed, kind of treatment received, rehabilitative services availed) and psychological factors (degree of interference in major life tasks, premorbid stress tolerance and coping skills, past history of psychiatric illnesses, social support) [9].

20.3 Mental Health Disorders

Psychosocial distress among women with breast cancer is estimated to range from approximately 20–40% [11]. According to research findings, the prevalence rates of a psychiatric disorder in cancer patients are found to be 45%, and the prevalence rate of anxiety and depressive diagnoses to be 42% [12]. Longer durations of depression may result in poorer quality of life and also shorter life expectancy [13]. A mandatory referral to a mental health professional should be considered for women with breast cancer who exhibit symptoms of depression or anxiety, suicidal thinking (attempts of self-harm), substance or alcohol abuse, confusional state (delirium), mood swings and/or insomnia.

Other risk factors that predict the requirement of psychiatric evaluation are family history of breast cancer, women who are very young, old, pregnant, nursing, single or alone, who are adjusting to multiple losses and managing multiple life stresses, who seem distressed by cancer treatment decisions or fear of death during surgery or who are terrified by loss of control under anaesthesia and who request euthanasia and seem unable to provide informed consent [9].

The following are the common mental health presentations:

20.3.1 Depression

The largest number of referrals of cancer patients to mental health professionals has always been due to depression. The prevalence of depression is greater among patients with greater impairment to physical functioning, more advanced stages of cancer, and those with severe pain [14]. The symptoms (i.e. body image disturbances and physical symptoms) secondary to the treatment procedures such as chemotherapy or surgery for cancer are also found to be an important causative factor for depression [15].

According to Rouchell, Pounds, and Tierney, the prevalence rates for depression are 20–38% for women with cancer, which is higher than many other chronic illnesses such as HIV, stroke and coronary heart disease [16]. In patients with early breast cancer, the prevalence of depression and anxiety is found to be as high as 33% at diagnosis and 45% at recurrence. The literature indicates that significant risk factors that predict depression in breast cancer patients are early stressors, long-standing sleep disturbances, poor social functioning and pessimistic thinking patterns.

Depression can have a negative impact on the patients' quality of life and are more likely to have lesser adherence to treatment procedures [15].

20.3.2 Anxiety Disorders

According to Massie and Holland, after depression and organic mental disorders, anxiety is the most common psychological problem arising in patients with cancer [17]. Research findings indicate that anxiety escalates during the discovery of tumour, during surgery and almost for a year after this period [18]. Severe anxiety can affect proper adherence to treatment and may result in the use of certain avoidance strategies in order to avoid the procedures they dread [19]. In a study by Maguire, Lee and Bevington, they found moderate-to-severe anxiety in 27% of the breast cancer patient group as compared to 14% in a control sample [20]. The surgical procedures such as mastectomy can worsen social anxiety [9].

The patients with cancer often spend too much time worrying about insignificant physical sensation and perceive them as signs of cancer, thereby causing more anxiety. High levels of anxiety are known to affect the patients' ability to problem-solve. Symptoms such as the use of avoidance strategies and hypervigilance also reduce the adaptation of the patient to stressful situations [21].

20.3.3 Suicide

The presence of other psychiatric disorders such as depression and anxiety are significant risk factors for suicidal behaviours. Research studies indicate that patients with breast cancer are at higher risk for suicide for about 25 years following the diagnosis [21].

During the course of treatment, the hospital stay, after discharge and on recurrence or instances of treatment failure are the times requiring monitoring for suicidal behaviours [22]. The risk for suicide is especially higher in advanced stages of the cancer and also in patients with symptoms of fatigue, or intense fear of recurrence of the illness [23–25]. However, one challenge for mental health professionals is that self-harm behaviours and suicides, especially in cancer, are under-reported due to the family's stigma and reluctance to report death by suicide [26]. The delay to seek any prompt psychological assessment and support might lead to worsening of mental health and increased risk of self-harming behaviours.

20.3.4 Body Image Disturbances

Body image disturbances are one of the most serious impacts of breast cancer treatment. A study by Sneeuw et al. found that 25% of women who had breast-conserving surgery had serious body image problems [27]. Mastectomy and breast reconstruction leaves behind scars that can serve as a constant reminder of loss of an important body part and distorted body image. The problems in body image and the insecure feelings that entail can often lead an individual to withdraw from social relationships. It affects sexual intimacy with a partner, causes feelings of reduced sexual attractiveness, restricts use of certain clothes, reduces self-esteem and causes an increased risk of presenting with psychological disorders.

20.3.5 Sexual Functioning Difficulties

Sexual function problems are quite common among cancer patients of both genders. Loss of interest in sexual activities is also a common symptom for patients of both sexes. The quality of life is largely impacted when these symptoms last for up to 1–2 years following the treatment [28, 29]. In patients with breast cancer, the surgical treatments, which result in a decreased sense of self-worth and decreased feelings of sexual attractiveness, also cause loss of sexual function. However, the patients undergoing immediate reconstructive surgery show higher levels of psychological well-being when compared to those undergoing mastectomy alone or delayed breast reconstructive surgery [30, 31]. Although treatment procedures for cancer, i.e. chemotherapy, radiation therapy, surgical interventions and medications for pain, can often result in sexual dysfunctions, the loss of sexual desire may be a result of fatigue or weakness secondary to the cancer treatment, depression, body image concerns and feelings of guilt or misbeliefs about the development and spread of cancer [32].

20.4 Psychological Interventions

Psychosocial interventions aim to decrease intense emotional distress and improve the quality of life in patients of different stages of coping with cancer, i.e. diagnosis, disease progression or recurrence [33–37].

The first step towards any clinical management is a detailed evaluation of the patient. The use of psychological assessments gives the therapist an opportunity to discuss the major concerns of patients and also to give precise and valid information regarding their psychological state.

The commonly used psychological assessment tools are shown in Table. 20.1.

Table 20.1 Psychological assessment tools

Psychological assessment
1. Assessment of psychosocial distress
• NCCN Distress Thermometer
2. Assessment of depression and suicidal intent
• Beck's Depression Inventory
• Hamilton's Depression Rating Scale
• Hospital Anxiety Depression Scale
• Beck's Suicide Intent Scale
3. Assessment of anxiety disorders
• Beck's Anxiety Inventory
• Hamilton Anxiety Rating Scale
• Hospital Anxiety Depression Scale
• State Trait Anxiety Inventory
4. Assessment of pain
• McGill Pain Questionnaire
• Visual Analogue Scale
5. Assessment of cognitive functions
• Mini-Mental Status Examination
• Addenbrooke's Cognitive Examination
6. Assessment of other psychiatric conditions
• Brief Psychiatric Rating Scale
• State Trait Anger Inventory

Table 20.2 Goals of psychological intervention

1. To validate the patient's feelings of distress, provide a safe environment to vent out the feelings
2. To help the patient to restore the personal, social and occupational functioning to maximum possible levels within the limits of the illness and treatment
3. To help the patient in making appropriate decisions regarding the treatment while at the same time encouraging autonomy
4. Enhancing support systems
5. To help the patient in conserving his/her sense of self-efficacy
6. To help the patient in smooth role transitions and shifting of responsibilities and make appropriate goals which are more plausible

The various factors to consider before beginning a psychological intervention are as below:

(a) Target population—patients recently diagnosed with cancer, or experiencing disease progression or recurrence, and survivors of cancer.
(b) Primary goal—to reduce psychological distress, to reduce secondary effects of cancer treatment or to modify lifestyle and risk factors (Table 20.2).
(c) Mode of treatment—individual therapy, group therapy, family therapy.

20.5 Psychological Interventions

20.5.1 Psychoeducational Interventions

Providing the information pertaining to the stage, progression, prognosis and treatment is crucial, and including these components in the psychosocial interventions is proven to be very effective in patients with cancer [38, 39]. These services may also include clarifying their various queries regarding the side effects, modifying the risk behaviours and maladaptive coping strategies and also facilitating further communication with their physician to clarify specific queries. Psychoeducation can be offered in an individual session or group session.

In patients with breast cancer, a significant improvement in the initial adjustment to the diagnosis was found following psychoeducational group intervention [40]. According to Devine and Westlake based on a meta-analysis of 116 studies, psychoeducational interventions resulted in significantly reduced pain, nausea and vomiting [41]. This could be as a result of their better tolerance of side effects due to effective communication and information sharing of the expected course and side effects during treatment. Hence, these approaches aimed at meeting the informational and educational needs of patients to improve their understanding of the illness and treatment options and prognosis increase satisfaction with health care and their compliance with treatment [42].

20.5.2 Individual Psychotherapy

Individual therapy focuses on renewing the psychological defences of an individual, improving coping mechanisms and reducing the sense of isolation [43]. Cancer patients are often seen to suppress their feelings and emotions out of fear of appearing weak, making it awkward for the family members and friends. It is during the individual therapy sessions that the patients often get chance to address these thoughts and to ventilate their feelings regarding the illness. They are also helped in a smooth shifting of responsibilities and reorganising their goals and values. The commonly offered individual psychotherapies are the following:

20.5.2.1 Supportive Psychotherapy

Supportive psychotherapy is a brief intervention aiming at restoring the emotional stability and normal functioning of a person who is temporarily staggering under severe life stressors [44]. The major strategies could be symptom control, controlling the external stress factors, giving proper guidance and reassurance, providing a safe environment for ventilation and brief interventions using art-based or music-based activities. Supportive psychotherapy sessions for cancer patients can be conducted in both individual and group sessions. Research evidence shows that it benefits the patients by reducing their feelings of isolation, strengthening coping skills [45, 46].

20.5.2.2 Cognitive and Behavioural Interventions

Cognitive behaviour therapy is a well-structured intervention, which is one of the most commonly utilised mode of treatment for a wide range of psychological problems. In cancer patients, problem-solving techniques, stress management and coping skills training are a few of the regularly used cognitive behavioural interventions.

In cancer patients, the cognitive behaviour therapist and the patient identify the perpetuating factors of the target problems. Later, using cognitive and behavioural interventions, the patient's negative beliefs and assumptions about themselves, their illness and the world are tested. The therapist usually sets agenda for each session. Homework assignments are given to test the beliefs, alter their maladaptive thoughts and then practice newly learnt coping skills. The behavioural interventions used are relaxation techniques, biofeedback, hypnosis, guided imagery, etc. These are aimed at reducing the intense physiological arousal experienced by the patients and enhancing their personal sense of control over bodily symptoms. These techniques are known to improve the immune response of the patients, thereby increasing the number of cases in remission.

20.5.2.3 Acceptance and Commitment Therapy (ACT)

Acceptance and commitment therapy (ACT) is one of the newer modes of cognitive and behavioural interventions, which emphasise that it is not always necessary to pursue one's thoughts and emotions. While other interventions focus on altering unpleasant thoughts and emotions, ACT aims at teaching skills to accept those experiences that are not subject to change. It is a therapy which makes use of metaphors, experiential exercises and mindfulness strategies. The skills necessary to cope with those thoughts, memories, physical sensations and feelings which are dreaded and avoided are taught. Through ACT, the patients also learn the ways to accept the unpleasant thoughts and feelings, understand their values and commit to take valued actions [47].

ACT is applied to a diverse set of problems and is seen to be effective in treating chronic pain, anxiety and depression [48].

20.5.2.4   Interpersonal Psychotherapy

Interpersonal psychotherapy (IPT) is a short-term therapeutic intervention, which has the objective of symptom relief and improving the interpersonal functioning of the patients. It is mainly concerned about the interpersonal factors that trigger and maintain psychosocial distress in an individual. The areas which IPT focuses are *grief*, *interpersonal disputes* (role disputes), *role transitions* and *interpersonal sensitivity* (interpersonal deficits) [49]. When treating the psychological problems in cancer, the therapist often focuses on the grief and role transitions areas. The strategies used in IPT include nondirective and directive exploration, clarification, encouragement of affect, communication analysis, role play, problem-solving (or decision analysis) and the therapeutic relationship.

20.5.3   Group Therapy

For over three decades, it has been found that, due to the availability of emotional support, sharing information with others who have similar experiences has a positive impact on emotional well-being and there is an improvement in coping skills and a significant decrease in emotional distress after group psychotherapeutic interventions [33]. The literature highlights that other benefits of group psychotherapy are positive feelings and positive growth [50–52].

Different types of group therapy include supportive-expressive group therapy, psychoeducational group therapy, cognitive behavioural group therapy, psychodynamic group therapy, interpersonal group therapy, etc. In all these group sessions, in common, a patient gets a chance to learn new skills with others and also to observe how others handle their stressors pertaining to the illness.

The patients with breast cancer often raise their concerns about body image problems, sexual difficulties and relationship issues during group sessions [53, 54]. In a study by Kissane et al., 227 metastatic breast cancer patients were assessed, and it was found that in those women who attended supportive-expressive group therapy and relaxation therapy, the new diagnoses of depression were prevented [55].

When forming groups for therapy sessions, it is important that the clinicians make sure that the therapeutic groups are as homogeneous as possible, since the concerns and needs of the patients can always vary according to their age, stage of cancer and cultural factors. Hence, for the patients to receive the expected benefits of therapy, these factors should be as common as possible among the group members.

20.5.4 Family Intervention

The loved ones of patients with cancer often display levels of distress comparable to that of the patient. Hence, it is recommended that when patients attend the psychosocial interventions, the carers are also to be assessed for any signs of burnout, caregiver burden or other clinically significant psychological disorders. There are numerous research findings indicating the positive effects of family-oriented interventions [56]. The diagnosis of cancer in one family member can disrupt the functioning of the entire family. For instance, if the person affected with breast cancer is the mother of the person who holds the maximum number of responsibilities, physically and emotionally, the entire household is very likely to be in significant distress. In such a situation, cancer becomes the primary problem of the family rather than the reactions of the individual members of the family.

Family therapy involves the patient, spouse and children or the patient's children and spouse, or children alone. The clinician should do a structured family assessment to understand their developmental level, interaction patterns, belief structure, etc. The clinician can further assist them by modifying certain familial factors, improving interaction patterns and thereby in the smoother shifting of responsibilities. By giving in-session and out-of-session tasks and assigning individual duties to each member, the maladaptive behaviour patterns of the system are altered.

20.5.5 Couple Therapy and Sex Therapy

The diagnosis of cancer in the spouse can be very devastating for the spouse. Couple therapy is a session where the psychosocial and emotional needs of both the patient and the spouse can be addressed. The major focus of this intervention could be to balance the intimacy needs of both the patient and spouse and help them in supporting each other while staying within the limits of the patient's diagnosis and treatment. In breast cancer, the couple therapy plays a crucial role in addressing body image disturbances and problems with sexuality resulting from mastectomy [57].

The sexual dysfunctions resulting from the physical and psychological impact of cancer and its treatment are addressed during sex therapy sessions. These sessions include components such as education, support and behavioural techniques, which are intended to reducing conflicts regarding sexual relationship and enhancing the sexual intimacy between the partners [43].

20.6   Future Direction

In view of the high prevalence of mental health co-morbidity following the diagnosis of breast cancer, the way forward would be to consider screening using the appropriate psychological assessment tools shown in Table 20.1 during the early stages of the diagnosis; the aim should be to offer early psychological intervention and support. It is also important to introduce support groups for caregivers, and the principle should be to offer comprehensive psychooncology service that supports and addresses psychological and sociocultural aspects of the individual and their families.

20.7 Conclusion

Breast cancer has been extensively researched in terms of the psychological impact; the prevalence of depression and anxiety is high among patients with breast cancer. As a result, there is a significant disruption in their personal, social and occupational functioning. This chapter highlights the need for a comprehensive oncology treatment provision, which includes routine psychological screening and intervention as standard clinical practice.

References

1. Andersen B, Anderson B, deProsse C. Controlled prospective longitudinal study of women with cancer. II: Psychological outcomes. J Consult Clin Psychol. 1989;57:692–7.
2. Nezu AM, Nezu CM. Psychological distress, depression, and anxiety. In: Feuerstein M, editor. Handbook of cancer survivorship. New York, NY: Springer; 2007. p. 323–38.
3. Chida Y, Hamer M, Wardle J, Steptoe A. Do stress-related psychosocial factors contribute to cancer incidence and survival? Nat Clin Pract Oncol. 2008;5:466–75.
4. National Breast Cancer Centre and National Cancer Control Initiative. Clinical practice guidelines for the psychosocial care of adults with cancer. Camperdown, NSW: National Breast Cancer Centre; 2003.
5. Carey MP, Burish TG. Psychological side effects in chemotherapy patients. Psychol Bull. 1988;104:307–25.
6. McCabe MS. Psychological support for the patient on chemotherapy. Oncology. 1991;5:91–103.
7. Holland JC. Historical overview. In: Holland JC, Rowland JH, editors. Handbook of psychooncology. New York: Oxford University Press; 1990. p. 3–12.
8. India State-Level Disease Burden Initiative Cancer Collaborators. The burden of cancers and their variations across the states of India: the Global Burden of Disease Study 1990-2016. Lancet Oncol. 2018;19(10):1289–306.
9. Rowland JH, Massie MJ. Breast cancer. In: Holland JC, Breitbart WS, Jacobsen PB, Lederberg MS, Loscalzo MJ, McCorkle R, editors. Psycho-oncology. 2nd ed. New York: Oxford University Press; 2010. p. 177–86.
10. Meyerowitz BE. Psychosocial correlates of breast cancer and its treatments. Psychol Bull. 1980;87:108–31.
11. National Cancer Policy Board, Hewitt M, Herdman R, Holland J, editors. Meeting psychosocial needs of women with breast cancer. Washington, DC: The National Academies Press; 2004.
12. Kissane DW, Clarke DM, Ikin J, et al. Psychological morbidity and quality of life in Australian women with early-stage breast cancer: a cross-sectional survey. Med J Aust. 1998;169:192–6.
13. Irwin MR. Depression and risk of cancer progression: an elusive link. J Clin Oncol. 2007;33:661–75.
14. Williamson G, Schulz R. Activity restriction mediates the association between pain and depressed affect: a study of younger and older adult cancer patients. Psychol Aging. 1995;10:369–78.
15. Newport D, Nemeroff C. Assessment and treatment of depression in the cancer patient. J Psychosom Res. 1998;45:215–37.
16. Rouchell AM, Pounds R, Tierney JG. Depression. In: Rundell JR, Wise MG, editors. Textbook of consultation liaison psychiatry. Washington, DC: American Psychiatric Press; 1999. p. 121–47.
17. Massie MJ, Holland JC. The cancer patient with pain: psychiatric complications and their management. Med Clin N Am. 1987;71:243–57.

18. Jenkins PL, May VE, Hughes LE. Psychological morbidity associated with local recurrence of breast cancer. Int J Psychiatry Med. 1991;21:149–55.
19. Patenaude AF. Psychological impact of bone marrow transplantation: current perspectives. Yale J Biol Med. 1990;63:515–9.
20. Maguire GP, Lee EG, Bevington DJ. Psychiatric problems in the first year after mastectomy. Br J Med. 1978;1:963–5.
21. Sareen J, Cox BJ, Afifi TO, et al. Anxiety disorders and risk for suicidal ideation and suicide attempts. Arch Gen Psychiatry. 2005;62:1249–57.
22. Passik SD, Breitbart WS. Depression in patients with pancreatic cancer. Cancer Suppl. 1996;78:615–26.
23. Chochinov HM, Wilson KG, Enns M, Lander S. Depression, hopelessness, and suicidal ideation in the terminally ill. Psychosomatics. 1998;39:366–70.
24. Breitbart W. Suicide in cancer patients. Oncology. 1987;1:49–53.
25. Valente S, Saunders J, Cohen M. Evaluating depression among patients with cancer. Cancer Pract. 1994;2:65–71.
26. Holland JC. Psychological aspects of cancer. In: Holland JF, Frei III E, editors. Cancer medicine. New York: Oxford University Press; 1982. p. 1175–203.
27. Sneeuw KC, Aaronson NK, Yarnold JR, Broderick M, Regan J, Ross G, et al. Cosmetic and functional outcomes of breast conserving treatment for early stage breast cancer. II: relationship with psychosocial functioning. Radiother Oncol. 1992;25:160–6.
28. Ganz PA, Rowland JH, Desmond K, Meyerowitz BE, Wyatt GE. Life after breast cancer: understanding women's health-related quality of life and sexual functioning. J Clin Oncol. 1998;16:501–14.
29. Marks DI, Friedman SH, DelliCarpini L, Nezu CM, Nezu AM. A prospective study of the effects of high dose chemotherapy and bone marrow transplantation on sexual function in the first year after transplant. Bone Marrow Transplant. 1997;19:819–22.
30. Atisha D, Alderman AK, Lowery JC, Kuhn LE, Davis J, Wilkins EG. Prospective analysis of long-term psychosocial outcomes in breast reconstruction: two-year postoperative results from the Michigan breast reconstruction outcomes study. Ann Surg. 2008;247:1019–28.
31. Al-Ghazal SK, Fallowfield L, Blamey RW. Comparison of psychological aspects and patient satisfaction following breast conserving surgery, simple mastectomy and breast reconstruction. Eur J Cancer. 2000;36:1938–43.
32. Schover LR. Sexuality and fertility after cancer. New York: Wiley; 1997.
33. Andersen BL. Psychological interventions for cancer patient to enhance quality of life. J Consult Clin Psychol. 1992;60:552–68.
34. Fawzy FI, Fawzy NW, Arndt LA, Pasnau RO. Critical review of psychological interventions in cancer care. Arch Gen Psychiatry. 1995;52:100–13.
35. Goodwin PJ, Leszcz M, Ennis M, Koopmans J, Vincent L, Guther H, et al. The effect of group psychosocial support on survival in metastatic breast cancer. N Engl J Med. 2001;345:1719–26.
36. Meyer TJ, Mark MM. Effects of psychosocial interventions with adult cancer patients: a meta-analysis of randomized experiments. Health Psychol. 1995;14:101–8.
37. Sheard T, Maguire P. The effect of psychological interventions on anxiety and depression in cancer patients: results of meta-analyses. Br J Cancer. 1999;80:1770–80.
38. Helgeson V, Cohen S, Schulz R, Yasko J. Education and peer discussion group interventions and adjustment to breast cancer. Arch Gen Psychiatry. 1999;56(4):340–7.
39. McArdle JM, George WD, McArdle CS, Smith DC, Moodie AR, Hughson AV, Murray GD. Psychological support for patients undergoing breast cancer surgery: a randomized study. BMJ. 1996;312:813–6.
40. Helgeson V, Cohen S, Schulz R, Yasko J. Long-term effects of educational and peer discussion group interventions on adjustment to breast cancer. Health Psychol. 2001;20(5):387–92.
41. Devine EC, Westlake SK. The effects of psychoeducational care provided to adults with cancer: meta-analysis of 116 studies. Oncol Nurs Forum. 1995;22(9):1369–81.
42. Anderson BL. Surviving cancer. Cancer Suppl. 1994;74:1484–94.

43. Wellisch DK, Surdam GB. Chapter 24: psychosocial care. In: Cancer treatment, 5th ed. 2001. p. 392–404.
44. Wolberg LR. Supportive psychotherapy. In: The technique of psychotherapy, 4th ed. 2013. p. 185–250.
45. American Psychosocial Oncology Society. Quick reference for oncology clinicians: the psychiatric and psychological dimensions of cancer symptom management. Charlottesville, VA: IPOS Press; 2006.
46. Spiegel D, Bloom JR, Yalom I. Group support for patients with metastatic cancer: a randomized outcome study. Arch Gen Psychiatry. 1981;38:527–33.
47. Seligman L, Reichenberg LW. Transpersonal therapy and emerging approaches emphasising mindfulness. In: Theories of counselling and psychotherapy, 3rd ed. 2011. p. 378–97.
48. Strosahl K. Acceptance and commitment therapy. In: Encyclopedia of psychotherapy. vol 1. 2002. p. 1–8.
49. Stuart S, Robertson M. Interpersonal psychotherapy—a clinician's guide. 2003.
50. Andryowski MA, Brady MJ, Hunt JW. Positive psychosocial adjustment in potential bone marrow transplant recipients: cancer as a psychosocial transition. Psycho-Oncology. 1993;2:261–76.
51. Antoni MH, Lehman JM, Kilbourn KM, Boyers AE, Culver JL, Alferi SM, et al. Cognitive behavioural stress management intervention decreases the prevalence of depression and enhances benefit finding among women under treatment for early stage breast cancer. Health Psychol. 2001;20:20–32.
52. Cordova MJ, Cunningham LLC, Carlson CR, Andrykowski MA. Posttraumatic growth following breast cancer: a controlled comparison study. Health Psychol. 2001;20:176–85.
53. Anillo LM. Sexual life after breast cancer. J Sex Marital Ther. 2000;26:241–8.
54. Carver CS, Pozo-kaderman C, Price AA, Noriega V, Harris SD, Derhagopian RP, et al. Concern about aspects of body image and adjustment to early stage breast cancer. Psychosom Med. 1998;60:168–74.
55. Kissane DW, Grabsch B, Clarke DM, et al. Supportive-expressive group therapy for women with metastatic breast cancer: survival and psychosocial outcome from a randomized controlled trial. Psychooncology. 2007;16:277–86.
56. Cohen MM. In the presence of your absence: the treatment of older families with a cancer patient. Psychotherapy. 1982;19:453–60.
57. Christensen DN. Post mastectomy couple counselling: an outcome study of a structured treatment protocol. J Sex Marital Ther. 1983;9:266–75.